OTHER TITLES OF INTEREST FROM GR/ST. LUCIE PRESS

Healthcare Book of Lists

Healthcaring: A Step-by-Step Prescription for Injecting Quality into Healthcare Systems

Utilizing Community Resources: An Overview of Human Services

Interdependence: The Route to Community

Healthcare Economics: Text, Cases and Readings

Healthcare Teams: Building Continuous Quality Improvement

The Textbook of Total Quality in Healthcare

The Handbook of Management and Organizational Behavior in Healthcare

Principles and Practices of Disability Management in Industry

The Disability Evaluation: Practical Guide for Physicians

Head Injury and the Family: A Life and Living Perspective

For more information about these titles call, fax or write:

GR/St. Lucie Press
100 E. Linton Blvd., Suite 403B
Delray Beach, FL 33483
TEL (561) 274-9906 • FAX (561) 274-9927

HOME

HEALTH

CARE

Principles and Practices

HOME

HEALTH

CARE

Principles and Practices

Editors
JOHN S. SPRATT
RHONDA L. HAWLEY
ROBERT E. HOYE

GR/St. Lucie Press
Delray Beach, Florida

Printed and bound in the U.S.A. Printed on acid-free paper.
10 9 8 7 6 5 4 3 2 1

ISBN 1-884015-93-X

Direct all inquiries to GR/St. Lucie Press, Inc., 100 E. Linton Blvd., Suite 403B, Delray Beach, Florida 33483.

Phone: (561) 274-9906
Fax: (561) 274-9927

Published by
GR/St. Lucie Press
100 E. Linton Blvd., Suite 403B
Delray Beach, FL 33483

Table of Contents

Preface

Home care. Each of our decisions to care for the sick in the home is based upon personal and professional experiences. As a boy, I (JSS) was a close observer of my grandfather, John Thomas Spratt, M.D., who finished Dallas Medical College of Trinity University in 1902 as valedictorian of his class and engaged in general practice in the small oil and coal towns of western Texas until his death in 1958. The nearest hospital of any quality was 75 miles away in Fort Worth, and he never worked in a hospital. His office was always a busy and interesting place. As a boy, I made house calls with him to witness firsthand a physician at work attending the sick in their homes with the assistance of family members.

His life and practice spanned a great period of medical as well as economic change. Blue Cross was born in the mid-1930s to cover hospital care. Blue Shield, to cover physician services, did not come into being until after World War II. Medicare and Medicaid came even later. The Hill-Burton program, to subsidize hospital development in communities across the land, was a child of the 1950s and 1960s.

Where the physician practiced was determined by the existence of payrolls. Without local industry providing a payroll, cash was always in short supply. Thus, some of my grandfather's fees were paid in kind. Most of us in medicine are aware of the great technological changes that occurred during this period. My grandfather, for example, acquired the first x-ray tube ever in Pecos, Texas, and ran it off a static generator. I still have the tube.

In addition to the profound technological changes, equally profound economic changes were occurring—the westward-moving frontier, the tapping of natural resources, industrialization, urbanization, and unionization. (My father, a professor of economics, later wrote two books [*The Road to Spindeltop*, 1957, and *Thurber, Texas—The Life and Death of a Company Coal Town*, 1986, both still available through the University of Texas Press] on the drastic economic changes that occurred over the span of my grandfather's life and practice, occasionally mentioning how these affected my grandfather's practice.

The home was the haven—people were born, lived, and died there and medical care came to them, except for an occasional office visit. People who were sick enough to go to the hospital were considered by their family and friends to be too sick to live and many never returned home. If "Doc" Spratt could not fix them up in their homes, many never made it.

My own professional experience with home care began to grow in spurts. As a junior medical student, I made home visits to postpartum patients with a visiting nurse (Parkland Hospital, Dallas). After my internship, I entered the Navy for two years, attending Field Medical School at Camp Pendleton and Cold Weather Survival School in the High Sierras in January of 1954. Then I spent 11 months of field duty with the First Marine Division in Korea.

Half of the period was spent as a battalion surgeon with the 1st Battalion, 7th Marines on Hill 495 north of Seoul and half on Paeng-nyong-do, an island off the North Korean coast. On Paeng-nyong-do, I had a nice dispensary with a small operating room. Field medicine provided home care in a tent or in the field. Home care in tents was possible with a buddy system replacing the family. The sicker patients were sent to a field hospital or the hospital ship. However, the truce was then signed and the Armed Forces Aid to Korea (AFAK) program was underway, and the military medical facilities became major contributors. Korean peasants with endless diversified pathology came from the farming and fishing villages on Paeng-nyong-do to my dispensary. The diversification of pathology and public health problems was endless. Kyu Fan Cho, a fourth-year medical student whose education had been interrupted by the Korean War, was my assistant and interpreter. With him, I went into the rice straw huts with dirt floors for the home care of the sick. Intestinal parasites and tuberculosis were very prevalent. Again, there was no hospital for these Koreans. I taught Kyu Fan Cho to administer drip ether anesthesia to permit needed surgery and transferred patients back to their homes for postoperative recovery. Through Cho, I learned to understand and respect the Korean culture and people—proud, but fatalistic. He told me that Koreans perceived themselves as people "with very large eyes, but very small feet." There was a pervasive fatalism among them, and the most important thing to them was the annual rice harvest and the catches of their fishing fleet. This fatalism had been brought home to me my first day on the island. Cho asked me to see his only son, age five, dying of tuberculosis meningitis. He was too far gone when I saw him and there were no antibiotics for tuberculosis on the island anyway. He died several days later. With the aid of AFAK, orphanages were built for children needing home care.

During 15 years as chief surgeon at the Ellis Fischel State Cancer Hospital, which served the medically indigent cancer patients of Missouri, I was witness to many still very ill patients who had to return home, often in the most rural parts of Missouri, after they had received maximum benefit from hospitalization. In many remote and very rural areas of the state, only the resources of the home were available, plus whatever resources and information patients and their families could take from the hospital. I found the same fatalism among the rural poor of Missouri as I had seen among the Koreans. If the crops were not seeded and harvested, the family would be left with neither food nor money. Operations, treatments, and clinic visits had to be scheduled to accommodate these basic needs, which often had precedence over medical needs thought urgent by the physicians. In these waiting intervals, home care had value. The unmet needs for better home care stimulated an ongoing interest in patient and family education about which I will comment later. Patient and family education is clearly an integral part of home care.

With the spiraling costs of health care and the mobility within society, there is continual study into what illnesses or aspects of illness can be attended in the home, potentially saving the "hotel" costs of hospitalization and many transportation and labor costs. Though home care services and technology are fueling a rapid-growth industry, the overriding philosophy has to be the containment of costs while maintaining high-quality care.

This text on home care is a first effort. It is incomplete, however, because the field of home care is potentially so large that a more comprehensive text will have to be built over time and experience as home care technology grows. We have tried to include some aspects of home health care that are unlikely to be found in most texts on the subject. The various contributors were assigned general areas, but how they perceive the use of their areas of expertise in a home care environment has been left up to each author. We have personally learned much from reading their contributions and their effort is greatly appreciated. We solicit feedback from our readers in terms of what should have been covered more extensively and what was left out.

John S. Spratt, M.D.

Having worked for surgical oncologists since 1976, I (RH) have seen home health care develop from obscurity into a multimillion-dollar industry. The motive behind the proliferation of home health care is probably more closely related to the dollar, but the benefit to the patient of care given in a loving, familiar environment cannot be underestimated.

Home health care was just another dimension of health care to me until its relevance became personal. Within a ten-month period, I lost two very special people in my life to cancer. Unfortunately, the terminal stage of one of my loved ones' cancer was tremendously sudden and swift. He died within six days in a hospital. The exact course of a terminal illness can never be predicted, yet when a loved one pleads with you to take them home from a hospital and you know they are dying, all the medical reasons for keeping them in the hospital become moot.

No one who has ever cared for a sick friend or relative in the home would tell you that it is easy. In fact, I am sure there are many in this situation who would readily place their loved one in a medical facility for care if circumstances or finances permitted. However, care in the home does provide the patient and the caregiver a certain amount of control and independence. These two commodities do not carry a price tag.

When exploring the possibilities of home health care, one must remove blinders. I have seen some of the surgeons with whom I have worked over the years do just that. Yet physicians who for the past 20 to 30 years have admitted patients to the hospital for infusion therapy are not going to miraculously think in terms of having this therapy done in the home. We all must be educated about home health care. I hope this text is a good beginning for that education.

Rhonda L. Hawley, B.S.

The Editors

John S. Spratt, M.S.P.H., M.D., F.A.C.S., F.R.S.S., F.A.A.M.A., is a Diplomate of the American Board of Surgery; Diplomate of the American Academy of Medical Administrators; Professor of Surgery and Professor of Health Systems at the James Graham Brown Cancer Center, University of Louisville; Clinical Professor of Surgery at the F. Edward Hebert School of Medicine, Uniformed Services University of the Health Sciences; and Captain (retired) in the Medical Corps U.S. Navy Reserve. Dr. Spratt is author of an extensive list of publications in his field and is a continuing student of health systems, medical economics, and medical education. He is a practicing surgeon in Louisville, Kentucky, where he resides.

Rhonda L. Hawley is a graduate of the University of Louisville College of Business and Public Administration. She brings fifteen years of medical office management expertise to this text. In 1994, she spent six months in intensive home health care research for a national home health care company as a special project coordinator. Her involvement in this project served as a catalyst for the publication of this text. She currently resides in Louisville.

Robert E. Hoye received his Ph.D. from the University of Wisconsin-Madison and recently retired from the University of Louisville, where he served as Professor (Emeritus) in the Department of Community Health, School of Medicine and Coordinator of the Graduate Program in Health Systems. He has been active in research and teaching in areas relating to health systems administration, planning and leadership. Dr. Hoye is a Diplomate and Fellow in the American Academy of Medical Administrators and a Fellow in the Royal Society of Health. He has served as delegation leader to five Delegations of Health Systems Administrators to the People's Republic of China. He is a Faculty Mentor and Professor of Health Services at Walden University and serves as a Visiting Professor at other universities. Among other activities, he serves as a Member of the Professional Advisory Committee for Alliant Home Health in Louisville.

Contributing Authors

Barbara M. Baker, Ph.D.
Associate Professor
Division of Audiology and Speech
    Pathology
Department of Surgery
University of Louisville School of Medicine
Louisville, Kentucky

Vanita Bellen, B.S., B.Comm., M.H.S
Director, Quality Management
Genesee Region Home Care Association
Newark, New York

Joanne Berryman, M.S.N.
Senior Vice President
Jewish Hospital HealthCare Services, Inc.
Louisville, Kentucky

Salvatore J. Bertolone, M.D.
Director, Division of Pediatric
    Hematology/Oncology
Professor of Pediatrics
University of Louisville School of Medicine
Louisville, Kentucky

Brian K. Brake, Esq.
Wright, Robinson, McCammon,
    Osthimer & Tatum
Richmond, Virginia

David R. Cunningham, Ph.D.
Professor and Director
Division of Audiology and Speech
    Pathology
Department of Surgery
University of Louisville School of
    Medicine
Louisville, Kentucky

M. Therese Dalton, R.N., M.P.A.
Assistant Vice President, Health Care
Technology Sector
Science Applications International Corp.
San Diego, California

Nemr S. Eid, M.D.
Associate Professor of Pediatrics
Department of Pediatrics
Director Pediatric Pulmonary Medicine
Director Cystic Fibrosis Center
University of Louisville
Frazier Rehab Center Pediatric Program
Louisville, Kentucky

Sofia M. Franco, M.D.
Associate Professor
Department of Pediatrics
University of Louisville
Louisville, Kentucky

Albert G. Goldin, M.D., F.A.C.P.
Associate Clinical Professor of
    Medicine
University of Louisville School of
    Medicine
Louisville, Kentucky

Rhonda L. Hawley, B.S.
Practice Manager and Research
    Associate
James Graham Brown Cancer Center
University of Louisville School of
    Medicine
Louisville, Kentucky

**Barbara Head, R.N., C.R.N.H.,
A.C.S.W.**
Director of Quality Improvement and
    Staff Development
Hospice of Louisville
Louisville, Kentucky

Margaret Hill, D.M.D.
Assistant Professor
Department of Periodontics,
    Endodontics, and Dental Hygiene
University of Louisville School of
    Dentistry
Louisville, Kentucky

Robert E. Hoye, Ph.D.
Professor of Education
University of Louisville
Louisville, Kentucky

Anna K. Huang, M.D.
Assistant Professor
Department of Internal Medicine
University of Louisville School of
    Medicine
Louisville, Kentucky

James Kolf, B.S.
Director of Sales and Business
    Development
Kelly Assisted Living
Troy, Michigan

Paul Mangino, Pharm.D.
Clinical Pharmacist
University of Louisville Hospital
Louisville, Kentucky

Regan L. Moore, D.D.S., M.S.D.
Associate Professor
Department of Periodontics,
    Endodontics, and Dental Hygiene
University of Louisville School of
    Dentistry
Louisville, Kentucky

Iris Phillips, M.S.S.W.
Kent School of Social Work
University of Louisville
Louisville, Kentucky

Hiram C. Polk, Jr., M.D.
Ben A. Reid, Sr. Professor and Chair
Department of Surgery
University of Louisville School of
    Medicine
Louisville, Kentucky

Benjamin M. Rigor, M.D.
Professor and Chairman
Department of Anesthesiology
University of Louisville
Louisville, Kentucky

David S. Robinson, M.D.
Associate Professor of Surgery
Sylvester Comprehensive Cancer Center
University of Miami Hospital and Clinics
Miami, Florida

Bibhuti K. Sar, Ph.D.
Assistant Professor
Kent School of Social Work
University of Louisville
Louisville, Kentucky

William J. Spanos, Jr., M.D.
Professor, Radiation Oncology
James Graham Brown Cancer Center
University of Louisville
Louisville, Kentucky

John S. Spratt, M.D.
Professor of Surgery and Health Systems
James Graham Brown Cancer Center
University of Louisville School of Medicine
Louisville, Kentucky

Danielle Turns, M.D.
Professor (retired)
Department of Psychiatry
University of Louisville School of Medicine
Louisville, Kentucky

David R. Watkins, M.D.
Medical Director
Frazier Rehab Center
Louisville, Kentucky

Paula Zelle, Pharm.D.
President
Infusion Consultant Services
Louisville, Kentucky

Home Health Care: A Physician's Perspective

John S. Spratt, M.D., Rhonda L. Hawley, B.S., and James Kolf, B.S.

Introduction

Directly or indirectly, all physicians are involved in home care. Their responsibilities precede and extend beyond office, clinic, hospital, and custodial care facilities. Maximizing the potential for home care requires knowledge, skills, and organization. The rapidly growing home care industry and the relationship the physician has with this industry is not without problems.[1]

Dr. Joseph Painter, during his tenure as president of the American Medical Association (AMA), was interviewed regarding the perception of the AMA on home health care. Painter discussed the AMA program directed by Joanne Swartzberg, M.D., which recognized that the aging population will require more home care in the future.

Painter emphasized that the AMA encourages medical schools "to teach the art and science of home care as an integral part of their curriculum." The AMA supports home care training and experience for medical students. Every home care program is believed to need a physician advisory board representing a broad range of insight that will be responsive to the needs of home care. As Painter points out, home care programs are continually requiring physician signatures and authorizations. The physicians who provide these signatures are responding to bureaucratic requirements and regulations. In many instances, these signatures also lay a burden of responsibility and potential liability on the signing physician. Painter considers that these rapidly expanding home care obligations of physicians are precisely the reason why home care is in the AMA spotlight. There has been and remains a need to improve the remuneration of physicians for home care activities. At the time of this interview, the AMA was in discussion with the Health Care Financing Administration (HCFA) regarding current procedural terminology (CPT) codes for physicians' home care activities and responsibilities. The 1995 AMA Physicians' Current Procedural Terminology[2] book contains the addition of two new CPT codes for "Care Plan Oversight Services." The service is to involve the physician's supervisory role of patients in specific outpatient settings (home health, hospice, or outpatient nursing facilities). The care should require complex or multidisciplinary modalities involving regular or recurrent physician review of patient status or reports, development or revision of care plans, review of lab or other diagnostic studies, and communication with other related health care professionals. The care must exceed 30 minutes of physician work in a 30-day period. The code (99375) is to be used for one physician per patient in a 30-day period only. If the supervisory care exceeds 30 days, then the same code (99375) may be used if there exists justification for at least 30 minutes of supervisory care in the succeeding month. The service is not to include the usual supervision of patients under the care of home health agencies requiring routine review of treatment plans or completion of routine forms and signatures, unless there is documented recurrent supervision of complex therapy.

Medicare began reimbursing physicians for home care on January 1, 1995. Following are some of the criteria for physician reimbursement (unpublished data):

- More than 30 minutes should be spent by the physician during a calendar month overseeing the patient's home care. This is the minimum time required for all activities related to home care. All time above this amount is included in the one fee.
- Payment will be made to only one physician during a calendar month for oversight of a patient's home care plan of treatment.
- The physician must have furnished a service requiring a face-to-face encounter with the patient during the past six months.
- The physician may not have a significant financial or contractual relationship with the home care company. (This does not include advisory board physicians or medical directors.)
- If a physician furnishes care plan oversight services during a postoperative period, payment for care plan oversight services is made if the services are documented in the patient's medical record as unrelated to the surgery.

This new policy is part of the HCFA Relative Value Unit (RVU) fee structure. The fee is approximately $60.00. Medicare will reimburse the physician 80%. The 20% co-pay may be billed to the patient if the physician desires to do so. Physicians should document the time spent in "medical decision making" related to a patient's home care services to justify the charge to Medicare. For more current information, physicians are encouraged to contact their professional society.

Discussions on physician participation in home care include reviewing the paperwork burden on physicians imposed by home care. Tort reforms are also under review that would make the use of home care by physicians less risky from the medicolegal standpoint. This is a very important area since patients managed by home care exist in highly variable environments not under the direct control of physicians, but with the physician often still responsible for various aspects of the care.

In relating to home care services, the physician also has to be concerned with other legal problems such as conflict of interest if the physician refers to a home care company in which he may also be a part owner. All such relationships require legal counsel to avoid problems. Arrangements between physicians and home care management are allowed some flexibility based on community need.

Val Halamandaris, president of the National Association for Home Care (NAHC),[3] has summarized commonly endorsed reasons for home care (Table 1.1). Not all these reasons are universally applicable and their implementation requires organization, education, and money, but they do constitute ideas. Home health agencies, home care aide organizations, and hospices are known collectively as "home care agencies." The NAHC identified a total of 15,027 home care agencies in the United States as of March 1994 (unpublished data).

In addition to traditional home care services (e.g., the Visiting Nurse Association), national home care companies that aggressively franchise their services in many communities are rapidly evolving.[4]

Many of these franchises are being acquired by people with no prior experience in health care. The exact number of franchises was not available, but the larger companies already had about 1,000 franchises in 1993 and were aggressively pursuing new markets. The only thing slowing down the process is government regulations and burdensome paperwork. However, larger organizations were seen as more capable of responding to this burden than were smaller or individual home care organizations. Many franchise offers are advertised in national newspapers. The cost of franchise ranged from $10,000 to $100,000. Proprietary agencies made up about one-third of the 6,617 agencies certified by the HCFA in 1993, an increase of 13% from 1992. Many legal turf battles are apparently in progress. Spin-off corporations such as the Medical Personnel Pool in Fort Lauderdale, Florida are appearing to service this industry.

Intense study of palliative home care, particularly for end-stage disease, is in progress in Canada.[5] The appendix of the study summarizing the recommendations of the expert panel assigned to study the problem is given in Table 1.2. The long-term results of these Canadian studies should provide insight into all aspects of home care and how to deliver it in the most effective way.

Table 1.1   Twenty Reasons for Home Care

1. It is delivered at home.
2. Home care represents the best tradition in American health care.
3. Home care keeps families together.
4. Home care serves to keep the elderly independent.
5. Home care prevents or postpones institutionalization.
6. Home care promotes healing.
7. Home care is safer.
8. Home care allows a maximum amount of freedom for the individual.
9. Home care is a personalized care.
10. Home care, by definition, involves the individual and the family in the care that is delivered.
11. Home care reduces stress.
12. Home care is the most effective form of health care.
13. Home care is the most efficient form of health care.
14. Home care is given by special people.
15. Home care is the only way to reach some people.
16. There is little fraud and abuse associated with home care.
17. Home care improves the quality of life.
18. Home care is less expensive than other forms of care.
19. Home care extends life.
20. Home care is the preferred form of care, even for individuals who are terminally ill.

From *Caring*, 4(10), 1985.

Table 1.2   Recommendations of the Expert Panel on Palliative Care to the Cancer 2000 Task Force—Home Care

1. Provincial governments should allocate a larger proportion of cancer funds to palliative care in the home setting.
2. Palliative home care should be administered as a distinct program designed as a palliative care unit (PCU) in-the-home project (a variant of the hospital in-the-home or extramural hospital) or as a separate division of the regional home care program.
3. A PCU in-the-home project should be administered regionally, contracting services from the regional home care program and regional palliative care centre. It would have a similar organizational structure to a health care facility with a board of directors and a medical advisory committee with responsibility for supervising patient care.
4. Specialized case managers are required to coordinate professional services in the home for palliative care to be successful. These case managers should have specialized training in palliative case management and have a caseload that reflects their time requirements.

5. A specialized team of visiting nurses are required for palliative care. In urban and semiurban areas, there should be a separate team of nurses that do only palliative care. These should receive special training for at least four weeks. The time allowed per home visit and the total number of visits per week must be increased over regular home care programs and be flexible to meet changing needs in the palliative care population.

6. At least one palliative care nurse must be available 24 hours per day. Many regions (even those with specialized palliative care nurse teams) arrange evening, night, and weekend coverage using nurses who are not trained in palliative care and who are not familiar with the patients. Often families calling for help only receive general telephone advice and this can lead to unrelieved symptoms and hospital admission.

7. Shift nursing must be made available (up to weeks in some cases). These nurses should also receive specialized palliative care training prior to being placed on a roster. Flexibility in using registered nurses, registered nurse assistants, and sitter staff levels will ensure optimal care.

8. Funding must be available to increase the number of hours of homemaking services. The acceptable hours for these homemakers must be expanded to include evenings and nights. All homemakers involved with palliative care must receive specialized training and support.

9. Physicians must become actively involved in the planning and implementation of palliative home care. There should be consideration of having some of the characteristics of the New Brunswick extramural hospital program introduced into palliative home care, with physicians having admitting privileges dependent on a set of responsibilities including 24-hour coverage by colleagues experienced in palliative care, CME requirements to maintain competence in palliative care, etc.

10. Physician reimbursement should be changed so that there are incentives to do home visits and to maintain good telephone management.

11. A regional consultation team consisting of a clinical nurse specialist in palliative care, a palliative medicine physician, and a social worker with special training in palliative care should be available as a quick outreach team. A family physician or visiting nurse could request that this team assess and give management advice on symptoms or problems. This should be available rapidly by home visit or by telephone. During evenings, nights, and weekends there must always be a physician and nurse with specialized training in palliative care available to assist the family physician and regular visiting nurses.

12. Governments should reimburse family members for lost income and expenses related to caring for cancer patients in the home.

13. The regional palliative care program (section 6) should try to coordinate the work of volunteers and organize a common regional training program. Community-based hospice groups that provide volunteers for patients in the home and less organized groups of church volunteers should be integrated into the care system.

14. Mechanisms to give family caregivers respite must be built into the system. Regional hospitals, both acute and long-term care, must utilize a small proportion of their beds for such respite admissions if a home care program is to succeed. The aggressive use of volunteers and periods of shift nursing could also give family respite while the patient remains at home.

Table 1.2   Recommendations of the Expert Panel on Palliative Care to the Cancer 2000 Task Force—Home Care (continued)

15. Day hospitals or hospices should be developed in some of the regions of Canada with appropriate evaluation of their effectiveness.
16. Palliative home care patients should have all prescription medication costs covered by provincial medical insurance.
17. In cooperation with regional pharmacists, the PCU in-the-home program must ensure rapid, 24-hour access to all palliative care drugs (including all parenteral forms) that may be needed in the home.
18. Palliative care patients in the home should have free access to all equipment that would be available to them if they were admitted to hospital including beds, pressure mattresses, infusion pumps, etc.
19. Insurance companies should be encouraged to review their policies to create a fast-track mechanism for urgent palliative care problems and increase flexibility in the type of staff that can be hired to assist a family.
20. Emergency services in each region of Canada should review their policy concerning the transportation of palliative care patients. Long waits and unpredictable service are often due to the fact that these patients are placed low on the ambulance priority system. These highly symptomatic patients with a short prognosis deserve a higher ranking in ambulance services.
21. While at home and during ambulance transfers, palliative care patients must have protection against inappropriate resuscitation efforts. Changes in provincial legislation and regulation must ensure that patients can be protected from CPR even if a family calls the emergency number for assistance.
22. Bereavement follow-up programs must be available to high-risk families following a death in the home.
23. Some patients may require less intense forms of palliative care in the home and therefore do not fit the eligibility criteria for a PCU in-the-home program. Therefore, a mechanism must also be in place throughout provincial home care programs to assist groups such as the elderly who are dying of multiple chronic illness in such a way that increased services and equipment can be provided without changing the regular case manager and visiting nurse whom they have come to trust.

From Roe, D.J., *J. Palliative Care*, 8:28–32, 1992. Reprinted with permission.

Home Health Care Patient Population

In 1992, the first annual National Home and Hospice Care Survey (NHHCS) was conducted as a segment of the Long-Term Care Component of the National Health Care Survey by the National Center for Health Statistics.[6] This survey was instituted in response to the rapid proliferation of home health agencies throughout the United States. The survey includes all types of agencies that

Table 1.3   First-Listed Diagnoses at Admission: United States, 1993

ICD-9-CM procedure category	*Home health patients*
Infectious and parasitic diseases	17,500
Neoplasms	94,900
Endocrine, nutritional, metabolic; immunity disorders	126,800
Diseases of the blood and blood-forming organs	36,700
Mental disorders	48,800
Diseases of nervous system and sense organs	93,600
Diseases of circulatory system	381,400
Diseases of respiratory system	87,100
Diseases of digestive system	50,800
Diseases of genitourinary system	35,100
Diseases of skin and subcutaneous tissues	44,200
Diseases of musculoskeletal system and connective tissue	122,200
Congenital anomalies	9,900
Certain conditions originating in perinatal period	12,700
Symptoms, signs, and ill-defined conditions	102,100
Injury and poisoning	132,200
All other or unknown	53,800
Total	**1,448,800**

Note: Figures may not add to total because of rounding.

Adapted from Strahan, G.W., An Overview of Home Health and Hospice Care Patients: Preliminary Data from the 1993 National Home and Hospice Care Survey, Advance Data No. 256, 1994.

provide home health and/or hospice care, whether they are Medicare or Medicaid certified or whether they are licensed.

In the 1993 survey, approximately 75% of the current home health care patients were 65 years of age or older.[7] Of these, 66% of the patients receiving home health care services were female. Married and widowed patients accounted for 67% of the patients receiving home health care services. Table 1.3 presents information on diagnoses at admission from the 1993 survey.

The Physician and House Calls

Since 1940 the number of physicians making house calls has decreased gradually.[8] A survey of the membership of the American Academy of Family Physicians revealed that only 53% of respondents made house calls. However, there are valid reasons for physician home visits. The physician visiting in the home

Table 1.4   Physicians' Reasons for Making a Home Visit

1. Assess home situation
2. Assess acute problems
3. Provide terminal care
4. Improve patient compliance
5. Manage chronic problems
6. Pressure from patient's family
7. Patient could not afford van or ambulance
8. Transportation available but inaccessible
9. Patient is long-term patient
10. Postsurgical care
11. To allow patient to stay home

Adapted from Keenan, J.M. et al., *Arch. Intern. Med.,* 152:2025–2032, 1992.

may gather information that will not be evident in the office environment. This information may include evidence of neglect, overuse of multiple prescription and over-the-counter medications, an unsanitary environment, and ordinary obstacles that may encumber patients in wheelchairs or patients who need high-tech medical equipment in the home. The physician who makes house calls is also able to monitor home health care services that are being utilized in the home. A physician who has a clear understanding of the patient's home environment is better able to direct the efforts of home health care workers in the home. The greatest benefit to the patient from physician home visits is the emotional support it provides from the knowledge that the patient is not cut off from the physician that he or she has depended upon in the past.

Table 1.4 illustrates physicians' reasons for making house calls.[9] The survey that provided this information also provided information on why physicians did *not* make house calls. Some of the reasons physicians gave for not making house calls included the physician's perception that house calls are a poor use of time, reimbursement rates for house calls are inadequate or nonexistent, and physician belief that house calls pose significant malpractice risks.

Keenan et al.[10] reported survey findings indicating that physicians who made house calls were more likely to utilize home health care agencies than their colleagues who did not make house calls. This would seem to indicate a relationship between education about home health care services and the use thereof. The Institute of Medicine has encouraged medical school residency programs to include at least six months of geriatric training by 1996 and nine months by 1999.[11] In a 1990 report by the AMA, ten competencies/goals for a home care curriculum were developed:

1. Physicians should acquire appropriate skills in home care patient assessment.
2. Physicians should be able to assess the adequacy of family caregivers and informal care resources.
3. Physicians should be able to evaluate the efficacy of home care efforts and contribute to improved quality assurance in home care.
4. Physicians should be able to apply home care principles and guidelines appropriately.
5. Physicians should know community resources.
6. Physicians should be knowledgeable about reimbursement policies in home care.
7. Physicians should be knowledgeable about home care technology.
8. Physicians should be able to integrate home, office, and hospital care for patients.
9. Physicians should play an active and major role on the home care team.
10. Physicians should demonstrate they value home care as a part of their practice.

Boston University's Home Medical Service is an excellent example of incorporating home health care education into a medical school curriculum.[12] Physicians at Boston University deliver medical care in the home while at the same time teaching senior medical students. The initial visit to the home is usually made by two medical students who do an extensive evaluation including thorough interview, physical examination, mental status examination, depression screen, functional assessment, nutritional screen, caregiver stress screen, and review of medications. They can also do an EKG and indicated lab work. This initial visit is followed by a team meeting involving the nurse coordinator and attending physician, and a management plan is developed. The attending physician and the students return to the home together within a week, which enables the attending physician to verify the information gathered by the students. Upon leaving the patient's home, the automobile becomes the classroom as the attending physician and the medical students discuss problems and possible remedies.

JCAHO Accreditation

The Joint Commission on Accreditation of Healthcare Organizations (JCAHO) established its Home Care Accreditation Program in 1988 (unpublished data). This program accredits organizations that provide any of the following services, either directly or indirectly:

- **Equipment management services**—Home medical equipment companies that deliver equipment for patients/clients and instruct same in the use of equipment in the home.
- **Home health services**—Organizations that provide professional health care services in the home such as nursing; physical, speech, and occupational therapies; medical social work; and nutrition/dietetics.
- **Personal care and support services**—Agencies that assist patients/clients in activities of daily living (ADL), including bathing services and household maintenance.
- **Pharmaceutical services**—Organizations that prepare and dispense drugs as well as monitor the clinical status of patients and their medication regime in the home.
- **Clinical respiratory services**—Services provided by respiratory care practitioners including, but not limited to, physical assessment, monitoring of vital signs, oximetry testing, and/or the administration of therapeutic treatments.

As of August 1994, the JCAHO had accredited over 3,800 home care service organizations. The advantages of accreditation to the organization include:

- Demonstration of the organization's commitment to provide quality services to patients/clients
- Enhanced community confidence
- Increased competitive edge in the marketplace
- Possible expedition of third-party reimbursement
- Enhancement of the organization's risk management program

Business Management in Home Care

From a business perspective, home care can provide a very attractive profit in specific market niches. It can also be fiercely competitive, thus limiting or, at the very least, driving profit margins in a downward direction.

As an example, on the upper end of profitability, the home infusion business enjoyed significant margins of profit at inception in 1979. During the following 10 to 12 years, margins remained very attractive until the payers began to better understand this not often dealt with entity.

As managed care organizations continued to emerge, consolidate, and control the health care direction of millions of lives, niches such as alternate site infusion therapies began to regroup, change strategies, and form much needed alliances in order to, at best, slow down the profit margin erosion.

Home care companies (not to be confused with home health care companies) remain at the lower end of the profit list, squeaking out 2 to 3% margins as compared to the mid-20% profits of home infusion organizations, and take considerably more effort and greater efficiencies than the "high-tech" alternatives. As a result, several home care and home health care agencies have made an attempt to enter these business arenas.

Home care agencies primarily provide services that are in great demand but generally not covered by government funding without waiver programs. These services include, but are not limited to, ADL:

- Meal preparation
- Housekeeping
- Transportation
- Dressing
- Bathing
- Toileting
- Live-in services

Home health care services can be loosely defined as services ordered on behalf of or by a physician. Some examples are:

- Wound care needs
- Infusion therapy
- Physical therapy
- Occupational therapy
- Social work counseling
- Enterostomy services

The first list of services can generally be handled by homemakers, certified nurse assistants (CNAs), or home health aides. The services in the second list are provided by RNs, LPNs, LVNs, or other professionally trained individuals. Training and accreditation of these workers are of variable quality throughout the industry and must be addressed more comprehensively in the future.

Several national organizations and hospital-based home health agencies provide both service levels. Home care agencies are limited to the ADL services previously stated unless they apply for and receive a license (on a state-by-state basis) to perform home health care services.

Both federal (Medicare) and state (Medicaid) regulations govern and change often enough to keep the service providers on a constant economic roller coaster. This statement is true for the majority of services that are provided outside the traditional hospital setting. The myriad of these services is far reaching and survival goes to the most adaptable organization.

Industry consolidations are also occurring almost weekly. As an example, over an 18-month period CORAM has grown from $0 to the largest alternative site infusion provider in the country. The original four consolidators (T^2, Curaflex, Medisys, and Health Infusion) additionally acquired HMSS and Caremark to form more than a billion-dollar organization with considerable networking potential for the growing managed care business (predicted to cover or insure 95%+ of the country's population by the year 2000). Thus, the home care industry's growth, both in profit attainment and overall revenues, has created a multibillion-dollar carrot that any and all payors would like to control.

Capitation is the critical determinant of agency survivorship. Capitation is a personification of the home care/home health care/universal health care dilemma in general. One entity may not only control its cost for services, but also may know what it is going to pay over a specific period of time. The opposing entity would like to ensure its top live revenue flow: assure cash flow and maintain or increase bottom-line profits.

Due to the myriad innuendoes which occur in providing alternative site products and services, capitation is a paradox regardless of the frequency of periodic review agreed upon by the two parties. Indeed, there is frequently considerable distrust among groups seeking to collaborate. Conflicts arise over services provided and payment received.

Of all the issues that are present in this health care environment, the only thing that is true is that no matter what is written today, it will be obsolete when it hits cyberspace and the Internet.

Again from a business perspective, consider the following quote from an article in *Modern Healthcare*, August 21, 1995:[13] "Physicians, especially in sunny regions such as Florida and Southern California, are taking disability leave in record numbers in a trend blamed on growing unhappiness in their work." This is reality? The same quote could probably be found in some medical news article that appeared in the 1700s (either A.D. or B.C.), but to have it appear now as fact could be very discouraging for future physicians.

In review of current trends vs. future trends, hospitals in the mid-1990s are heavily recruiting the primary care specialties.[14] Family practice and internal medicine are being sought out 73.5 and 53.1% of the time, respectively, closely followed by pediatrics (41.6%) and ob/gyn (32.7%). The primary reason for this goes back to our earlier discussion of the influence of managed care. The more primary care physicians on staff, the greater the chance of working within the managed care system. Thus, this green-eyed monster has also raised its head in directing the recruitment activities of physicians in every community across the nation.

A decision for a physician may very well be to choose a new course of studies or pick a health care stock to invest in. But be careful, and watch the Internet, because you can be sure that the government will decide retroactively that physicians cannot do that due to potential conflict of interest.

The physician's first priority with respect to home care is not to enhance the profitability of home care agencies. It is to extend the patient care possibilities to the home environment, ideally to continue good care and not increase the economic morbidity of illness.[15,16]

During 15 years (1961 to 1976) as chief surgeon at the Ellis Fischel State Cancer Hospital, I (JSS) had the challenge of sending cancer patients home to many rural communities where there was no organized home care available. The Social Service Department directed by Miriam C. Hoag did a remarkable job of identifying and utilizing what services were available. In those days, the Missouri Division of the American Cancer Society provided much assistance through local service committees. In completing the requirements for a master's in public health, I completed a credited course reviewing the operation of that society, which included interviewing chairwomen of these local service committees. I was amazed at the remarkable efforts of these committees in mobilizing community services on behalf of the homebound. Now the Cancer Society has, to its loss and society's as well, largely removed itself from the service area. The Social Service Department also maintained 100% follow-up on these patients, permitting the completion of many longitudinal studies.

While working on my master's degree, I also completed a course in health education. The insight derived totally changed my perspective on the importance of patient and family education at the hospital before discharge. To facilitate the planning, implementation, and evaluation of patient and family education, a health educator was added to the hospital staff. This educator worked directly with the professional staff to develop, implement, and evaluate the efficacy of patient and family education programs. This experience was published.[17]

The results were remarkable. Many responsibilities for home care can be provided by patients and families if appropriate education is provided at the hospital, clinic, or doctor's office. Appropriate equipment for specialized needs was provided by the hospital. The program made the entire hospital run more efficiently by earlier discharge and fewer return visits to the clinic and hospital. There undoubtedly was better patient care and less anxiety among patients and families over not knowing what to do without "asking the doctor."

With respect to current home care, one of the most important aspects is to evaluate what patients and families can do for themselves if they are provided education appropriate to their needs. Any hospital or home care agency that does not have such an educational program is not taking advantage of the possibilities. Education is a humane cost-containing strategy. It is essential in rural environments.

The physician must also be educated in home health care services. In a 1992 study, Keenan et al.[18] surveyed Minnesota home care agencies to assess family and other primary care physicians' practices, knowledge, and skills with regard to home health care services. Physicians were most frequently thought to be deficient in the following areas: home care clinical skills, knowledge of home care technology and capabilities, and knowledge of reimbursement policies and practices.

Rural home care is a special area since many rural environments do not have the population density to support a comprehensive home care agency. Planning for rural care requires social workers, discharge planners, and rural physicians most knowledgeable about the resources available in specific regions. Where none is available, education of patient, family, and available caregivers is particularly essential.

Home health care agencies in rural areas increased 37% in number in 1993,[19] but the distribution of services remains spotty and of variable completeness. Regional and national agencies have expanded into rural areas through acquisition, merger, or new market entry.

Conclusion

Provision of home care is one of the most rapidly expanding areas of health care delivery. Home care is an integral part of the total health care delivery system. Maximizing its full potential will require an expansion of responsive educational and research programs, quality assessment and cost-containing programs, and realignment of many hospitals and clinics to outpatient services and home care networking and management.

References

1. Remington, L., Exclusive interview with Dr. Joseph T. Painter: President of the American Medical Association (AMA), *The Remington Rep.*, Feb./Mar.:25–31, 1994.
2. American Medical Association, Physicians' Current Procedural Terminology CPT 95, 1994.
3. Halamandaris, V. J., Twenty reasons for home care, *Caring*, 4(10), 1985.
4. Lutz, S., Home-care franchises soar in popularity, *Modern Healthcare*, June:34–36, 1993.
5. Roe, O. J., Palliative care 2000—home care, *J. Palliative Care*, 8:28–32, 1992.
6. Haupt, B. J., Hing, E., and Strahan, G., The National Home and Hospice Care Survey: 1992 Summary, National Center for Health Statistics, *Vital Health Stat.*, 13(117), 1994.
7. Strahan, G. W., An Overview of Home Health and Hospice Care Patients: Preliminary Data from the 1993 National Home and Hospice Care Survey, Advance Data No. 256, 1994.

8. Knight, A. L. and Adelman, A. M., The family physician and home care, *AFP*, 44:1733–1737, 1991.

9. Adelman, A. M., Fredman, L., and Knight, A. L., House call practices: a comparison by specialty, *J. Fam. Practice*, 39:39–44, 1994.

10. Keenan, J. M., Boling, P. E., Schwartzberg, J. G., Olson, L., et al., A national survey of the home visiting practice and attitudes of family physicians and internists, *Arch. Intern. Med.*, 152:2025–2032, 1992.

11. Mauch, V. L., Physician education in home care, *Caring*, Sept.:24–28, 1994.

12. Champney, K. J., The physician's role in Boston University's Home Medical Service, *Caring*, April:48–51, 1994.

13. Disability figures show more docs sick of work, *Modern Healthcare*, 25:85, 1995.

14. Burda, D., Legal fears force some changes in recruiting tactics, *Modern Healthcare*, 25:88, 90, 1995.

15. Spratt, J. S., The relation of "human capital" preservation to health costs, *Am. J. Econ. Sociol.*, 34:295–307, 1975.

16. Spratt, J. S., The physician's obligation to minimize the economic morbidity of cancer, *Semin. Oncol.*, 2:411–417, 1975.

17. Monaco, R. M., Salfen, B. J., and Spratt, J. S., The patient as an education participant in healthcare, *Missouri Med.*, 69:932–937, 1972.

18. Keenan, J. M., Hepburn, K. W., Ripsin, C. M., Webster, L. W., and Bland, C. J., A survey of Minnesota home care agencies' perceptions of physician behaviors, *Fam. Med.*, 24:142–144, 1992.

19. Monier, M. G., Strategies for marketing home care in rural America, *The Remington Rep.*, Feb./Mar.:32–35, 1994.

Systems Approach Needed for Home Health Care

2

Robert E. Hoye, Ph.D. and
M. Therese Dalton, R.N., M.P.A.

We are at the beginning of a revolutionary change in health care delivery as the health care system moves toward greater integration and greater use of information technology to manage health care and costs. Without considering the home as part of the health care system, health care in the last 50 years has omitted a crucial component in maintaining the wellness of the American population. In a study by the American Medical Association's Council on Scientific Affairs, it was found that home care is an increasingly important aspect of medical practice in the continuum of health care settings.[1]

Home health care can be defined as the provision of services and equipment to the patient in the home setting for the purpose of restoring and maintaining his or her maximum level of health, function, and comfort. The key to utilizing this aspect of health care, however, is coordination of the services in the health care system available to the patient in the community. In the United States, there are more than 16 health workers for every physician as part of the teamwork needed in the health care system.[1] In the typical patient-flow scenario (Figure 2.1), the patient moves through the health system beginning with the primary care physician and on to home health care when needed. The information that needs to flow with the patient through the health care system has many facets, including clinical data and financial aspects.

©GR/St. Lucie Press CCC 1-884015-93-X 1/97/$100/$.50

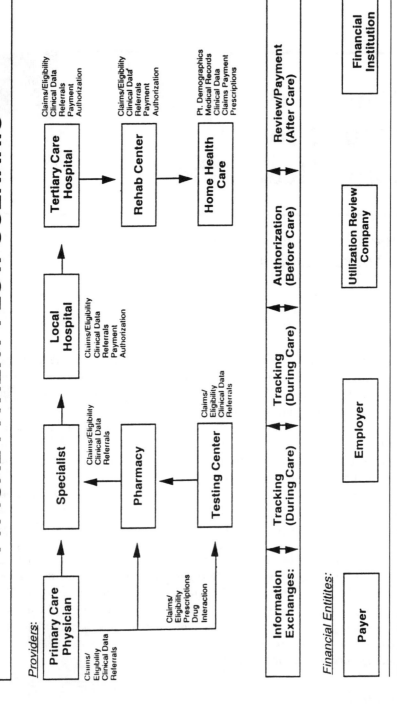

Figure 2.1 Systems flow scenario.

Home Health Care a Is Component of the Health Care System

Home care has been one of the more underutilized aspects of the health care system and is beginning to attract greater physician interest and participation. Home health care is a rapidly growing field that can be most effective when used in conjunction with hospital- and community-based services. Whereas hospital beds and utilization have declined in recent years, the home health industry has seen growth in the trend toward delivering care in the home. In the past, few considered the linkage between the health care system and home health care, but with the potential for significant savings and improved patient quality of life, home health care is no longer a minor component of the health care system. Many primary care physicians see preventive home care as an extension of their office practice and, indeed, it can be that and much more. Medical care at home can be preventive, diagnostic, therapeutic, rehabilitative, or long-term maintenance care for many age ranges from infants to the elderly.[1]

There is an ever-growing plethora of both services and equipment available for home health to assist patients. The technology and equipment being adapted for home health care range from blood glucose monitoring for the diabetic through mini intensive care units with ventilators, central venous lines, and long-distance telemetry for the acutely ill. There are even devices to improve communication, socialization, and recreation for the homebound. Emerging information system technologies can make home health care surprisingly effective. Information from computer-based medical records can be used to identify effective therapies and treatments, and automatic alert and monitoring systems, body function monitoring, teleconsulting, and health coaching will provide the feedback link needed between patients and health care providers.[2]

The health care system from the patient's perspective has been viewed as the hospital, the clinic, and the emergency room—all generally impersonal and not geared to the patient's comfort. However, the least traumatic form of medical care and the most efficient and effective is seen as home health care. The diagnostic value of home visits, especially for geriatric and chronically ill patients, is seen in improved assessment and diagnosis of functional status and environmental characteristics.[1] This shift from hospital to home care appears to be spurred by several factors, with economics and technology being the predominant "push and pull" factors in this emerging facet of the health care system.

With the evolution from private pay to managed care and the host of technological innovations, the home health industry is rapidly being overhauled. The coordination of home care services coupled with the daily demands and requirements placed on the home health caregiver are complicated when the primary caregiver is a family member. When the caregiver is a visiting nurse, clinical data can be captured with mobile computers or hand-held systems that can send data to a central repository and support integration with the agency, resulting in better outcomes. Some managed care environments are turning toward home health care divisions that rely on wireless computing and contain costs.[3]

So what is the health care system? Most observers of the health care system agree that it deals primarily with the diagnosis and treatment of disease and not with health. Much of the present-day medical practice in health care is based upon old, unproven technology handed down in the education of health professionals and focused upon the physical pathology of the patient. Health is a term used often without thinking about the definition. In fact, health and disease are not simply opposites. The Greek physicians believed that health was a condition of perfect equilibrium of the body's humors or whatever constituted the human body. According to H.D. Banta, *Webster's Unabridged Dictionary* defines health as "physical and mental well-being" and "freedom from defect, pain or disease."[4]

Analyzing the Health Care System

What is the American health care system and who does it serve? To answer the first question, let's begin by answering who it serves—the U.S. population of a little more than 250 million Americans who reside in an area of about 3.6 million square miles. Based upon either population or area, the United States is one of the largest countries in the world. Unlike most European and other developed countries, the American population is heterogeneous, with a wide variety of cultures, races, and ethnic groups dispersed over a large land mass. This has significant implications for the types of health care provided and the ways in which health care is delivered.[5]

Health care is provided by physicians, nurses, and more than 200 different occupational groups that range from physical therapists to lab technicians. Health care is increasingly provided in larger, more complex organizations, the leading types being ambulatory care, hospitals, long-term care, and mental health. Another important way of analyzing the health care system is to assess how the system and its services are financed. According to Kovner, "Containing health care costs has been an important national problem for at least 25 years."[5] Coupled with the financing of the health care system is the government's role in regulating the providers and providing health services directly. Planning health care and measuring health status, analyzing consumer preferences, evaluating utilization, quality control, and cost effectiveness of technology all contribute to the underpinnings of the health care system and how it works.

Strategic Change and Systems Theory

Futurist John Naisbett sees many paradoxes in the dramatically changing world. The paradox he focuses on is the larger the system, the smaller and more powerful and important the parts.[6] The recent explosive developments in telecommunications are the driving forces behind creating the global economy and empowering its parts. One of the biggest trends in recent years has been the move from "economies of scale" to "diseconomies of scale," where the smaller, speedier, and more innovative organizations are prevailing because as more information becomes available to the individual through telecommunications systems, individuals become more empowered.

With this in mind, another major trend is the formation of strategic alliances, where competitors agree to cooperate and carve out business for each competitor. One of the unarticulated reasons for the growth of strategic alliances is that organizations can avoid getting bigger and small/medium-sized organizations can innovate faster and take advantage of new technologies.[6] Naisbett believes that this strategic change, which is now occurring, is the creation of the information age based upon the blending of technologies, computers, telephones, and televisions into one telecommunications industry. The telecommunications technology has triggered a dramatic change in information sharing and in the way we communicate. Just as we are globally moving to one economic marketplace, we are moving in telecommunications to a worldwide network of information networks linked together.[6]

The essence of systems thinking, according to Senge,[7] lies in a shift of mind, which perceives interrelationships rather than linear cause–effect chains and processes of change rather than snapshots. The two types of processes are (1) reinforcing or amplifying feedback and (2) balancing or stabilizing feedback. This "shift of mind" made possible through systems thinking propels the individuals in the organization to grasp the capacity for subtle interconnectedness, which is what gives living systems their unique character. Senge's approach to systems theory emphasizes that organizations and societies resemble complex organizations because they too have myriad balancing feedback and reinforcement processes that can change or kill an organization.[7] The new angle, though, is that individual empowerment is possible once systems thinking is embraced and implemented, such as in home health care situations.

Beckhard and Harris[8] see the organization as a system that has various forces in its environment that affect it, such as competitors, societal issues, global location, and the explosion of technology. For example, use of technological innovations has changed the actual shape and character of many organizations by giving access to information in seconds rather than weeks. In any organizational change, there is always a future state or "to be achieved" condition, the present state, and the transition state during which the actual changes take place. Managing complexity involves a strong ability to deal with ambiguity, managing conflict, a concern for people and their potential, a balance between planning skills and intuition, and, most importantly, a strategic vision. Successful intervention in complex systems is becoming more of a science than an art, but it is still not an unambiguous process.[8]

Comparisons of Systems View, Strategic Change, and Organizational Transitions

In looking at systems theory from the perspective of the systems view of the world, strategic change, and organizational transitions, there are various approaches to managing change and meeting the demands of the shifting environment. The complex organizational change now being felt in organizations and systems today was the subject of Senge's systems thinking approach, which is that as the world becomes more interconnected and complex, people need to become more of a learning community. The essence of this fifth discipline of systems thinking lies in a shifting of the mind to perceive interrelationships rather than linear cause–effect chains.

Beckhard and Harris emphasize the management of complex changes and the dilemma of achieving or managing change in an organization. They see the organization as a system that has various forces in its environment, such as competitors, societal issues, and the explosion of technology which is changing the shape and character of organizations. Senge's approach is learning organizations, where individual empowerment is possible once systems thinking is embraced. Beckhard and Harris's assessment is more of a top-down management mapping of the mission, goals, priorities, and ability to deal with ambiguity and manage conflicts.

In another view, Boulding perceives the world as a total system that will evolve with advanced communications to the point that no one is in charge. This spread of information and knowledge through better communication within and between systems is a major change from before this information technology was available. Empowerment of individuals through better communication is expected to happen to a greater extent with information technology, and even the interdependency of smaller organizations with their outside environment will be influenced through the feedback and forces of the system.[9] It is this linkage between system thinking and feedback as it applies to the health care system and home care that will be explored further here.

Systems Thinking and Health Care

Reisman's[10] notable explanation of a systems approach as it applies to the study of health care organizations is that a system is an organization of man and machine components that have coordinated and goal-directed activities, which are linked by information channels and affected by the external environment. The range of system types in health care can be represented by three extremes within which all systems fall. The points on this multidimensional triangle of systems are (1) a stationary individual system doing repetitive tasks; (2) a complex, fully automated self-regulating system process; and (3) a large, high-technology socioeconomic system performing a one-of-a-kind function.

The concept of a system involves a number of observed variables coming into and leaving the system; the input quantities are called independent or exogenous variables and the output quantities are called dependent or endogenous variables. To relate this concept to the health care system, the "inputs" in a clinic, hospital, or home setting are the patients; the conversion process could be the examination, surgery, or physical therapy; and the "outputs" are serviced patients now healthy. The concept of an information feedback system is a key component of the health care system because it exists whenever the environment leads to a decision, which results in action that affects the environment and influences future decisions. In a feedback-control system, control ensures that what the system produces is sensed, measured, or counted at the point of output and is consistent with the goals of the system. Controls allow the system to recognize deviations and make the necessary corrections whenever a discrepancy between the actual and desired output is detected.[10]

Finally, the concept of health as a right is different from health care as a right because health is primarily the concern of the individual and the health care system cannot provide health. As society changes, its state of health changes and its view of health and health care itself changes. A balance between personal freedom and public health can be difficult to obtain, but dramatic savings in lives have occurred due to safe drinking water, vaccinations, air bags in cars, and less fat in beef, when both personal and governmental action was taken. Banta[4] states that "This country needs a health policy that deals with the four elements seen to affect health: human biology, environment, lifestyle, and the health care organization."

Recognition of Needs and Statement of Problem

Health care is on the threshold of a crisis that will both push it and pull it into change. We have developed a health care system characterized by large institutions and specialists practicing narrow, expensive medicine that is failing to meet many human needs and is largely ignoring disease prevention and health promotion. The recent trends toward massive mergers and for-profit conglomerates in the health care sector may only exacerbate these problems, while the physician is expected to be a gatekeeper who takes care of the sick and contains the costs of care.[4] Under the auspices of the technological medical system, predicted advances include human gene therapy, understanding the genetic origin of many diseases, regeneration of tissues, slowing of aging, and increased epidemiological knowledge resulting from databanks. However, this technological system is failing to meet many human needs and has ignored opportunities for disease prevention and health promotion through home health care.

Health care is a very personalized service, with both physical and psychological elements that are interrelated with the consumer's motivation to seek service, cooperate with the physician and the health care team, and change behavior to improve health.[4] Caring for the human lives entrusted to the health care system implies a dynamic process that needs to be responsive to more than treating diseases; it must also create health. The transition to the new paradigm of health systems will need to include better, faster, and more effective modes of containing costs, controlling clinical decisions, monitoring patient health, educating patients, improving education, and addressing inadequacies in the health systems, such as lack of continuity of care by various health care providers. There are new efforts to examine practice patterns and medical outcomes to improve the quality of care. In the current period of uncertainty and experimentation, many areas of the United States are moving toward more managed care in a regulated market, which regulates what the doctor gets paid, what the doctor does, and the care a patient receives.[4] It is this elusive balance in the health systems that seems to keep the decision makers constantly reacting to the changing environment and then readjusting to meet the needs of the systems.

Health Care Shift and Health Systems

There are many problems in today's health care system and still many more approaches to solving these problems that are being considered in the shifting health care scenarios. One of the fundamental concepts of the systems approach is feedback, and it is this feedback which has been an important element missing in the U.S. health systems. Achieving this missing feedback to provide needed input and output in our fragmented health care system can be accomplished through better use of information technology in health care.

According to Senge,[7] the essence of systems thinking is in: (1) seeing the interrelationships rather than linear cause–effect chains and (2) seeing the processes of change rather than snapshots. If the separate interests of health providers (mainly hospitals, physicians, and health plans) continue to fuel adversarial relationships, then the health care systems will continue to have problems. On the other hand, focusing on the health status of the community may serve as the bridge needed to share information and power so that the health system can survive.[11] Use of systems thinking in evaluating and addressing the issue of home health care is most appropriate because the workings of the health care system have become so complex.

Information technology can play a key role in transforming health systems to include home health care. The failures of the current system are not the result of spending too little; rather, the problems stem from spending too much on the wrong things, thereby producing practice patterns and organizations ill-suited for primary care, public health, and prevention. We need to shift the emphasis of health care systems away from overspending, overspecialization, and over-building by using information technology to support a deeper understanding of the effects, the costs, and outcomes of actions taken that could support better decisions. In peeling back the onion of complexity in the U.S. health care system, it appears that many aspects in the current crisis of health care are symptoms of deeper discord. We have a complex health care system that is so preoccupied with its advanced technology and maintaining the institutional autonomy of its elements that it has neglected the population that it is meant to serve.

System Failures Can Be the Impetus Necessary for Change

Overall, there are a number of failures in the health care system that may serve as the impetus needed to produce change. First, the health care system has failed to take responsibility for the spiraling cost of care, which caused cost-containment measures to be imposed from outside the system and exacerbated discord. Second, the health care system has failed to address the class of problems associated with the proliferation of advanced technology and has failed to address the relationship of medical practice to public health and to growing social problems linked to teenage pregnancy, substance abuse, and domestic abuse. Third, the system has failed to take responsibility for wellness and prevention and has failed to provide leadership in coping with many bioethical issues. Fourth, the most active component of the system, the physician community, has failed to lead in regulating itself as a profession by taking responsibility for the number, specialty training, distribution, professionalism, and quality of practice of its members. Finally, the health care system has failed to use any but the most rudimentary tools and techniques of systems and management sciences, including information technology, to keep its complex house in order.[12]

The U.S. health care system is so complex and interlocked that the costs realistically can only be contained by cooperative planning and action. It is the awakening of some sectors to the impact of competition that is forcing change even before health care reform legislation is mandated by Congress.[13] Managed care is believed to be the most likely mechanism available capable of reducing health care delivery costs.[14] Managed care plans are fundamentally altering the paradigm of health care delivery by rapidly eroding the traditional fee-for-service referral system, where health care providers are reimbursed based upon resources used without regard for appropriateness of the health services consumed.

The New Health Care Approach

Even before the notion of health care reform was politically popular, there were significant changes well underway throughout the United States. The pioneering efforts of a number of leading health care providers are pointing the way to the "new health care." This concept is now being recognized by several innovative health care organizations which are structured to reward providers who maintain the health of the population they serve. Payment mechanisms, technology, lifestyle, and customer expectations are outside forces that have begun to converge to motivate providers to integrate health care systems in order to maintain the health of defined populations, prevent disease, and foster early detection and treatment. As noted in Figure 2.2, the pendulum on the continuum of care has begun to swing toward greater emphasis on achieving and maintaining health through primary care screening and preventive care with immunization, education, and wellness.[15]

Collaboration is the underpinning of this new health care approach. Customers' expectations and economic reality are forcing replacement of the freestanding health facility or independent practitioner with a new order of networks and mega-health systems that recognize the potential of integration or at least cooperation. It is this recognition which is changing the adversarial relationships that often existed between providers and purchasers. Further, this integration of providers is facilitated by combining information and telecommunications technologies to allow accessible delivery of appropriate health care data to the customers in the systems.

Understanding the concept that the health of the population served is the ultimate measure of accountability has propelled forward-thinking providers in the direction of clinical pathing, using appropriateness of care methodologies, and providing optimal lifestyles information. The current focus on clinical outcomes, which serves to assess internal quality management, will give way to

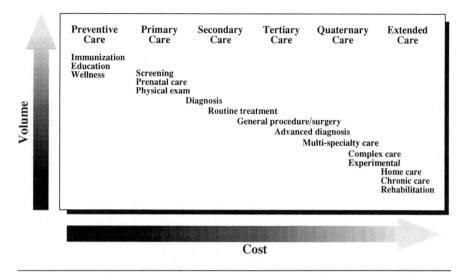

Figure 2.2 Continuum of care.

measures of wellness and customer satisfaction that are measured against expectations and actual costs.

This new health care is led by providers that have recognized that "managed care" means predictability, risk management, appropriateness of care, and accountability to the purchasers of the health care. This patient focus and gatekeeper approach accomplished by using a primary care physician is illustrated in Figure 2.3. Here, the team cooperates to support the primary care physician, who has

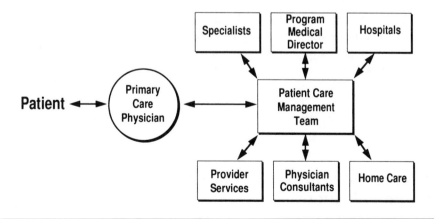

Figure 2.3 Health care system.

immediate contact with the patient and identifies the care needed. Through this teamwork, the primary care physician can better coordinate patient encounters and interaction with the health care team and home health caregivers.

Finally, the new health care is competitive in that the health care systems that survive will seek to preserve the free enterprise of American medicine in a socially and economically responsive fashion.[15] Thus, the newly focused and redesigned health care systems that emerge will be more than reformed; they will be redirected to meet the needs of their customers. A major thrust for this new direction emanates from the effects of information technology which make possible the communication, integration, and competitive edge in the health care systems of today and tomorrow.

In analyzing the U.S. health care system in term of systems thinking, it becomes evident that our health system deals primarily with the diagnosis and treatment of disease and not with health itself. The health system evolved as it did for various reasons but was primarily driven by financial incentives to build and expand itself. However, the health system has gotten out of control in terms of costliness and its purpose for existence. The formulation of a better value model for the health system is difficult to envision and to effect when there are so many competing entities that will be affected by any change through health care reform. What we see happening is the health care system beginning to take some corrective actions even without the push from legislation, and this is encouraging. While it is unlikely that any comprehensive national health insurance plan will be enacted in the near term, the consolidation of formerly direct competitor health service organizations is precipitating new forms of communication within and among these health services.

The shift toward greater use of information technology in health care systems reflects the changes emanating from the organizational and social changes in the health care environment. Health care has entered one of the greatest periods of consolidation and upheaval faced by any major industry in recent memory. Compounding this period of change, the health care system, which has been one of the last holdouts to computerize its data, is beginning to accept information technology as an approach to systems integration. The cost of health care and payer pressures are compelling hospitals and doctors to collaborate much more closely than before as all parties are moving to shape an information networked future.

Missing Link in Health Care Today Is Communications

Information management systems and telecommunications are critical to build the information infrastructure for health care reform and communications. These information technologies are needed at all levels to obtain and share clinical and cost data throughout the continuum of care.

Today, the health care system environment can be described as follows:

- Vast majority of patient information resides in doctors' offices
- Legacy hospital information systems exist in most hospitals and HMOs
- Paper medical records in hospitals and doctors' offices do not link care provided to cost
- Nonexistent patient feedback loop through the continuum of care
- Little empirical data exist on clinical outcomes measurements
- Limited communications between health care team members
- Outdated business practices in administering care, purchasing from suppliers, and reimbursement
- Negative incentives to be cost effective in providing care
- Only some pressures for measuring quality and accountability exist

The health care system is information rich, but communications poor. It has hundreds of millions of patient records, thousands of textbooks, hundreds of periodicals, and several online information services such as MEDLINE, yet the information is not readily accessible. In an information-liberated system, information of all kinds would be available to all parts of the health care system.[12]

Dissonances in the Health Care System

The hallmark of a system in crisis is dissonance, and this abounds in the current health care system. The crisis in health care is foremost a crisis of mission, with confusion about the values and goals of caregivers and consumers. The crisis is also to a large extent a crisis of expectation, where the expectations of consumers of health care diverge from the capabilities of the diverse health care delivery system. Finally, it is a crisis of unmet responsibilities of each party involved. For example, new considerations for the aging population have largely been ignored by the system, and promising new tools such as information systems and techniques for quality are being adopted too slowly.[12]

It is not enough to identify the kinds of crises and dissonances that are plaguing the health care system. Before effective solutions can be proposed, it is necessary to understand the underlying causes and forces at work. The health care system is extraordinarily complex in size and scope, reaching into every corner of the country and society. By taking the classic systems approach of examining relevant aspects of the health care system, we can decide what the underlying causes and problems are before looking for solutions. The underlying causes of dissonance in the health care system fall into three areas. First, the system does not have an infrastructure within which it can govern itself and set policy. Second, as problems have developed, the health care system has been unwilling to take the lead in finding solutions. Third, health care providers, consumers, educators, researchers, and policymakers do not have the information they need for the effective functioning of the health care system.[12]

Much of the information needed to bring the health care system into the next century exists but is not readily available. The major blockage is information flow, which is hampering achievement of potential modern medical and communications technology. Information that could be used for clinical decision making, health education, research, and policy formulation is trapped at its origins. It is trapped in patient records stored somewhere in clinics or hospitals or trapped in research laboratories, textbooks, and journals. Information is trapped in files of third-party payers and in the minds of providers and consumers. As a result, the information is inaccessible to the health care team who could be guided by its collective wisdom.[12]

Operationally, the tools exist to deliver information where it is needed and to support the effective use of information. However, the health care system has not taken full advantage of these tools, which include information technology, practice management techniques, and biostatistical methodologies. In the absence of national leadership from within the health system, each stakeholder group or geographic region has devised its own disconnected solutions, such as standards of care. A systems approach would require that all stakeholders collaborate in designing the solutions, but this is not easy for a system that has no infrastructure and is unaccustomed to providing leadership for solving its problems. Solutions for information-based problems, such as those caused by lack of good information, can be addressed by information technology and establishment of an infrastructure.[12]

Communication of Information

It has been said that "an individual without information cannot take responsibility; an individual who is given information cannot help but take responsibility."[16] There are few greater liberating forces than the sharing of information because information motivates in several ways. Information is seen to flatten the organizational pyramid and shift skill and responsibility to the front line by facilitating needed communications across functional barriers (horizontal management). It provides critical confirmation that the organization sees the worker as a partner and problem solver; it also stirs the combative juices for problem solving and continuous improvement.[16] To achieve information liberation, the health care system must have an infrastructure to communicate from one health care provider or element of the system to another and must make a conscious choice to shift from individual interests to that of the system as a whole. With this type of integration, information could flow in several directions as needed.

Optimally, information would flow in several directions, as described in the following examples of localized flow, upward flow, and downward flow. At the local level, appropriate information would be shared by doctors, patients, and hospitals by sharing a single health record; patient education based upon individual health status would begin; and local public health planning groups would correlate data on environmental and industrial pollution with variations in types of hospital admissions. In regions and states, as well as diverse national organizations, upward-flowing information could be used from the local level for regional planning, research, and policy-making. Thus, the local level would contribute to the refinement of the medical knowledge base. Downward flow of information, especially medical knowledge, policy guidelines, and drug warnings, could be distributed directly to the local caregiver. Public health advisories and treatment for specific patient problems would be disseminated to all caregivers who wanted and needed such information. Also, clinical research information would be readily available to researchers, clinicians, or consumers.[12]

Scope of Information Networking Needed

For the regional-level functions, information networking would include:

- Maintaining health-related databases on health status, costs, and facilities
- Creating medical and consumer educational programs for the region
- Coordinating and managing a payment system
- Assessing quality of care, including evaluating institutions, monitoring quality, and options for improvement[12]

The regional level may facilitate a downlink for clinical guidelines and educational material from the national level and at the same time act as an uplink for medical records from the local level.

The local level of information networking provides data from individual health care facilities, which are critically important to the system. The kinds of information functions at the local level include:

- Maintaining longitudinal medical records for a population that received health care at diverse locations, including the home and workplace
- Offering consumers access to medical knowledge and educational programs
- Coordinating the scheduling of patients for multiple providers

- Tracking patient compliance with preventive care and treatment programs
- Providing informal communication, consultations, and referrals
- Offering clinicians up-to-date information about new clinical guidelines, research findings, and local health care statistics
- Providing software to health care providers and researchers for modeling, specialized database search strategies, and compliance monitoring[12]

Conclusion

Just as the use of a computer-based patient record implies and involves cultural changes in health care organizations, so too is its adoption more than a technology issue; it is a business issue.[17] Just as a patient moves through an integrated health care system from office visits to inpatient care to ancillary services such as home health, the information collected and used at each point should travel with the patient through the process. Then, the effect or outcome of the clinical intervention can begin to be assessed and the quality of care given linked to the costs. In order for useful outcomes research studies and for the clinical decision makers to understand the dynamics driving the health care system and its costs, patient data need to be obtainable and usable by all involved in the health care team.[18]

As society moved from hometown family practitioners to the monolithic health care superstructure and health care specialists and from privately paid health care to third-party insurance coverage, communications with and for the patient did not keep pace with this system expansion. Huge health conglomerates built empires and medical technology became infatuated with the space age possibilities, ignoring the mounting national fiscal deficit. To further complicate matters, the health care system focused on patient illness instead of patient wellness and continued system operations in almost complete isolation of each other. The dissonance in the health care system smoldered due to the lack of a self-governing policy-making infrastructure, lack of leadership, and lack of necessary information for providers and consumers to make appropriate decisions.

Effective communication of information will contribute to the improvements needed in the U.S. health care system; however, in and of itself, information will not solve the fractionation of the current health care system. Information can, however, expedite identification of feasible solutions to providing better health care and promotion of wellness through integrated health care systems. Comprehensive cradle-to-grave health care that is accessible, effective, appropriate, and provided at a reasonable cost may become a reality in the 21st century. Until then, we will be evolving the health care system and information infrastructure needed for near-term clinical and administrative decision making. Information systems technology offers the bridge necessary for the Tower of Babel in health care to communicate information effectively so that the health system can continue, can make improvements, and can better serve its intended purpose.

References

1. Home Care in the 1990's, Council on Scientific Affairs Report, *JAMA*, 263(9):1241–1244, 1990.
2. Institute for Alternative Futures and Consumer Interest Research Institute, *21st Century Learning and Health Care in the Home: Creating a National Telecommunications Network*, Washington, D.C., 1992, pp. 12–18.
3. Rollins, S., Trends and imperatives for home healthcare information systems, *Healthcare Informatics*, 11(9):40–50, 1994.
4. Banta, H. D., What is health care? in *Health Care Delivery in the United States*, 4th edition, Kovner, A. R., Ed., Springer Publishing, New York, 1990, pp. 8–26.
5. Kovner, A. R., Ed., *Health Care Delivery in the United States*, 4th edition, Springer Publishing, New York, 1990.
6. Naisbitt, J., *Global Paradox: The Bigger the World Economy, The More Powerful Its Smallest Players*, William Morrow, New York, 1994.
7. Senge, P., *The Fifth Discipline: The Art and Practice of the Learning Organization*, Doubleday/Currency, New York, 1990, pp. 72–83.
8. Beckhard, R. and Harris, R. T., *Organizational Transitions: Managing Complex Change*, 2nd edition, Addison-Wesley, Reading, Massachusetts, 1987.
9. Boulding, K. E., *Three Faces of Power*, Sage Publications, Newbury Park, California, 1990, pp. 109–123.
10. Reisman, A., *Systems Analysis in Health-Care Delivery*, Lexington Books, Lexington, Massachusetts, 1979.
11. Grayson, M., Sharing the power, *Hospitals and Health Networks*, 68(15):36–43, 1994.
12. Duncan, K. A., *Health Information and Health Reform: Understanding the Need for a National Health Information System*, Jossey-Bass, San Francisco, 1994.
13. Morone, J. A., The health care bureaucracy: small changes, big consequences, *J. Health Politics, Policy and Law*, 18(3):723–739, 1993.
14. Miccio, J. A., Ed., Managed care spells change, *Competitive Insight*, 1(4):1–25, 1994.
15. Weaver, F. J., The new health care, *J. Health Care Marketing*, 14(2):10–11, 1994.
16. Peters, T., *Thriving on Chaos*, Harper & Row, New York, 1987, pp. 609–618.
17. Bergman, R., Health care in a wired world, *Hospitals and Health Networks*, 68(16):28–36, 1994.
18. Marwick, C., Using high-quality providers to cope with today's rising health care costs, *JAMA*, 268(16):2142–2145, 1992.

Home Intravenous Antibiotic Therapy

3

Anna K. Huang, M.D. and Hiram C. Polk, Jr., M.D.

Introduction

In the past two decades, the American medical industry has seen the growth of home health services, due in part to the recognition that certain conditions can be treated effectively and to some extent less expensively than in the acute or chronic care facility.[1-3] Infectious processes in which the clinical response is rapid and the treatment course is prolonged are well-suited for outpatient management. Serious infections often require parenteral therapy which can be provided in an ambulatory setting. In those many instances when repeated antibiotic administration is not possible in a doctor's office or hospital infusion unit, home infusion is a good alternative, especially when other nursing or ancillary therapies are needed. The benefits of home intravenous antibiotic therapy, the various types of infection for which this approach is reasonable, and the criteria for patient and antibiotic selection are discussed in this chapter. In addition, adaptations of infusion equipment for home use, laboratory monitoring, and complications of home antibiotic therapy are described.

Benefits

There are some specific benefits from antibiotic therapy in relation to other home health services. In many instances of infection, it is the length of drug therapy that determines the duration of hospitalization. Therefore, the ability to transfer care to the home setting saves that portion of the cost of hospitalization, which mainly consists of the hospital room charges.[4,5] Many patients with endocarditis, osteomyelitis, and cryptococcal meningitis will resolve the signs and symptoms of their infection long before an adequate treatment course is completed. For these people, prolonged hospitalization may be psychologically detrimental to their full recovery. One aspect of prolonged hospitalization is the increased risk for nosocomial, or hospital-acquired, complications, especially other infections. While superinfections with *Clostridium difficile* or *Candida* species will not be avoided in the patient on home antibiotic infusions, exposure to multidrug-resistant pathogens, such as methicillin-resistant *Staphylococcus aureus* and *Pseudomonas aeruginosa*, will be reduced in the home setting.

Conditions Amenable to Home Infusion Antibiotic Therapy

The types of infections requiring parenteral antibiotic therapy that can be treated in the ambulatory or home setting have expanded in the past 15 years. While the amount of published data remains small, clinical experience has proven the efficacy, safety, and cost savings of this approach. Technological developments have aided in providing infusion equipment adaptable to the home setting. In all instances, medical stabilization must occur before consideration of continuing antibiotic therapy at home.

Bone and Soft Tissue Infections

Bone and soft tissue infections were some of the earliest sites that provided data for the feasibility of home infusion therapy.[6] The diagnoses of osteomyelitis and septic arthritis have traditionally meant very long (6 or more weeks) courses of intravenous antibiotics to deliver adequate drug levels into bone or joint space. Patients remained in the hospital or nursing home for the duration of therapy until the late 1970s when Antoniskis et al.[6] demonstrated the efficacy of outpatient parenteral therapy for osteomyelitis. Eisenberg and Kitz[4] performed a cost analysis of patients discharged home on once-daily antibiotic therapy, after stabilization in the hospital, and found that it would save at least several hundred dollars per case. This analysis compared hospitalization costs from several different sources, including the New Jersey diagnosis-related group (DRG) program where hospital costs may be reimbursed at a minimum level. With the introduction of quinolone antibiotics that provide high serum and tissue concentrations with oral administration, many patients with osteomyelitis can avoid or shorten long-term parenteral antibiotic therapy. Oral therapy can begin as soon as pathogen susceptibility patterns are found to include ciprofloxacin or ofloxacin.

In the case of prosthetic device infections, prolonged courses of antibiotics are utilized to sterilize the surgical site both when the prosthesis remains and when hardware is removed and future reimplantation is contemplated.[7-10] Home infusion therapy can assist the patient in coping with this lengthy treatment plan. For a small group of patients who are not candidates for further joint replacement, infection may need to be suppressed chronically in the home setting with parenteral antibiotics. Other soft tissue infections requiring only 1 to 2 weeks of intravenous therapy can also be managed outside of the hospital. When diagnosed with cellulitis or diabetic foot infections which do not require surgical debridement, patients can receive one dose of parenteral antibiotic in the physician's office or hospital outpatient unit to ensure no immediate hypersensitivity reaction and then complete the therapy at home with a referral to a home health agency.[11]

Abscesses

Home antibiotic therapy for infections involving abscess formation in such sites as the brain, lung, and abdomen is becoming more frequent. Since these diagnoses are often the result of multiple tests and invasive procedures, patients will initially be started on antibiotic therapy in the hospital. When the patient's overall medical condition requires less intensive nursing skills, home infusion can be arranged for the remainder of the 4- to 6-week course of antibiotics. The combination of drugs that is often necessary to eradicate these frequently polymicrobial infections can be administered by various routes, such as intravenous β-lactam plus oral metronidazole, thus simplifying the home care regimen.

Endocarditis and Intravascular Infection

Another infection whose therapeutic approach has been changed dramatically is the intravascular infection or endocarditis. These cases often required prolonged hospitalizations to complete 4 to 6 weeks of antibiotic therapy. Since the growth of the home health industry, patients with intravascular infections can receive most of their therapy at home, once medical stabilization has been achieved. Close monitoring in the outpatient setting will help the clinician recognize the late complications of endocarditis (e.g., embolization, mycotic aneurysm, and myocardial abscess). Successful treatment has been most frequently seen when pathogens can be controlled quickly, e.g., streptococci, enterococcus, and HACEK (*Haemophilus, Actinobacillus, Cardiobacterium, Eikenella*, and *Kingella*) organisms.[12] In addition to the conventional regimens for these particular bacteria, other, newer antibiotics, especially ceftriaxone, have been used successfully for outpatient treatment of endocarditis.[13,14]

Large numbers of immunocompromised and seriously ill patients have led to the increased use of chronic venous access devices. There is now extensive experience with curing intravascular infection without removing the indwelling catheter.[15] Patients with reticuloendothelial neoplasms and infection associated with Hickman catheters apparently had sterilization of their catheters with 6 to 8 weeks of intravenous antibiotics. Failure was most often associated with bacteria producing adhesive substances or slime layers (e.g., *Staphylococcus aureus*, *Staphylococcus epidermidis*, and *Candida* species). Given circumstances where central venous access must be maintained, such as for chemotherapy or total parenteral nutrition, one should treat bacteremia aggressively. If the catheter is replaced, 4 weeks of antibiotics may be sufficient to protect the new device from being contaminated. If replacement would be difficult (e.g., secondary to thrombocytopenia), then an 8-week course through the catheter lumen may be attempted for cure.

Meningitis

The introduction of new broad-spectrum antibiotics in the past 15 years has aided physicians tremendously in the treatment of meningitis. The third-generation cephalosporins—ceftriaxone, cefoperazone, ceftizoxime, and ceftazidime—have simplified the standard regimens for bacterial and atypical meningitis. These drugs, having both Gram-positive and Gram-negative coverage, achieve therapeutic concentrations in the cerebrospinal fluid via the intravenous route, thereby minimizing the need for intrathecal aminoglycoside therapy. In addition, by giving them in two to three daily doses, these are preferred agents over penicillin derivatives with similar microbiologic activity. A variety of situations will allow home therapy following diagnosis of meningitis. The patient with bacterial meningitis without serious neurologic deficits acutely and whose symptoms respond rapidly may complete his antibiotic course outside of the hospital.[16] Pathogens with a more subacute presentation (e.g., *Borrelia burgdorferii* [Lyme disease] or tertiary or neurosyphilis [or late latent disease in the person with human immunodeficiency virus infection]) may also be eradicated with outpatient intravenous antibiotic therapy.[17,18] Cryptococcal meningitis will be discussed in the next section.

Fungal Infection

In the era of acquired immunodeficiency syndrome (AIDS) and bone marrow transplantation, growing numbers of invasive fungal infection are being encountered and successfully controlled, if not cured, by long-term antifungal therapy. This has led to greater experience in the use of amphotericin B, in both the hospital and ambulatory settings. Sepsis with true yeast, as in *Candida* or *Torulopsis*, is often a result of extensive antibiotic use or secondary to spread from a colonized site, such as the bladder or skin. Patients with these infections will require only short courses of therapy, especially if done in conjunction with cessation of systemic antibiotics, parenteral nutrition, and indwelling foreign bodies.[19] In contrast, cryptococcus meningitis is seen mainly in patients with underlying immunosuppression resulting from AIDS, chemotherapy, or transplantation. Neurologic abnormalities, such as altered mental status, portend a poor outcome and must be addressed aggressively with amphotericin B.[20,21] Many patients with such abnormalities will require long-term, often lifelong, antifungal maintenance therapy. Following stabilization with amphotericin B, these patients can be switched to alternative oral agents. Dimorphic fungi, such as *Histoplasma*, *Coccidioides imitis*, and *Blastomyces*, while often controllable with imidazoles, may exhibit drug resistance and require treatment with amphotericin B. In the case of opportunistic fungal infection, such as *Aspergillus* or *Mucor*, even prolonged amphotericin B therapy may not be curative until the underlying immunosuppressive condition is corrected.

Greater experience with the nuances and multiple side effects of amphotericin B administration in the past decade has allowed its use for home infusion. Even a short course of amphotericin B with a goal of 1 gram cumulative dose will require 3 to 4 weeks. Protracted treatment for the more refractory fungi (with a goal of 2 to 3 grams cumulative dose) must be given over several months. Nephrotoxicity due to this drug can be managed with salt loading and adjustment of dosing intervals.[22,23] The frequent side effects associated with drug administration, which are due to the solubilization of amphotericin B in bile salts, can be controlled with premedications such as acetaminophen and diphenhydramine and parenteral meperidine. In the future, the availability of liposomal amphotericin B and other modified preparations will drastically reduce these acute side effects.[24–26]

AIDS-Related Conditions

The permanence of immunosuppression with human immunodeficiency virus (HIV) infection has meant that as therapies for the secondary opportunistic infections have developed, patients can expect to be on lifetime maintenance regimens for many of these infections. This may lead to chronic home infusion therapy when no effective oral alternative is available. In addition to cryptococcal meningitis and disseminated histoplasmosis, cytomegalovirus retinitis has necessitated long-term intravenous antiviral therapy with either ganciclovir or foscarnet sodium to prevent blindness.[27] In many instances, hospitalization following diagnosis lasts only long enough to establish chronic venous access and home health referral. The recent Food and Drug Administration approval of oral ganciclovir may reduce this aspect of home infusion if efficacy similar to the intravenous route can be shown.

Antibiotic Administration

Several factors must be considered before initiating home intravenous antibiotic therapy, including appropriate patient selection, choice of antibiotic, dose frequency, and route of administration.[3,28] Fortunately the development of drugs and device technology in the last decade offers the clinician multiple options for home therapy.

The patient first must require intravenous antibiotic therapy and must be stable enough to be at home. There are several quinolone antibiotics that permit oral therapy for even chronic infections, such as osteomyelitis. Patients with poor gastrointestinal absorptive function or who require β-lactam antibiotics are good candidates for home infusion therapy. Malnourished patients or those with little muscle mass will not tolerate prolonged courses of intramuscular antibiotic injections. Diabetics with variable microcirculatory perfusion of muscle, and therefore unpredictable pharmacokinetics, are poor candidates for intramuscular therapy. Sites of infection that rely upon high peak antibiotic concentrations to eradicate pathogens such as meningitis and endocarditis are best managed with intravenous antibiotic therapy.

In addition, patient selection should focus on the physical and psychological support systems available in the home as compared with the hospital or outpatient infusion center.[29] The ability to train family members, friends, or even the patient in the safe administration of antibiotics will enable compliance with recommended therapy in the home setting. The management of the patient with multiple medical problems and nursing needs at home will likely require intensive home nursing services as well as the intensive involvement of household members. The shorter hospitalizations that result from home therapy will lower exposure to nosocomial complications and offer psychological benefit, especially in patient perception of quality of life.

In the past decade, two factors have increased the feasibility of home therapy for many patients: new antimicrobial agents with long half-life and innovations in both access and delivery devices. Table 3.1 summarizes commonly used antibiotics in home infusion, with dosage ranges, dose frequencies, and antimicrobial spectrum. Heading the list of new broad-spectrum antibiotics are

Table 3.1 Commonly Used Antibiotics in Home Infusion Therapy

Antibiotic	Indications	Comments
Nafcillin/ oxacillin	Infections with *Staphylococcus aureus*	Use 2 grams every 4 hours for endocarditis, meningitis
Cefazolin	Infections with *Staphylococcus aureus,* Enterobacteriaceae	Use 2 grams every 8 hours for endocarditis, osteomyelitis
Cefotetan	Intra-abdominal or gynecologic infections involving Enterobacteriaceae and anaerobes	Typical dose is 1 to 2 grams every 12 hours
Ceftriaxone	Infections with *Staphylococcus aureus*, Gram-negative bacilli other than *Pseudomonas*, spirochetes including *Treponema pallidum* and *Borrelia*, and gonococcus; good central nervous system penetration	For bacterial meningitis, use 2 grams every 12 hours; treatment for Lyme meningitis is 2 grams/day; dose for neurosyphilis is 1 gram/day
Ceftazidime	Infections with *Pseudomonas aeruginosa*	Use 2 grams every 8 hours for meningitis, endocarditis
Vancomycin	Infections with *Staphylococcus aureus,* coagulase-negative *Staphylococcus,* and *Enterococcus*	Starting dose of 1 gram every 12 hours should be adjusted by following serum levels
Ciprofloxacin	Infections involving *Pseudomonas aeruginosa*	Not to be used in children or for meningitis

cephalosporins, such as ceftriaxone, cefonicid, and cefotetan, and quinolones, such as ciprofloxacin and ofloxacin. These drugs are given once or twice daily and, in the case of the cephalosporins, can be given intramuscularly or intravenously. Additional advantages of the cephalosporins include good activity against *Staphylococcus aureus*, a low incidence of phlebitis as compared with antistaphylococcal penicillins, and good central nervous system penetration, with ceftriaxone. There has been extensive experience with using cefonicid in patients with osteomyelitis, especially after prosthetic joint implantation.[30,31] Ceftriaxone has been effective in treatment of meningitis (bacterial, Lyme, syphilitic) and endocarditis.[14,16–18] Cefotetan provides coverage against many Gram-negative organisms (except for *Pseudomonas aeruginosa*), as well as anaerobes, and is useful in the treatment of intra-abdominal or pelvic infections.[32–34]

Quinolones have had a significant impact on the treatment of serious infections. Long half-life and equivalent serum concentrations with oral or intravenous administration have meant early switching to oral therapy for many patients. Ciprofloxacin has good activity against *Pseudomonas aeruginosa* and other Gram-negative bacteria. Since the mechanism of action for these drugs is to inhibit DNA gyrase function, there are essentially no crossover allergic or antibiotic resistance problems for patients unable to use β-lactam agents.

The choice of dose size and frequency is dependent upon the site of infection being treated, the antibiotic used, and the ability of the home health nurse and the patient's family to manage the prescribed dose frequency. For example, patients with *Staphylococcus aureus* intravascular infections (i.e., endocarditis) can be treated adequately with cefazolin given at a dose of 2 grams three times daily, as compared with nafcillin, which must be given at a dose of 2 grams six times daily and is associated with phlebitis.

The expanded and safe options for long-term intravenous access have made home therapy available to a wider population.[35] The low complication rate associated with subcutaneous devices, such as the Infuse-A-Port and Mediport, and tunneled catheters, such as the Hickman and Groshong catheters, in the administration of chemotherapy and total parenteral nutrition has led to their use in home infusion therapy. The major problem is the requirement of insertion and removal by a physician, often in the operating room. The peripherally inserted central catheter (PICC) has gained favor in the past decade because it enables nursing personnel to insert and remove these catheters in the home as well as in the health care setting. In addition, the treatment of complications, such as thrombosis, catheter puncture, and insertion site infection, can be easily managed by home health personnel in consultation with the treating physician. All of these venous access devices can be maintained and utilized for drug administration without complications for long periods of time. Shorter lasting percutaneous central venous catheters have been modified in attempts to reduce infection rates, offering yet another alternative.[36,37]

Advances in drug delivery systems have also substantially benefited the home health industry. Infusion pumps, cassettes, and other user-friendly devices have facilitated self-administration of antibiotic doses.[35,38] The pumps allow for fixed infusion rates that decrease reactions associated with rapid delivery of certain drugs, such as vancomycin and amphotericin B. By adding a cassette containing multiple doses, a pump can be programmed to deliver doses on a set schedule, which enhances compliance with medications given frequently (e.g., penicillin and nafcillin/oxacillin) and limits the nursing supervision necessary for the administration of such drugs. Small balloon infusers and cassettes that can be hung on a belt increase patient mobility by eliminating poles and pumps.

Monitoring

After the patient and/or the family receive training in antibiotic administration, home nursing personnel must monitor for appropriate use of infusion equipment, sterile technique in handling the venous access, compliance with ordered dose frequency, and potential drug reactions. Initially this monitoring may occur daily to several times a week; eventually, weekly nursing evaluation should be the goal.

There are few guidelines for the laboratory monitoring of home antibiotic administration. For drugs with narrow therapeutic/toxic windows (e.g., vancomycin and aminoglycosides), frequent drug levels may be necessary until a dosing schedule that provides therapeutic serum concentrations is established. At that point, once-weekly monitoring may be adequate. In the case of vancomycin, the peak level helps determine therapeutic concentrations, and the trough level determines the dose frequency. While aminoglycoside use in the outpatient setting may be limited to infections due to drug-resistant pathogens, such as *Staphylococcus epidermidis* and *Pseudomonas aeruginosa*, these infections often occur in patients who are at most risk for nephrotoxicity. Renal insufficiency due to aminoglycoside therapy is reflected in rising drug trough levels and serum creatinine levels. In patients with normal baseline renal function and stable body weight, determining serum creatinine levels serially may be a less expensive alternative to aminoglycoside trough levels as a means of monitoring antibiotic-associated nephrotoxicity.[39]

Other laboratory tests can help in following the course of an infection or monitoring for known organ toxicities associated with certain agents in the ambulatory setting. The erythrocyte sedimentation rate, if elevated at the time of diagnosis of endocarditis or osteomyelitis, can be checked every 2 weeks for normalization that signals adequate antibiotic levels suppressing the infection-induced inflammatory response. In addition, the serum bactericidal test can be used in situations where cure requires high drug concentrations over a long period, as in endocarditis or osteomyelitis.[10,40] This test measures the effectiveness of the antibiotic dose *in vivo* against the specific pathogen cultured from the patient. Serum obtained at peak or trough concentrations of antibiotic is serially diluted. The highest serum dilution that demonstrates bactericidal activity against the infecting microorganism is determined. In cases where curative therapy is important, such as infections involving prosthetic valves or joints, the peak serum should be bactericidal at 64 or more dilutions.[41]

Weekly or biweekly monitoring of the complete blood count will alert the clinician to the bone marrow suppression that occurs with medications such as ganciclovir for cytomegalovirus retinitis. Patients receiving amphotericin B for fungal infections or foscarnet sodium for cytomegalovirus retinitis should have a weekly chemistry profile to measure electrolytes, blood urea nitrogen, and creatinine to detect any of the commonly associated renal derangements.

Other forms of monitoring include an electrocardiogram, every 1 to 2 weeks in cases of endocarditis, to reveal the development of arrhythmias or heart block which may signal an occult myocardial abscess. Radiographs or computerized tomographic scanning may be useful in judging the adequacy of antibiotic therapy for an abscess.

Failures and Complications

Some subsets of patients experience a higher rate of treatment failure with home parenteral antibiotics. Those of advanced age, with obesity, diabetes, or peripheral vascular disease, may exhibit poor peripheral drug distribution even with intravenous therapy. Infections with a greater likelihood of early complications, such as endocarditis with *Staphylococcus aureus*, may not be safely treated at home shortly after diagnosis. Intravenous drug abusers should rarely be offered outpatient intravenous antibiotics because of their high risk of noncompliance and misuse of venous access.

The complications associated with home intravenous antibiotic therapy are the same as those encountered in the hospital setting, with the additional factor of possible time delay in the evaluation of a newly recognized problem. Home health nurses or personnel will rely on the patients' or families' descriptions of the acute situation to determine the urgency of a visit on the same day versus the next day.

Reported incidence rates for catheter-related infection vary with type of catheter and catheter usage, such as parenteral nutrition, antibiotic infusion, or blood sampling. For short-term percutaneous central venous catheters, the incidence of infection with line-associated sepsis is between 4.7 and 35%.[36,37,42] A better comparison tool is reporting by number of catheter days, with a reported rate of 2.39 to 5.60 catheter-related infections per 1000 catheter days. The use of catheters manufactured with infection-reducing features (e.g., silver impregnation, iodinated compounds, and antibiotic bonding) has apparently reduced infection rates to the range of 1 to 2%. Infection rates associated with the PICC are only slightly higher than the range of 0.76 to 1.4 infections per 1000 patient days reported with use of long-term central venous catheters, such as Hickman, Infuse-A-Port, and Mediport.[35,43]

Secondary infections of the venous access often occur in immunocompromised hosts, such as those patients with neoplasms or AIDS, in patients who do not consistently use sterile technique in the care of their access, and in patients receiving highly concentrated sugar solutions, such as with total parenteral nutrition. With subcutaneous reservoirs, infections extend from the skin into the port site and are very difficult to eradicate without port removal. Antibiotic therapy is necessary for at least 4 weeks in either case. The treatment of tunneled catheter-associated infections depends upon the site of involvement. Insertion-site infections can be treated with aggressive local care and a brief period of antibiotics. Infection within the tunnel is rarely curable and is best managed with immediate catheter removal. Intraluminal or catheter tip infection can be treated like other intravascular infections, with prolonged intravenous antibiotic therapy. In comparison, PICC-related infections are often local and treatable with immediate removal of the catheter and a short course (5 to 7 days) of antibiotic therapy if there is secondary bacteremia.

The rate of catheter obstruction by thrombus is estimated at 5 to 10%.[42] Intraluminal thrombosis can sometimes be lysed using standard protocols of streptokinase or urokinase injections. Initiation of antibiotic therapy in a controlled setting such as the hospital or physician's office will identify patients with anaphylactic reactions to the selected agent. Upon continuation of therapy at home, home health personnel should be trained to keep careful records of symptoms and physical findings. This will assist in the early recognition of side effects or late allergic reactions secondary to antibiotic therapy. Good communication can alert the treating physician to the possibility of more serious allergic complications, such as Stevens-Johnson syndrome.

Summary

Home infusion therapy has expanded the options of patients who require prolonged parenteral antibiotic therapy for serious infections. Clinicians have gained valuable experience in the outpatient treatment of a wide variety of infectious conditions. New advancements in drug development, venous access devices, and infusion equipment have contributed to the greater utilization of home health services in the past decade.

References

1. Stiver, H. G., Telford, G. O., Massey, J. M., et al., Intravenous antibiotic therapy at home, *Ann. Intern. Med.*, 89(5, Part 1):690–693, 1978.
2. Kind, A. C., Williams, D. N., Persons, G., et al., Intravenous antibiotic therapy at home, *Arch. Intern. Med.*, 139(4):413–415, 1979.
3. Rehm, S. J. and Weinstein, A. J., Home intravenous antibiotic therapy: a team approach, *Ann. Intern. Med.*, 99(3):388–392, 1983.

4. Eisenberg, J. M. and Kitz, D. S., Savings from outpatient antibiotic therapy for osteomyelitis: economic analysis of a therapeutic strategy, *JAMA*, 255(12):1584–1588, 1986.

5. Balinsky, W. and Nesbitt, S., Cost effectiveness of outpatient parenteral antibiotics: a review of the literature, *Am. J. Med.*, 87(3):301–305, 1989.

6. Antoniskis, A., Anerson, B. C., Van Volkenburg, E. S., et al., Feasibility of outpatient self-administration of parenteral antibiotics, *West. J. Med.*, 128(3):203–206, 1978.

7. Amstutz, H. C. and Kass, V., Management of the septic total hip replacement, in *The Hip, Proceedings of the 5th Open Scientific Meeting of The Hip Society*, C.V. Mosby, St. Louis, 1977, pp. 152–169.

8. Brause, B. D., Infected total knee replacement, *Orthop. Clin. North Am.*, 13(1):245–249, 1982.

9. Insall, J. N., Thompson, F. M., and Brause, B. D., Two-stage reimplantation for the salvage of infected total knee arthroplasty, *J. Bone Joint Surg.*, 65A(8):1087–1098, 1983.

10. Rand, J. A., Morrey, B. F., and Bryan, R. S., Management of the infected total joint arthroplasty, *Orthop. Clin. North Am.*, 15(3):491–503, 1984.

11. Lindbeck, G. and Powers, R., Cellulitis, *Hosp. Pract. Off. Ed.*, 28(Suppl. 1):10–14, 1993.

12. Durack, D., Endocarditis, *Hosp. Pract. Off. Ed.*, 28(Suppl. 1):6–9, 1993.

13. Stamboulian, D., Bonvehi, P., Arevalo, C., et al., Antibiotic management of outpatients with endocarditis due to penicillin-susceptible streptococci, *Rev. Infect. Dis.*, 13(Suppl. 12):S160–163, 1991.

14. Francioli, P., Etienne, J., Hoigne, R., et al., Treatment of streptococcal endocarditis with a single daily dose of ceftriaxone sodium for 4 weeks, *JAMA*, 267(2):264–267, 1992.

15. Press, O. W., Ramsey, P. G., Larson, E. B., et al., Hickman catheter infections in patients with malignancies, *Medicine*, 63(4):189–200, 1984.

16. Bradley, J. S., Meningitis, *Hosp. Pract. Off. Ed.*, 28(Suppl. 1):15–19, 1993.

17. Luft, B. and Mariuz, P., Spirochetes, *Hosp. Pract. Off. Ed.*, 26(Suppl. 4):34–39, 1991.

18. Dowell, M. E., Ross, P. G., Musher, D. M., et al., Response of latent syphilis or neurosyphilis to ceftriaxone therapy in persons infected with human immunodeficiency virus, *Am. J. Med.*, 93(2):481–488, 1992.

19. Stone, H. H., Studies in the pathogenesis, diagnosis, and treatment of *Candida* sepsis in children, *J. Pediatr. Surg.*, 9(1):127–133, 1974.

20. Saag, M. S., Powderly, W. G., Cloud, G. A., et al., Comparison of amphotericin B with fluconazole in the treatment of acute AIDS-associated cryptococcal meningitis, *New Engl. J. Med.*, 326(2):83–89, 1992.

21. Powderly, W. G., Therapy for cryptococcal meningitis in patients with AIDS, *Clin. Infect. Dis.*, 14(Suppl. 1):S54–59, 1992.

22. Heidemann, H. T. H., Gerkens, J. F., Spickard, W. A., et al., Amphotericin B nephrotoxicity in humans decreased by salt repletion, *Am. J. Med.*, 75(3):476–481, 1983.

23. Fisher, J. A., Talbot, G. H., Maislin, G., et al., Risk factors for amphotericin B-associated nephrotoxicity, *Am. J. Med.*, 87(5):547–552, 1989.

24. Moreau, P., Milpied, N., Fayette, N., et al., Reduced renal toxicity and improved clinical tolerance of amphotericin B mixed with intralipid compared with conventional amphotericin B in neutropenic patients, *J. Antimicrob. Chemother.*, 30(4):535–541, 1992.

25. Ralph, E. D., Barber, K. R., and Grant, W. M., Clinical experience with multilamellar liposomal amphotericin B in patients with proven and suspected fungal infections, *Scand. J. Infect. Dis.*, 25(4):487–496, 1993.

26. Hay, R. J., Liposomal amphotericin B, AmBisome, *J. Infection*, 28(Suppl. 1):35–43, 1994.

27. Polis, M. A., Foscarnet and ganciclovir in the treatment of cytomegalovirus retinitis, *J. Acquired Immune Defic. Syndr.*, 5(Suppl. 1):S3–10, 1992.

28. Smego, R. A., Home intravenous antibiotic therapy (Editorial), *Arch. Intern. Med.*, 145(6):1001–1002, 1985.

29. Brown, R. B., Selection and training of patients for outpatient intravenous antibiotic therapy, *Rev. Infect. Dis.*, 13(Suppl. 2):S147–151, 1991.

30. Kunkel, M. J. and Iannini, P. B., Cefonicid in a once-daily regimen for treatment of osteomyelitis in an ambulatory setting, *Rev. Infect. Dis.*, 6(Suppl. 4):5865–5869, 1984.

31. Wagner, D. K., Collier, B. D., and Rytel, W., Long-term intravenous antibiotic therapy in chronic osteomyelitis, *Arch. Intern. Med.*, 145(6):1073–1078, 1985.

32. Bohnen, J. M. A., Solomkin, J. S., and Dellinger, E. P., Guidelines for clinical care: anti-infective agents for intra-abdominal infection, *Arch. Surg.*, 127(1):83–89, 1992.

33. Soper, D. E., Infections following cesarean section, *Curr. Opinion Obstet. Gynecol.*, 5(4):517–520, 1993.

34. Hemsell, D. L., Little, B. B., Faro, S., et al., Comparison of three regimens recommended by the Centers for Disease Control and Prevention for the treatment of women hospitalized with acute pelvic inflammatory disease, *Clin. Infect. Dis.*, 19(4):720–727, 1994.

35. Kravitz, G. R., Advances in IV delivery, *Hosp. Pract. Off. Ed.*, 28(Suppl. 1):21–27, 1993.

36. Kamal, G. D., Pfaller, M. A., Rempe, L. E., et al., Reduced intravascular catheter infection by antibiotic bonding, *JAMA*, 265(18):2364–2368, 1991.

37. Maki, D. G., Wheeler, S. J., Stolz, S. M., et al., Clinical trial of a novel antiseptic-coated central venous catheter, presented at the 31st Interscience Conference on Antimicrobial Agents and Chemotherapy (ICAAC), Abstract #461, Chicago, 1991.

38. New, P. B., Swanson, G. F., Bulich, R. G., et al., Ambulatory antibiotic infusion devices: extending the spectrum of outpatient therapies, *Am. J. Med.*, 91(5):455–461, 1991.

39. Gilbert, D. N., Aminoglycosides, in *Principles and Practice of Infectious Diseases*, Vol. 1, 4th edition, Mandell, G. L., Bennett, J. E., and Dolin, R., Eds., Churchill Livingstone, New York, 1995, pp. 279–305.

40. Reller, L. B., The serum bactericidal test, *Rev. Infect. Dis.*, 8(5):803–808, 1986.

41. Woods, G. L. and Washington, J. A., The clinician and the microbiology labora-

tory, in *Principles and Practice of Infectious Diseases*, Vol. 1, 4th edition, Mandell, G. L., Bennett, J. E., and Dolin, R., Eds., Churchill Livingstone, New York, 1995, pp. 169–199.

42. Sitzmann, J. V., Townsend, T. R., Siler, M. C., and Bartlett, J. G., Septic and technical complications of central venous catheterization, *Ann. Surg.*, 202(6):766–770, 1985.

43. Clarke, D. E. and Raffin, T. A., Infectious complications of indwelling long-term central venous catheters, *Chest*, 97(4):966–972, 1990.

Pain Control in Home Care

4

Benjamin M. Rigor, M.D.

Historical Background

> *We cannot minister to others in pain*
> *unless we first acknowledge our own pain.*
>
> Nouwen, 1979

The first home health care program in the United States was started at the Boston Dispensary in 1796, allowing the indigent to receive this type of service. By 1800, home nursing service was organized, and graduate nurses employed by the Women's Board of the New York Mission cared for the sick at home. The first government agency to allow home visits for the poor was the Los Angeles County Health Department in 1898.

The Montefiore Hospital in New York established a hospital-based home care program in 1947 and in 1949 expanded its services to provide medical, social, nursing, housekeeping, transportation, nutrition, occupational therapy, and other services.[1] In 1960, the Community Health Services and Facilities Act authorized the surgeon general to grant funds to public and nonprofit agencies to develop out-of-hospital health services, with emphasis on projects that would prevent, detect, or treat diseases and disability and improve care for persons who were not in the hospital.

The Medicare Act of 1965 included health benefits for Medicare beneficiaries living at home, such as nursing, physical therapy, speech therapy, occupational therapy, home health aid, and social work services. These services must be ordered by a physician and the patient must be homebound; the services can be part time or intermittent.[2] Many health insurance carriers incorporated portions of the Medicare services into their policies. They varied significantly in their coverage; some require co-payment or cover only specific services with prior preauthorization.

The prominent and exceptional work of Dr. Elizabeth Kübler-Ross in the 1960s influenced the development of palliative care. She emphasized that health care professionals isolated dying patients due largely to their own ineffectual coping with the subject of death. She demystified the dying process by using the radical teaching technique of interviewing dying patients in front of a group of health care professionals. This provided an excellent role model for other health care professionals and the lay public to deal with and understand the intricacies and complexities of the dying process.[3]

Meanwhile, Dame Cecily Saunders founded the St. Christopher's Hospice in London, England in 1967. She began her career as a nurse and went on to become a medical social worker prior to attending medical school. The word "hospice" was derived from *hospitia* to designate a temporary shelter for travelers and sick pilgrims. The hospice care concept in the United States was patterned after the one at the St. Christopher's Hospice. In 1974, Florence Wald resigned as dean of the Yale School of Nursing to participate in the development of the first American hospice, the Connecticut Hospice, Inc.[4] This was followed by the establishment of the National Hospice Organization, whose purpose was to provide support and care for persons in the last phases of their illness or disease so that they could live as fully and comfortably as possible. It affirms life and regards dying as a normal process in life. It neither hastens nor postpones death and believes that, through personalized services and a caring community, patients and families can attain the necessary preparation for a death that is satisfactory to them.[5]

In 1971, Medicaid made home health care benefits mandatory, and the Medicare statutes required home health care agencies to provide nursing services and one additional service (i.e., physical therapy, occupational therapy, speech therapy, or medical, social, or home health aid services). In 1974, the Health Care Financing Administration reported that 392,700 persons (16% of those enrolled) received an average of 21 covered Medicare home visits, which increased to 24 in 1986.

In 1982, the political factor that significantly impacted the use of home health care services was the enactment of the Prospective Payment System on the Medicare diagnosis-related group for hospital care as an attempt to curb Medicare spending. It resulted in shortened hospital stays, discharge of acutely ill patients, and the shift from hospital- to community-based care.

In 1990, the reported home health care expenditure by all payors was $16.2 billion, which was 2.8% of the total home health care expenditure reported by the National Association for Home Care.[6] Total health care expenditures reached $666.2 billion and absorbed 13.3% of the gross national product. About 15% of

Americans, or 37 million people, still are not covered by any insurance plan and another 20% have inadequate health insurance. Despite these enormous expenditures, Americans are not healthier than citizens of other countries of similar or lesser wealth.[7]

Basic Concepts and Perspectives of Home Care

The acceptance of home care for patients with cancer with stable medical conditions or several stages of terminal events has been most gratifying and also has proven to be an effective and rational choice. The major areas of need for home care include palliation of symptoms, management of pain and self-care difficulties such as colostomy and laryngectomy, managing side effects of treatments, and caring for patients who require treatment at home.[8] However, home care can also be extended beyond the cancer patient to the aged and infirm and other specific patients with unique and special needs (viz., infants and children, known substance abusers, minorities and non-English-speaking patients, HIV-positive or AIDS patients, and those with overwhelming psychiatric problems). The concept of home care therapy is changing, not only because of the variety of patients but also due to the advent of high technology; changing fees and reimbursement schedules by federal government agencies and third-party or commercial payors for home therapies; changes in societal expectations; consumer advocacy; and, above all, the recognition and realization by physicians, patients, and relatives of the advantages of home care therapies and services. This enhanced modality of health care provided in homes is widely accepted and heavily endorsed by patients, families, advocacy groups, and even the health care regulatory agencies.

The advantages of home care are numerous and far-reaching. They include the prevention of or decreased exposure to hospital-acquired nosocomial infections in patients who are extremely vulnerable because they are emaciated, immunosuppressed, and debilitated from disease or complications of therapeutic modalities. Hospital beds can be utilized for patients needing acute and in-hospital care. There are also numerous reports of cost effectiveness, with savings up to 50% during this era of economic restraints and dwindling resources. Home care also provides better and improved psychological gratification, establishment of family ties and bonding, and nurtured relationships in the safety, comfort, and convenience of a friendly and familiar atmosphere. There is less disruption of family activities and relationships, and, with the advent of computers, advanced telecommunications, and mass media, it is possible for the patient and the family caregiver to continue working, schooling, receiving wages, and earning a living. These are virtually impossible in an in-hospital setting.

There are also inherent risks in being confined to a hospital, such as iatrogenesis, medication errors, neglect or lack of vigilance, a nonsympathetic attitude from some health providers (especially toward the terminally ill patient), excessive laboratory examination and tests, electrical hazards of monitoring modalities, and accidents such as falls, etc. Isolation and solitary confinement also impact those who are immunosuppressed in isolation rooms, which can cause chronic depression and feelings of helplessness. For this group of patients, the "I's" of cancer therapy and confinement include the following:

Iatrogenesis	Inanition	Insomnia
Immobility	Inattention	Intractability
Immunodeficiency	Infections	Isolation
Impecunity	Infirmity	

Intensive therapeutic regimens, such as total body radiation, steroids, and chemotherapy, and conditions such as granulocytopenia can cause transfer of patients to protective isolation or placement in laminar air flow rooms or micro-organism-free environments. Among 815 consecutive admissions to a hospital's general medicine service, an overall rate of 497 iatrogenic events developed, involving 36% of patients; 9% of patients had complications classified as major, and in 2% the complications contributed to death![9] Malnutrition that leads to inanition is the result of anorexia, diarrhea, fistulas, infections, malabsorption (short bowel) or damage to absorbing surfaces, mucositis, nausea and vomiting, and other side effects of radiation and chemotherapy. Insomnia can be due to recurrent and uncontrolled pain, medications, routine hospital or care proce-dures, or worries about impending death, financial problems, etc. Immunodefi-ciency is due to cytotoxic chemotherapy, immunosuppressive drugs, and the effect of the disease on the immune process and system of the body. Immobi-lization can result from excessive pain, application of braces and/or casts, and the effects of exhausting and intensive forms of cancer therapy. Lack of vigi-lance and inattention are common problems among some care providers, espe-cially in patients who are terminal and possibly those with DNR (do not resus-citate) orders. The financial impact of long-term care on family resources is so devastating that impecunity is always an unending problem for patients with cancer.

Intractability of pain as the disease progresses and uncontrolled pain are important factors contributing to feelings of hopelessness, suicidal ideation, and requests for clinician-assisted suicide or euthanasia. On the average, nearly 75% of patients with advanced cancer have pain. At the time of diagnosis and at intermediate stages, 30 to 40% of patients experience moderate to severe pain.[10] These issues are overwhelming, and home care provides a better, if not the best, alternative for cancer patients at certain stages of their disease on an individual basis.

As the in-hospital course of the patient stops and home care is the next step, there must be a discharge plan that is properly organized and coordinated to ensure a smooth transition in the provision of cancer care. Emphasis must be on early assessment and management of pain, including changes in pain pattern or development of new pain. Development of new pain should initiate and trigger diagnostic evaluation and modification of treatment, which can be summarized as the "ABCDE" of cancer management:[11]

A = Ask about pain or other symptoms regularly. Assess pain systematically.

B = Believe the patient and the family in their report of pain and other symptoms and what relieves or intensifies it.

C = Choose pain control options or treatment modalities appropriate for the patient, the family, and the home care setting.

D = Deliver interventions in a timely, logical, and coordinated fashion.

E = Empower patient, families, and the home care team or professionals. Enable them to control their course to the greatest extent possible within therapeutic and financial constraints.

The objectives of a good home health care program include providing the finest quality medical care to the cancer patient in a home environment; supporting the patient and the family in dealing and coping with the philosophical, emotional, and spiritual aspects of impending death or terminal care; assisting the patient's family, relatives, friends, and associates in handling interpersonal, social, domestic, and financial problems; providing a valuable program with continuity, comprehensiveness, and adaptability to specific circumstances; allowing the patient to deal with health care needs and terminal illness with dignity; and, as much as possible, providing the patient freedom from pain and complications. The program must also provide for ongoing education in the care of the infirm and the terminally ill. This must be financially feasible and must have a positive impact on the remainder of the health care system.[12]

The complexity of home care has been shown in that caregivers or providers experience burdens or hardships associated with home pain management. These include sleep disturbances, giving medications frequently, and physical strain. Psychological and social burdens include confinement, family relationship adjustments, changes in personal plans and itineraries, demands on time, emotional and work adjustments, financial strains, and feelings of being overwhelmed.[13] These have been associated with negative mood states in the caregiver, such as anxiety, depression, and chronic fatigue.

Therefore, in order for home care to succeed, there must not only be commitment in terms of time, effort, and the will to succeed but also the provision of unending help to the terminally ill. The reward and gratification are that we belong to a noble and humane profession that offers help, assistance, compassion, and dedication for the duration.

Discharge Planning and Organization

The degree of discharge planning and organization will vary from patient to patient depending upon the stage of the disease; the need for specific therapies and services; the patient's educational and cultural background, activity level, family relationships and bonding, home structure and atmosphere, and financial resources; and governmental agency support as well as other logistical factors relevant to a successful home care program. Discharge planning is always a team responsibility that includes physicians, nurses, hospital staff, social workers, family/relative/guardian/surrogate, therapists, pharmacists, dietitians, and other paramedical professionals. The patient should be given a written home chore or pain management plan (Figure 4.1) which is easy to read and to understand. The plan should cover the patient's expected functional deficits and health care needs and, if possible, whether these are persistent, progressive, or reversible, as well as the anticipated time course over which the plan should be assessed and reassessed. The plan should be made known not only to the health care team but also to family members.

The discharge plan must include *assessment parameters* such as the diagnosis, age, treatments, care requirements, functional limitations, cognitive abilities and disabilities, intrapersonal relationships with family members, concurrent illnesses of the patient or family members, usual coping mechanisms, financial and insurance resources, knowledge of the disease and treatments, cultural factors, and social support system.[14]

Patients with special needs and requirements, as stated previously, present different challenges and require special and specific consideration for home care therapies and services (i.e., bilingual instructions or use of an interpreter for the non-English-speaking patient, or encouraging the elderly and the handicapped to use visual or hearing aids to read or hear discharge instructions and plans). It must be anticipated that patients who are not naive to narcotics, those with a history of chemical dependency, and suspected or known drug abusers will require higher opiate dosages with probable increases in frequency of administration. The child receiving home care for cancer pain needs proper parental guidance and supervision for intake of opioids and analgesics or for using patient-controlled, or parent-assisted, analgesia (PCA).

Before the patient is referred to a home health agency, the following requirements must be satisfied or accomplished:

1. Adequate admission or transfer information, including the diagnosis that makes the continuation of care at home a medical necessity.
2. Justification that home care is more cost effective and logistically feasible.

Pain control plan for

At home, I will take the following medicines for pain control:

Medicine	How to take	How many	How often	Comments
_____	_____	_____	_____	_____
_____	_____	_____	_____	_____
_____	_____	_____	_____	_____
_____	_____	_____	_____	_____

Medicines that you may take to help treat side effects:

Side effect	Medicine	How to take	How many	How often	Comments
_____	_____	_____	_____	_____	_____
_____	_____	_____	_____	_____	_____

Constipation is a very common problem when taking opioid medications. When this occurs, do the following:

❑ Increase fluid intake (8 to 10 glasses of fluid)
❑ Exercise regularly
❑ Increase fiber in the diet (bran, fresh fruits, vegetables)
❑ Use a mild laxative, such as milk of magnesia, if no bowel movement in 3 days
❑ Take _____ every day at _____ (time) with a full glass of water
❑ Use a glycerin suppository every morning (this may help make a bowel movement less painful)

Non-drug pain control methods:

_____
_____

Additional instructions:

_____
_____
_____

Important phone numbers:
Your doctor_____   Your nurse_____
Your pharmacy_____   Emergencies _____

Call your doctor or nurse immediately if your pain increases or if you have a new pain. Also call your doctor early for refill of pain medicines. Do not let your medicines get below 3 or 4 days' supply.

Figure 4.1   Pain management plan.

3. The comprehensive care plan, which addresses the patient's social, financial, philosophical, psychological, emotional, and religious or spiritual needs.
4. Prior to initiation of home care services and therapies, prescriptions of medications necessary to treat symptoms and the medical condition should be available and up-to-date.
5. An ongoing education program, both formal and informal (videotapes, audio cassettes, TV programs, etc.), for the patient, the family, and the health care providers.
6. Documentation of adverse effects or complications of therapy, with report to the primary physician or leader of the home health care team.
7. Interventional protocols for managing adverse reactions, including options of emergency room or in-hospital admission or care.
8. Early and rapid response by the home health care team to diminish and treat morbidity and complications.
9. Schedule of laboratory studies and pharmacological evaluation as part of the long-term care.
10. List of consultants and experts, including those for specific therapies and behavioral medicine.
11. Delineation of the level and intensity of care needed.
12. An evaluation of the patient's living environment and proper use of social service consultants.
13. Feedback from the patient care team as to satisfaction and quality of health care, therapies, and services rendered.

The members of the home health care team, including the family, must be accessible. If they are employed or have other responsibilities, their whereabouts and telephone numbers must be posted for immediate availability on a 24-hour basis. Substitutes or surrogates must also make their home addresses and phone numbers available. It is counterproductive if the health care provider is not likable or amiable and friendly at all times. He or she must be acceptable to the patient, the immediate family, other relatives, and other members of the health care team. Availability is not necessarily the same as accessibility, but a variety of therapeutic modalities and services should be available, including an adequate supply of opiates, other analgesics, and adjuvant drugs. Adaptability is essential because of the changing pattern of the disease, changing family situations, the need for advanced high-technology treatments, the variety and changes in composition of the health care team, and the unpredictability of the course of the disease. Accountability refers to total quality management of the patient up to the time of death and should include asking the following questions: What went wrong? What can we do about it? Did we intervene in a timely manner? Can we do better? Services, therapies, and other modalities of care must be available at all times, not only in the appropriate quantity and intensity but also in the appropriate quality of care that produces tangible results and a better and more satisfactory outcome. The "A's" of a successful home care program are *accessibility, amiability, acceptability, availability, adaptability,* and, last but not least, *accountability.*

Therapies, Services, and Other Modalities of Home Care

Home care provides short-term, intermittent, or continuous services and therapies, depending upon the needs of the patient and the family, that enhance the knowledge and skill of the caregiver in managing care. This also depends upon the patient's financial arrangement or type of health insurance coverage and the availability of family and community support. Funding can be obtained from the Public Health Department's Medicare-Medicaid home health agency, intermediaries and/or third-party or private duty agencies, or a combination of all the available resources which the patient is qualified to receive. It is also possible for some patients to pay the expenses of these modalities of care out of pocket; however, this is usually the rare exception.

The various services for patients with cancer include skilled nursing care (oncological clinical nurse specialist), psychiatric care, dietary services, psychosocial care, speech therapy, physical and occupational therapy and rehabilitation, pastoral care, pharmacy services, respiratory therapy, home health aide/volunteer services, and pain control and management teams. A variety of specific therapies and services are also provided to the cancer patient, such as total enteral or parenteral nutrition or feeding; chemotherapy; antimicrobial therapy; infusion and hydration therapy; antiemetic therapy; management of constipation; administration of biologic response modifiers; immunosuppression; wound, ostomy, and laryngectomy care; and administration of blood and blood products or elements.

Nursing is the foundation of home care, and federal legislation has emphasized the role of nursing in home health care in order to receive Medicare-Medicaid funds. The responsibilities of nursing include assessment; direct physical care; evaluation of patient's progress; patient and family education, training, supervision, and coordination of patient care; and the provision of psychosocial support.[15]

The advances over the last 20 years in the technology and concepts of vascular access and other specialized techniques of drug delivery systems have been phenomenal. Long-term venous/vascular access devices (VADs) are available as external devices such as the Hickman™, Broviac™, or Groshong™

catheters or implantable ports such as the Port-A-Cath™ and Infusaport™ with single- or double-lumen catheters; there are also external catheters with triple lumen. Most infusion therapy can be administered through central VADs which are totally implantable, small, lightweight, and easy to operate and maintain at home. For patients who have VADs and cannot physically travel, infusion therapy can be done at home. VADs can be used for administration of chemotherapy, hydration therapy, total parenteral nutrition, antibiotic therapy, and blood and blood component transfusion. In patients where the oral route is not feasible, VADs are also the preferred route for opiate/opioid maintenance. Patients who are capable can be taught to care and manage their own VADs, and with regular follow-up, the efficacy, efficiency, and integrity of VADs can be trusted and maintained. Toward the terminal course of a patient, VADs can be used for intravenous opioid administration and for PCA. There is a learning curve in the use of VADs, and education and training should be conducted regularly and should be ongoing for the family, relatives, health care providers, and the patient.

Cancer rehabilitation involves assisting the person with cancer to attain maximum physical, social, psychological, and vocational functioning within the limits of the treatment and disease. The goal of cancer rehabilitation is to improve the quality of life by maximizing functional ability and independence regardless of life expectancy and, when appropriate, reintroducing the patient into the socioeconomic life of the community.[16]

Physical therapy provides maintenance as well as preventive and restorative treatment at home so as to promote functioning at optimal levels. Occupational therapy assists the patient to achieve his or her highest functional level and to be as self-reliant as possible. The patient is taught adaptive techniques and the use of adaptive equipment to perform tasks essential for daily living, is provided preprosthetic and prosthetic training, and is provided assistance in the selection and construction of splints to prevent or correct a deformity.

Speech therapists and language pathologists provide therapy to individuals with communication problems (speech, language, or hearing) or those with swallowing disorders after radical neck dissection, laryngectomy, esophageal surgery, and other head and neck procedures. The respiratory therapist provides oxygen therapy or supplemental oxygen needs, tracheobronchial toilet, suctioning, incentive spirometry, arterial blood gas determination, chest physiotherapy, mechanical ventilation, and limited choices of pulmonary function tests.

Malignant wounds are difficult to take care of because of the large amount of necrotic tissue and eschar that contributes to infection and odor and requires debridement regularly with special cleansing and dressing. Other routine surgical wounds require meticulous care, especially in the immunosuppressed patient. The aim is to prevent the spread of infection and the consequent septic shock resulting from overwhelming and uncontrolled infectious processes.

Studies have shown that ostomy patients have low self-concept because of their anger at having the ostomy, grief and revulsion at losing bowel or bladder control, fear regarding sexuality, and feelings of ugliness and worthlessness.[17] These feelings make the expert care of ostomies essential, as is helping to prevent the patient from developing an inferiority complex and a low self-image or concept through repeated counseling and teaching, positive regard, genuineness, and concreteness. Postoperative teaching on the care of colostomy should begin immediately, and for home care, educational materials should accompany the patient as part of discharge planning.

Home care must promote these varieties of services, therapies, and modalities of care in an environment of love, caring, concern for others, teamwork, and empathy. The provision of these types of care to cancer patients must rely not on economic or financial factors but on the desire to make dying effortless, nonritualistic, and humane, where the patient maintains his or her dignity up to the last day.

Goals and Objectives of Home Care and Therapy

The major goals of home care are to promote, maintain, or restore health; to minimize the effects of illness and disability; to provide the patient relief from pain and other distressing symptoms; to provide a support system to help the patient live as actively as possible in the face of impending death or to allow for peaceful death; and to provide psychological care for the patient and the family during periods of illness and bereavement.[18]

The scope of this comprehensive care includes features such as coordinated home and inpatient-like care. The patient and the family are regarded as a unit of care and physician-directed services. Care is provided by an interdisciplinary team of well-trained and competent professionals. Both physical and psychological symptoms must be controlled. Medical, nursing, and paramedical services must be available round-the-clock, 365 days a year, and on an on-call schedule. There must also be a structured staff support and communication system, as well as acceptance of the total patient and family on the basis of need instead of ability to pay. When the end comes, bereavement follow-up for the family is a medico-moral obligation and not a funded or compensated service.

A home care program must provide the finest available medical and nursing care for the patient's organic, biologic, psychologic, and spiritual problems. It must support the patient and the family in dealing with the philosophical and religious aspects of the illness and impending death. It must also assist the patient and the family in handling interpersonal, social, and financial problems. The care should be rendered in an optimal home setting with the usual family activities, traditions, ties, mores, culture, etc. The program must also have continuity, be comprehensive, and be adaptable to individual circumstances. It must also provide ongoing education in the care of the terminally ill. Lastly, its impact on health care must be positive, and, as emphasized earlier, it must be financially feasible and affordable.

Selection of Patients for Home Care

Cancer patients who can benefit from home care are those with advanced disease who require pain and/or symptom management and those with treatment-imposed self-care deficits (i.e., ostomies, VADs, etc.), all of which require education and follow-up in the home. Some patients have treatment-related side effects, such as mucositis, gastrointestinal problems, neuropathies, etc. Others are homebound yet still in need of treatment and follow-up (i.e., chemotherapy, immunotherapy, etc.) that can be given appropriately and adequately in a home setting.

The prerequisites and general criteria for selection and acceptance of patients for home care are as follows:

1. The patient should have a home environment that is amenable to support the treatment program or protocol of care.
2. The patient must want and request therapy or services at home.
3. The patient and/or the caregiver must be knowledgeable about the therapy, including names, dosages, side effects, and adverse reaction to drugs; action to prevent or minimize side effects; and proper procurement, storage, handling, and disposal of drugs, as necessary.
4. The patient must have the financial means to pay for home care, treatments, therapies, and services.
5. The patient and/or the caregiver must have an understanding of the technology and operational aspects of the devices, equipment, etc. used, including their mechanisms, use of alarms and limits, troubleshooting, and routine maintenance and upkeep.
6. The diagnosis, prognosis, and course of the disease must be determined through a reasonable, logical, and thorough workup.
7. A physician or practitioner with expertise in oncology and pain management and control must be responsible and available for frequent reevaluation and monitoring of the patient's condition.

8. The patient's medical condition must be stable (i.e., absence of congestive heart or respiratory failure, uncontrolled diabetes, severe sepsis, fluid and electrolyte imbalance, recent myocardial infarction, uncontrolled coagulopathy, etc.); if not, the patient is better off as an in-hospital patient.

9. There must be access to communication among the patient, physician, home care providers or team, pharmacy, hospital (emergency medicine and oncology), and health insurance payors (i.e., Medicare/Medicaid or third-party or commercial health insurance carriers).

These general prerequisites and criteria are not inclusive and will vary from patient to patient based on stage of the disease, indications for home care, conviction of family members, and available resources in the community. Financial capability must never be the sole determinant for the provision of home care; the determinant should be the desire to treat the patient better in his or her home environment with the expert care of a team of sincere, cohesive, trustworthy, and dedicated professionals, volunteers, and family members.

As the disease progresses or escalates, the level of care must be more intense, including the degree of vigilance from the providers. Successful cancer therapy and pain management require frequent skilled assessments; consistent and precise pain management and intervention; physician collaboration; and frequent changes in dosages and drug choices or selections, schedules, and routes of administration.[19] This will indeed help to promote health, prevent disease, and restore and maintain health in a friendly and natural atmosphere of love and camaraderie.

Reported problems or difficulties in posthospital or home care include inadequate or no support or backup system, inadequate financial resources, poor environmental conditions (viz., an immunosuppressed patient who lives in a dirty home), inability to carry out treatment and medication regimens, inability to carry out activities of daily living (ADL), poor socialization, and other unanticipated problems resulting from these factors.[20] Although these hindrances are not insurmountable, it is essential that they be resolved before initiating a home care program for a patient with cancer.

Modalities of Home Care and Therapies

The modalities for home care, including services and therapies mentioned earlier, can be applied to postoperative management of pain and care after same-day or ambulatory surgery, to patients who are dying or terminally ill due to cancer or other diseases such as HIV/AIDS, to care of the elderly (Home

Eldercare) and the infirm, and to patients who require services and therapies outside a hospital setting in the environment of a home or a house setting.

Postoperative or Postsurgical Pain and Care of a Cancer Patient

Many patients with cancer require one-day or same-day surgery for procedures such as insertion of a central VAD for chemotherapy, hydration, nutrition, etc.; revision of arteriovenous shunts for home care dialysis; laser therapy for tumors in the air passages and other parts of the body; insertion of high-technology modalities for pain control such as intraspinal (intrathecal) or epidural (peridural) continuous infusion devices; placement of an intraventricular catheter with an Ommaya chamber for infusion or administration of opioids; neurosurgical modalities for pain control such as neuroablation or neuroaxial opioid infusion; procedures for pain control such as neurolytic blocks; and regional blocks such as sympathectomy (celiac plexus block for pancreatic neoplasms, etc.).

In many cancer centers, children and infants are treated daily with irradiation while under the care of their parent or guardian and return home after a series of radiation therapy. In these patients, the importance of discharge planning is again emphasized. If the patient receives a high-technology gadget, such as a continuous or intermittent infusion pump for pain therapy, the caregiver at home must be trained in managing, maintaining, and assuring functional operation of the equipment or device. The patient must be discharged with full instructions (package inserts and literature) about the device, drug, or medications to be infused, as well as dosages, side effects, and telephone numbers of the physician, pharmacy, and other resource personnel.

To reduce postoperative pain in patients who undergo a surgical procedure, a preemptive form of analgesia is recommended. Preemptive analgesia with local anesthetics, nonsteroidal anti-inflammatory drugs (NSAIDs), or opiates is capable of modifying central sensitization, analgesic requirements, and other associated changes such as C-Fos expression. Postoperative pain is associated with inflammatory changes elicited by tissue damage and the release of inflammatory mediators, resulting in peripheral and central sensitization, which causes the increased sensitivity of nociceptors (pain-sensitive receptors). In addition to the traditional inflammatory mediators, there is also release of purines, cytokines, leukotrienes, nerve growth factor, and various neuropeptides. Central sensitization changes the excitability of neurons in the spinal cord, resulting in an increase in the receptive field for sensitized dorsal horn neurons, increase in the duration of response (prolonged pain), and reduction of pain response threshold. This progressive change, starting with the creation of the peripheral "sensitizing soup" and followed by central sensitization, progressively increases spinal cord excitability, which is called "wind up."

In a patient who is presently in home care therapy, a preemptive form of analgesia can be initiated by administering a NSAID preoperatively and providing regional or conduction anesthesia with local anesthetic for the surgical procedure with or without general anesthesia. If the patient has excessive anxiety, benzodiazepine is given. Patients who experience nausea and vomiting should be treated accordingly with standard antiemetics at home; if venous access is not available, rectal suppositories can be used. The patient can resume his or her home care opiate therapy as soon as possible, knowing that the surgical procedure can provoke or cause breakthrough pain which should be treated properly with rescue doses of morphine sulfate, as needed, by whatever route of administration is available.

Home Care Pain Therapy and Management

In home care pain management, health professionals and caregivers should ask about pain, and the patient's self-report should be the primary source of assessment. The assessment tool used must be brief, easy to use, and must reliably document pain intensity and relief and must relate these factors to other dimensions of pain such as mood, anxiety, despair, etc. This initial pain assessment should elicit information about changes in ADL, including work and recreational activities, sleep patterns, mobility, appetite, sexual functioning, and mood. The patient should be observed for cues that indicate pain (e.g., distorted posture, impaired mobility, guarding or splinting painful areas, restricted movement of the limbs, anxiety, and attention seeking or depression). Absence of these behaviors should not be interpreted to mean that the patient has no pain.

There must be ongoing pain assessment and documentation at regular intervals after the start of the treatment plan. Each new report of pain or changes in its distribution, character, duration, and intensity must be documented at suitable intervals after each pharmacologic and/or nonpharmacologic intervention. With factual reporting, stoicism and exaggeration are avoided. It has been shown that prompt recognition and treatment of pain, pain syndromes, and neuropathies can minimize and possibly even prevent neuralgia and impairment and disability.[21]

In a home care pain management program, problems related to the health care professional include inadequate knowledge, poor pain assessment, excessive concerns about regulation of controlled substances, fear of patient addiction, and exaggerated concerns about the side effects of opiates, such as respiratory depression and the patient becoming tolerant to analgesics. Problems related to the patient include reluctance to report pain and take medications. These are compounded by problems related to the health care system, such as inadequate reimbursement for home care, low priority given to cancer patients in an era of possible or existing health care rationing, restrictive and prohibitive regulation of controlled substances, and limitations on access to and availability of different treatment modalities.

Low-income patients experience greater pain and suffering than do other Americans, and a disproportionate share of people with little or no insurance are minorities. Health care professionals and agencies must assure these patients and their families that most pain can be relieved safely and effectively.

Effective home care management should adhere to the World Health Organization's three-step analgesia ladder (Figure 4.2), which portrays a progression in the doses and types of analgesic drugs for effective pain management. When the noninvasive approach is ineffective, alternative modalities in-

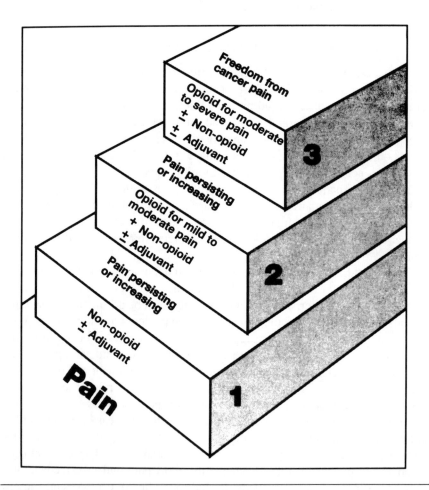

Figure 4.2 The WHO three-step analgesic ladder. (Reprinted with permission from World Health Organization.)

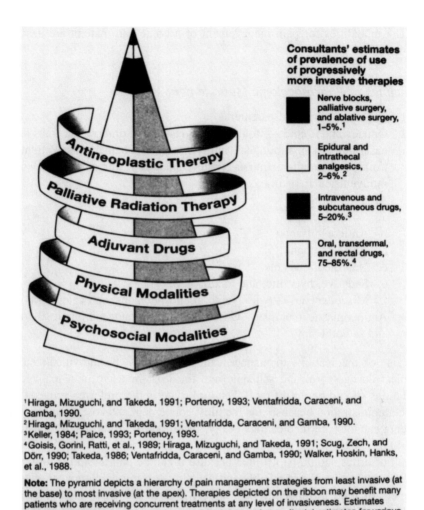

Consultants' estimates of prevalence of use of progressively more invasive therapies

Nerve blocks, palliative surgery, and ablative surgery, 1–5%.[1]

Epidural and intrathecal analgesics, 2–6%.[2]

Intravenous and subcutaneous drugs, 5–20%.[3]

Oral, transdermal, and rectal drugs, 75–85%.[4]

[1]Hiraga, Mizuguchi, and Takeda, 1991; Portenoy, 1993; Ventafridda, Caraceni, and Gamba, 1990.
[2]Hiraga, Mizuguchi, and Takeda, 1991; Ventafridda, Caraceni, and Gamba, 1990.
[3]Keller, 1984; Paice, 1993; Portenoy, 1993.
[4]Goisis, Gorini, Ratti, et al., 1989; Hiraga, Mizuguchi, and Takeda, 1991; Scug, Zech, and Dörr, 1990; Takeda, 1986; Ventafridda, Caraceni, and Gamba, 1990; Walker, Hoskin, Hanks, et al., 1988.

Note: The pyramid depicts a hierarchy of pain management strategies from least invasive (at the base) to most invasive (at the apex). Therapies depicted on the ribbon may benefit many patients who are receiving concurrent treatments at any level of invasiveness. Estimates presented in the sidebar are based on published data and consultants' estimates for various clinical populations in industrialized nations but may not reflect all settings and do not necessarily reflect what is optimal.

Figure 4.3   Pain management strategies: a hierarchy.

clude other routes of drug administration, nerve blocks, and neuroablative therapy. Patients receiving treatment of varying degrees of invasiveness may benefit from other modalities either separately or in combination (Figure 4.3). These modalities include pharmacologic management, physical and psychosocial modalities (nonpharmacologic), and invasive therapies, which are used as a last resort.

The modalities for pain management of a home care patient are described below.

Principles of Pharmacologic Management

1. NSAIDs—Oral and parenteral.
2. Opiates and opioids—Route of administration: oral, rectal, transdermal, nasal/transnasal, sublingual, intravenous, or subcutaneous. Patient-controlled, or parent- or nurse-assisted, analgesia; intraspinal, epidural, or intraventricular (neuraxis opiates).
3. Adjuvant drugs—
   a. Corticosteroids
   b. Anticonvulsants
   c. Antidepressant
   d. Neuroleptic agents
   e. Sedative, hypnotic, and anxiolytic
   f. Miscellaneous—hydroxyzine, biphosphonates, and calcitonin
4. Antineoplastic therapies—Chemotherapy, hormone biologic therapies, and radiotherapy.

The use of medications to manage cancer pain must be individualized. The simplest dosage form and schedule and the least invasive pain management modalities should be used first.[11] The oral route is the preferred route of analgesic administration because it is the most convenient and cost effective. When patients cannot take medications orally, rectal and transdermal administration should be considered as they are relatively noninvasive. Intramuscular administration of drugs should be avoided because it can be painful and inconvenient, and the absorption is not reliable and usually is erratic.[11] Pharmacologic management of mild to moderate pain should include NSAIDs, such as acetaminophen, unless there are contraindications. Acetaminophen does not affect platelet function and is relatively inexpensive but has lesser anti-inflammatory effects than other NSAIDs. Nonacetylated salicylates such as salsalate, sodium salicylate, and choline magnesium trisalicylate do not affect platelet aggregation or bleeding time and can be used on patients who are thrombocytopenic or who have clotting abnormalities. Other NSAIDs can cause major gastrointestinal problems such as perforation, ulceration, and bleeding, and minor gastrointestinal problems such as dyspepsia, heartburn, nausea and vomiting, abdominal pain, etc. Because of their extensive binding to plasma proteins, they can displace other protein-bound drugs such as methotrexate, cyclosporine, coumadin, digoxin, oral antidiabetic drugs, etc. Since they have a ceiling effect, the use of doses higher than those specified is not recommended. NSAIDs can be administered orally, rectally, intramuscularly, and intravenously. They do not result in tolerance or physical or psychological dependence. When pain persists or increases in intensity, an opioid should be added. Treatment of persistent or moderate to severe pain should be based upon increasing the opioid potency and/or the dose and/or the frequency of administration. Medication for persistent cancer-related pain should be administered on an around-the-clock basis with additional "as needed" or rescue doses for breakaway pain, because regularly scheduled dosing maintains a constant blood level and helps prevent the recurrence of pain. Opioid tolerance and physical dependence are expected with long-term opioid treatment and should not be confused with addiction.

For home care, the progressive and sequential route of opioid delivery is sublingual, rectal, transdermal, subcutaneous, and intravenous (Table 4.1). The sublingual route generally is not considered because of the lack of a specifically formulated opioid for this route and because most opioids, except for buprenorphine, are poorly absorbed through the oral or buccal mucosa. Buprenorphine is an agonist-antagonist synthetic derivative of thebaine and is about 25 to 50 times more potent than morphine. A 0.4-mg sublingual dose (equianalgesic to 0.2 to 0.3 mg intramuscularly) has an onset of action of 30 to 120 minutes and a duration of analgesia of 6 to 9 hours. It has a low abuse potential, but can promote withdrawal symptoms, and its respiratory depressant effect can be partially reversed by naloxone. Recently, a fentanyl transmucosal preparation (Fentanyl Oralet™—oral transmucosal fentanyl citrate) was released. This solid formulation of fentanyl citrate is intended for oral transmucosal administration. It consists of a medicated lozenge on a plastic holder and is consumed by sucking the dosage form. It is supplied in three dosage strengths of fentanyl citrate equivalent to 200, 300, or 400 μg fentanyl base. The onset of effect begins 5 to 15 minutes from start of administration, with peak analgesia within 20 to 30 minutes, and it is totally consumed in 10 to 20 minutes. Its possible use for rescue doses or breakthrough has not been studied in the home care environment. Although it is only indicated for an in-hospital setting, there are possible indications and implications for the home care patient who is properly watched and cared for at home.

The rectal route is ideal for patients with nausea and vomiting or those who are fasting either pre- or postoperatively, unless contraindicated in patients with anal or rectal lesions, diarrhea, and the elderly patient who physically cannot insert the suppository. Assistance can be obtained from caregivers or the home nursing team. The medication can also be applied to the colostomy or similar stoma provided the flow of affluent is slow enough to allow absorption via the mucosa.[22] The rectal dose is the same as the oral dose. Commercially available opioid suppositories are oxycodone (Roxicodone™), hydromorphone (Dilaudid Rectal Suppositories™), oxymorphone (Numorphan Suppositories™), and morphine, which is available as suppositories (Rexanol Suppositories™, MS/S Suppositories™) or as controlled-release morphine tablets (MS Contin™).

Table 4.1   Routes of Administration

Route	Comment
Oral	Preferred in cancer pain management.
Buccal	Supporting data meager; generally impracticable.
Sublingual	Buprenorphine effective but not available in U.S. Efficacy of morphine controversial. No clinical studies of other drugs.
Rectal	Available for morphine, oxymorphone, and hydromorphone. Few studies available. Used as if dose is equianalgesic to oral dose.
Transdermal	Viable route with some drugs. Currently available for fentanyl.
Intranasal	May be efficacious with some drugs. Butorphanol formulation available.
Subcutaneous Repetitive bolus Continuous infusion Continuous infusion with PCA	Advent of ambulatory infusion pumps permits outpatient continuous infusion with or without PCA. Can be accomplished with any drug with a parenteral formulation.
Intravenous Repetitive bolus Continuous infusion PCA with or without infusion	Intravenous route seldom used for long-term management, but feasible if venous access device present.
Epidural Repetitive bolus Continuous infusion Intrathecal Repetitive bolus Continuous infusion	Clearest indication is pain in lower body with poor relief and intolerable side effects from systemic opioids. Epidural catheter can be percutaneous (from lumbar region or tunneled to abdomen) or connected to subcutaneous portal. Intrathecal usually administered via subcutaneously implanted pump. Morphine most common drug, but has risk of delayed respiratory depression; other opioids, such as hydromorphone and methadone, also in use, despite little supporting data. Equianalgesic doses not known. Usual starting doses equivalent to 5 to 10 mg intramuscular morphine for epidural and 0.5 to 1 mg intramuscular morphine for intrathecal.
Intracerebroventricular	Rarely indicated.

From Portenoy, R. K., *Semin. Oncol.*, 20:19–35, 1993. Reprinted with permission.

Transdermal fentanyl (TDS-Fentanyl™) comes in four patch sizes and provides delivery of fentanyl at 25, 50, or 100 μg/hour. This is usually ideal for patients who are already on opioid therapy but have relatively constant pain and infrequent episodes of breakthrough pain such that rapid increases or decreases in pain intensity are not anticipated. Each patch contains a 72-hour supply of fentanyl and plasma levels rise slowly over 12 to 18 hours. Elimination half-life is 21 hours. The maximal recommended daily dose is 300 μg/hour, and doses up to 550 μg/hour have been reported.[23] The most commonly reported side effects are nausea, mental clouding, and skin irritation. The home care patient who requires large doses via the transdermal route should be switched to subcutaneously administered opioids.

Subcutaneous or intravenous opioids for home care are indicated in patients with nausea and vomiting, those with severe dysphagia or swallowing disorders, those who have obtunded or altered mental states (e.g., delirium, confusion, or stupor), those who are taking excessive or high doses and numerous tablets for oral and suppositories for rectal medication, those who require rapid escalation of doses for pain relief, those who suffer from undesirable side effects, and patients whose permanent or temporary intravenous access is nonfunctional. The opioid used for continuous subcutaneous infusion should be soluble, well-absorbed, and nonirritating to the tissues (viz., hydromorphone, oxymorphone, morphine, heroin, levorphanol [Levo-Dromoran™]). Opioids with a short half-life are preferred because of the ease of titration. Patients receiving continuous subcutaneous infusion around the clock may require rescue doses for breakthrough pain; the size of the rescue dose is equivalent to approximately 50 to 100% of the hourly dose. When using portable infusion devices for home care, it is very important to be familiar with several devices (Baxter Infusor System™, Pharmacia 5800™, Abbott Management Provider™) which vary in complexity, functional capability, and cost. Pump characteristics must include the following:[24]

1. Ability to administer a continuous basal infusion or intermittent bolus dose, or both
2. Ability to program the pump either in terms of volume per hour (milliliters per hour) or dose per hour (milligrams per hour)
3. Simple programming algorithms
4. Availability of a "lockout" function to prevent an inadvertent change in programming
5. Simple alarm to indicate malfunction
6. Modest overall weight (light and portable)

Subcutaneous opioids can be accomplished with insertion of a 27-gauge "butterfly" pediatric scalp vein needle (Figure 4.4) or a silastic needle under the

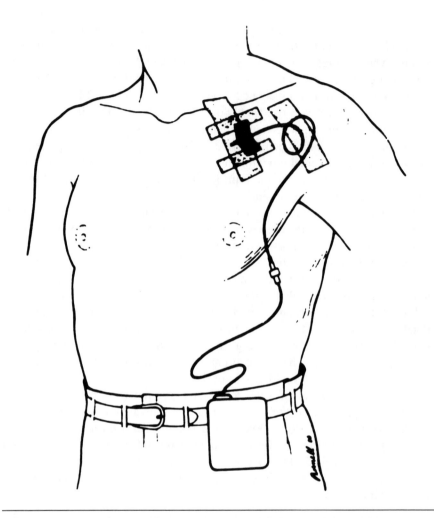

Figure 4.4 Needle placement for a continuous subcutaneous infusion. (From Coyle, N. et al., *Oncology*, 8:21–37, 1994. Reprinted with permission.)

skin. This can be maintained for up to a week or longer depending upon the condition of the skin. Blood levels are the same for the intravenous or subcutaneous route. Using hydromorphone, the analgesic outcome was the same and 78% of the drug was bioavailable with the subcutaneous route.[25] Most patients can absorb a volume of 2 to 5 ml/hour or up to 125 ml/hour with hyaluronidase (Wyadase^TM). The needle site should be inspected twice daily for any signs of irritation, leakage, or infection. The needle and needle site can be changed every week by a trained family member or the home care nurse. Once initiated, the availability of a 24-hour resource person is mandatory. It is important to anticipate side effects associated with opioids (i.e., constipation, sedation, nausea and vomiting, and respiratory depression), and they should be treated promptly. Respiratory depression occurs when pain is abruptly relieved and the sedative effects of opioids are no longer opposed by the stimulating effect of pain.[26] In some patients, physical stimulation or a "stir-up" regimen may be enough to prevent or reverse significant hypoventilation. Slowing or stopping the rate of infusion for a period of time prior to pharmacologic reversal can also be tried. An opioid antagonist should be given cautiously to patients receiving opioids on a long-term basis. The respiratory depression should be treated carefully, when needed, by using a dilute solution of naloxone (0.4 mg in 10 ml of saline), administered at 0.5-ml (0.02-mg or 20-μg) boluses every minute based on the patient's respiratory rate but not to reverse analgesia.

The intravenous route provides the most rapid onset of analgesia, but the analgesic effect is of short duration. For the home care patient who has a temporary or permanent VAD, continuous intravenous infusion provides the most constant and consistent level of analgesia. PCA provides the terminal patient with an enhanced sense of control and self-participation in the administration of medication for proper level of functioning, which varies from patient to patient.

Portability of pumps allows mobility for participation in and accomplishment of daily activities or duties. The pump can be programmed to provide a continuous basal rate or administration with or without bolus dosing.[27] The pump is ideal for treatment of both acute and chronic pain (i.e., continuous infusion for consistent or persistent chronic pain and bolus doses for acute, new, or breakthrough pain). For example, the physician can order 5 mg morphine sulfate per hour continuously, 2-mg bolus doses every 20 to 30 minutes if needed, and a limit of 2 to 4 boluses per hour. The advantages of a PCA pump for home pain management include a built-in safety mechanism (lockout function) to prevent accidental overdose of narcotics, maintained analgesic efficiency due to steady-state plasma level of the drug, optimal drug titration based upon need and level of activity, decreased overall narcotic requirement, minimal lag time for onset of effect, decreased dependence upon others, and effective pain control.[28] It must again be emphasized that the intravenous route is utilized only for severe pain after the oral, rectal, and transdermal routes have failed. When the intravenous route becomes inadequate or causes additional side effects, then the neuroaxial, spinal, or epidural route is the last resort.

Prior to initiation of intraspinal or neuroaxial opioids, it is very important to document the failure of maximal doses of opioids and other analgesics through other routes. Patients who have a high degree of tolerance to systemic opioids may require large or larger doses of spinal opioids.[29] Before implantation of permanent intraspinal or epidural access, a temporary percutaneous catheter is mandatory to test its efficacy and to establish baseline doses of opioids, which vary widely among patients depending upon the intensity of pain, stage of the disease, and degree of tolerance. All patients treated with intraspinal or intraventricular analgesics should have access to rescue medications (oral or parenteral) for periods of breakthrough pain or in case of equipment or device failure or catheter malfunction. Tolerance to opioids can be delayed by initial concurrent use of low concentrations of local anesthetics (bupivacaine) and opioids. Although other drugs can produce pain relief when administered epidurally or intrathecally (i.e., NSAIDs, clonidine, somastatin, ketamine, etc.), their efficiency for home care cancer pain has not been explored. Morphine sulfate is the standard drug used for spinal, epidural, or intraventricular administration. The drug must be preservative free (Duramorph™ or Astramorph™), 0.5 or 1.0 mg/ml, 10-ml ampules, or prepared by the pharmacy, which when compounded aseptically is stable for 13 to 30 days. For short-term treatment of weeks to a few months, externalized catheters (tunneled or untunneled) can be used, but for prolonged treatment the delivery system (catheter plus port or pump) can be internalized. For resistant or recalcitrant head and neck pain, intraventricular morphine is administered via an intraventricular catheter connected to a subcutaneous (Ommaya) reservoir for intermittent or continuous infusion.[30] With these methods, relief can be expected in up to 90% of patients. Adverse effects include the development of tolerance, urinary retention, nausea and vomiting, constipation, pruritus, device failure, and infections.

The adjuvant drugs enhance the analgesic efficacy of opioids, treat some side effects, alleviate concurrent symptoms that exacerbate or aggravate pain, provide independent analgesia for specific types of pain, and probably enhance or augment the coping process.

Principles of and Recommendations for Physical and Psychological Modalities

1. Physical modalities—
   a. Cutaneous stimulation—Thermotherapy (superficial heat), cryotherapy, massage, pressure, and vibration
   b. Exercise
   c. Counterstimulation—Transcutaneous electrical nerve stimulation (TENS), acupuncture, etc.
2. Psychological interventions—
   a. Relaxation and imagery
   b. Distraction and reframing

    c. Patient education
    d. Hypnosis and psychotherapy
    e. Pastoral counseling
    f. Improvement of coping skills

The previously discussed pharmacologic treatment can be enhanced and supplemented by physical, psychological, and nonconventional pain control and coping mechanisms. Cutaneous stimulation techniques, including application of superficial heat and cold, massage, pressure, vibration, etc., should be offered to alleviate pain associated with muscle tension or spasm. Patients should be encouraged to remain active and participate in self-care when capable and if possible. Home caregivers and physicians should reposition patients on a scheduled basis during long-term bed rest and/or provide passive range of motion (ROM) exercises. Patients with acute pain can exercise, but this is limited to self-administered ROM. Prolonged immobilization should be avoided whenever possible to prevent joint contracture, muscle atrophy and paralysis, cardiovascular deconditioning, and other untoward effects such as deep venous thrombosis, bed sores, hypostatic pneumonia, etc. Psychosocial intervention should be introduced early in the course of the illness as part of the multimodal approach to pain management, but it should not be used as a substitute for analgesics. Clinicians and caregivers should offer families and patients the means to contact peer and support groups. Pastoral care team members should participate in home health care meetings where the needs and treatment of the patient are discussed. They should develop information about community resources that offer spiritual care and support for patients and their families.*

Principles of and Recommendations for Invasive Therapies (Nonpharmacologic)

    1. Radiation therapy*
    2. Anesthetic techniques*—Nerve blocks, sympathetic blocks, spinal/epidural opiates, neurolytic blocks (phenol or alcohol)
    3. Neurosurgery* and neuroablation*
    4. Neuroaugmentation* dorsal column and spine cord stimulation
    5. Neuroaxial opioid infusion therapy* (Ommaya chamber)

As emphasized before, noninvasive treatment modalities must precede invasive palliative approaches, with very few exceptions.[11] Many of the invasive proce-

---

* These types of therapies are performed in the hospital or on an outpatient (ambulatory) basis, and continuation and follow-up are done at home for home care patients.

dures are done, applied, or initiated in an in-hospital setting, and after careful and extensive discharge planning, these modalities are continued, maintained, and managed in a home environment. Patients on home care can have palliative radiation therapy for treatment of symptomatic metastasis in sites where tumor infiltration has caused pain, obstruction, bleeding, or compression and can have radiopharmaceuticals for pain of bone metastasis shown by bone scintigraphy. Neurolytic blocks and intraspinal opioids with or without pumps should be reserved for those rare exceptions and for those instances where other therapies (pharmacotherapy, TENS, palliative radiation, etc.) are ineffective, poorly tolerated, clinically inappropriate, or have failed completely.[11] When a patient is pain free after neurolysis (neurolytic blocks), opioids should not be stopped abruptly because a withdrawal syndrome may be provoked. After the patient is discharged, the surgeon or physician must recognize the interactions of chemotherapy, radiation, and surgery to avoid or anticipate iatrogenic complications. The surgeon or physician should recognize and treat characteristic pain syndromes following specific surgical procedures or those resulting from the cancer and the coexisting disease process or associated diseases.

Home Care for Cancer Patients with Special Problems and/or Needs

Home Care for Infants, Children, and Adolescents

The discharge planning for this age group must be more detailed and elaborate because of the difficulty in pain assessment and interpretation of the manifestations and behaviors related to pain. Pain perception and reaction in children are influenced by the child's developmental level; emotional and cognitive states; personality traits; physical condition; past experience; the meaning of pain for the child; stage of the disease; the child's fears and concerns about illness and death; issues, attitudes, and reactions of the family; cultural background; and environment.[31]

The written and verbal instructions given to the child, parents (guardian), and caregiver must be clear, concise, to the point, and very easy to understand. A room other than the child's room should be used for treatment(s) whenever possible. Anything that reminds the child of the hospital-like environment (i.e., syringes, alcohol, needles, beepers, etc.) can escalate stress and bring memories of pain and suffering in the hospital.[32] Because it is more difficult to assess pain in children, open communication is essential. The use of flow sheets reduces redundant questioning and can provide the means for keeping up with the child's coping skills, learning disabilities, developmental delays, and language barriers.

The self-report method provides the most reliable and valid estimate of pain intensity and location. Children rarely fabricate pain, but they may deny or underreport pain if their admission of pain means more painful procedures (pain shots), they are unaware that pain can be treated, they want to protect parents/ guardian from the reality of disease progression, or they want to please or placate others.

The treatment options must be optimized and adjusted according to the patient and the family's needs and preferences, the procedure, and the context. Pharmacologic and nonpharmacologic options must be integrated in a complementary style. The child and the parents should be informed about what can be expected and how the child might respond. During nonpharmacologic procedures, the parents should be allowed to be with the child. The presence of the parents is a source of great comfort for most children, and very young infants can benefit from sensory motor intervention (e.g., pacifiers, touching, stroking, and patting).[33] During pharmacologic interventions, analgesics should be administered by a painless route (i.e., oral, transdermal, or intravenous) if possible, especially for patients with VADs. The wide variability of opioid dose requirements mandates more frequent assessment of pain and vigilance for side effects. In infants, where opioid clearance is prolonged and the blood–brain barrier more permeable, close monitoring and early intervention are necessary. This might make home care less ideal for infants less than 1 year of age. Most children over the age of 7 can use a PCA, because they are old enough to understand the relationship between a stimulus (pain), a behavior (pressing the button), and a delayed response (pain relief). It is also possible that epidural morphine can be used successfully in children with cancer, but this requires more extensive and intensive expertise and close monitoring if applied in a home care situation. Adjuvant drugs should be used when needed to smooth the course of therapy and to relieve some of the undesirable side effects.

Although children have no clear understanding of death in the prelanguage age, they have intense reactions to separation. Rudimentary ideas and feelings about death take shape in preschool age, and death is viewed as sleep, as temporary, or as personified. Between 7 and 13 years, most children come to regard death as universal and irreversible.[34] The uniqueness and special qualities of children require a different attitude and mindset characterized by patience, understanding, competence, and skill.

Home Care for the Elderly Patient with Cancer

About 51% of cancer deaths are individuals between 55 and 74 years old; 36% are ages 75 or older, and 71% of patients in long-term care facilities had pain. These patients have subtle signs of ominous medical events (i.e., sepsis without fever and leucocytosis, shock without tachycardia, and myocardial infarction without pain [silent myocardial infarctions]).

Elderly patients should be considered an at-risk group for undertreatment of cancer pain because of improper beliefs about their pain sensitivity, tolerance, and ability to use opioids properly and safely.[11] The misconceptions and myths about pain in the aged are aggravated by their cognitive impairment; multiple organ-associated diseases; dementia; polypharmacy or multiple drug use; high prevalence of visual, hearing, and motor impairment; and their altered pharmacokinetics and pharmacodynamics. These physiological alterations in the aged (i.e., low serum protein, decreased hepatic and renal perfusion and function, decreased enzymatic detoxification mechanisms, etc.) result in higher and more sustained blood levels for opioids and other analgesics and adjuvant drugs. They are also more sensitive to the sedative and respiratory depressant effects of opioids, and their altered detoxification mechanisms can lead to accumulation of biologically active metabolites and intermediate products of opioid metabolism, such as morphine-6-glucuronide and normeperidine. Supplemental use of local anesthetics (for nerve blocks and epidural/spinal opioids) can cause cognitive impairment, clumsiness, postural or orthostatic hypotension, etc., leading to falls, fractures, etc. In the presence of reliable, young relatives and caregivers, the use of PCAs and other high-technology pain treatment modalities, such as continuous or intermittent epidural or intraspinal analgesics, can be continued from the hospital to a home care environment. The following are recommendations for management of medications in the elderly (Eldercare) in a home care program:[35]

1. Evaluate thoroughly and carefully for treatable and associated medical conditions (i.e., diabetes, hypertension, angina, etc.).
2. Differentiate between acute, chronic, and breakthrough pain.
3. Avoid drug interactions by using fewer drugs and less polypharmacy.
4. Start with the lowest effective dose (i.e., usually one-third to one-half of the usual adult dose) but tailored to the stage of the disease, intensity of pain, and activity of the patient.
5. Individualize and simplify the regimen; use analgesics one at a time.
6. Provide perceptual and sensory aids (i.e., hearing aids, prescription lenses) for better adherence to and understanding of instructions.
7. Monitor toxicity, efficacy, and compliance.
8. Use drugs with short half-lives.
9. Additive effects are shown by multiple drugs, especially other analgesics and sedatives.
10. Maximize drug dosages and allow enough time for drug action before changing to another drug prematurely.

The most effective and efficient home care for the elderly requires frequent assessment, attention to details, understanding the limitations of altered physiology, and allowing the natural course of the disease to progress in the most comfortable and economically feasible manner.

Home Care for Patients with AIDS/HIV

Pain is a common symptom experienced by patients with HIV infection, even in the absence of Kaposi sarcoma. About 40 to 60% of HIV-infected individuals have pain, and pain intensifies as the disease progresses; 53% of patients with far advanced AIDS in a home care situation have pain. The pain can be due to peripheral sensory neuropathies, invasive and extensive Kaposi sarcoma, arthralgias and myalgias, and painful dermatological conditions.[36] Drug-induced pain usually results from neuropathies induced by chemotherapy and antiviral drugs.

As the disease progresses, more pain is due to other causes, such as intestinal infections, hepatosplenomegaly causing abdominal distention, oral and esophageal candidiasis causing pain on eating, severe painful spasticities from encephalopathy, headaches from sinusitis and otitis media, and very severe neuritic pain from herpes zoster (shingles). Depression is a significant element of intractable and recurrent severe pain, and those with pain are twice as likely to have suicidal ideation. The principles of pain assessment and treatment for these patients are not fundamentally different from those for patients with cancer. If pain medications are withheld from these patients, they are liable to obtain drugs from illicit and unclean sources. Home and ambulatory care under a properly supervised and nurtured environment can make the dying process peaceful, serene, and more acceptable.

The Psychosocial Aspects of Home Care

Cancer is no longer considered to be a disease that affects only the patient; rather, it affects the entire family. Attention to the needs of the family is an integral part of care of the dying. Communication and understanding between the physician, the patient, the family, and the caregiver(s) should be maintained throughout the entire process of caring for the dying and beyond it.[38] A contented family increases the likelihood of a fully satisfied patient. Caring for a loved one with cancer has inherent physical and psychosocial burdens. It involves adjustments in daily schedules and finances and realignment of family priorities, traits, hopes, and aspirations. Caregivers must be versatile because they are required to treat multiple symptoms; administer a variety of medications; manage tube feedings, intravenous infusions, and high-technology pain infusion pumps; change wound dressings or take care of ostomies; and address a multitude of other physical, psychological, and spiritual demands of the patient.[39] They must be "jacks-of-all-trades" and masters of all.

The categories of family interventions provided to the cancer patient include managing physical care and treatment regimens; assisting with household duties and finances; coping with the unpredictable and ever-changing expectations of the health care system; coping with alterations in the well-being of the spouse/caregiver and in the patterns of living; exercising constant vigilance and anticipating future needs; dealing with cancer itself; and adjusting to cyclical alterations in the patient's mood, temperment, and demeanor.[40]

Interventions to enhance the quality of life at home include accurate assessment of the family, such as family routines, roles, health status, and the presence of any barriers to effective care; symptom control at home, including treatment of nausea, fatigue, nutritional disturbances, etc.; psychological needs such as changes in moods and the presence of anxiety or depression; enhancement of the quality of life and the continuity of care; and the appropriate use of technology at home.

During the provision of home care, a variety of conflicts may occur between the physician and the patient, the patient and the caregiver, the patient and family members, the physician and the family, the caregiver and the physician, etc. These conflicts can be related to treatment or medication issues, financial problems, spiritual and religious biases, interpersonal relationships, personal decisions, etc. Unresolved conflicts result in guilt, anxiety, and, eventually, the personal resignation that everything is hopeless or futile. Such conflicts can be worse than the physical aspect of pain, and it is mandatory that they be resolved promptly.

The impact of pain on the quality of life must be identified. The quality of life is conceptualized as including the components of well-being, absence of symptoms, psychological well-being, social concerns, and spiritual gratification.

We must learn to provide hope, which is defined as an expectation greater than zero of achieving a desired goal. Hope diminishes the patient's mental isolation or state of quandary. Communicating the truth, no matter how unpleasant and stressful it may be to the patient and the caregiver, does not destroy hope. Such frankness and candor provides realism tinged with optimism and, in the last few days, submission to the eventualities of the disease process.

Members of the healing profession must decide when life sustenance is essential, when modalities of care are futile, and, finally, when to allow death to occur without further impediment. If we have the know-how and the technology to prolong life, do we have the moral responsibility to prolong death? Physicians tend to underestimate the life expectancy of patients with terminal illnesses. They should not, however, overlook the fact that a significant minority of patients has outlived initial estimates, usually by months and occasionally by years. Thus, the key points to remember are the patient's biologic prospects, the therapeutic goals of each treatment, and the need to prescribe not a lingering death but a death free from pain with dignity and honor.

Before the final day, the home care team must provide for all the needs of the dying patient (i.e., physiologic needs such as good symptom and pain control and treatment of side effects of therapeutic modalities; safety or the feeling of security; belonging or the need to be needed and the need not to feel like a burden; love or the expression of affection and human contact (touch); understanding of the disease and its symptoms; the opportunity to discuss death or dying; acceptance regardless of mood, sociability, or state of mind; and, lastly, self-esteem by involving the patient in decision making). It is necessary for physicians, nurses, and other caregivers to establish a common baseline of intent relating to the terminally ill, enriched by mutual trust, respect, and common goals. This is the basic foundation of effective terminal care and the best care we can offer the dying.[41]

Summary and Conclusions

Medicare has recently approved reimbursement to physicians for supervising patient care at home or in a hospice.[37] Doctors have successfully argued that they deserve payment for telephone coordination of treatment efforts provided by home and hospice care. The conditions under which physicians can receive payment are as follows:

1. The patient must be receiving Medicare-covered home health and hospice services.
2. The physician must have provided a service requiring a face-to-face encounter with the patient in the previous 6 months.
3. The physician does not have a significant financial relationship with the home care agency or hospice.

This is indeed a step forward, and hands-on involvement of the physician in a home care program should benefit the cancer patient. If home care and hospice care are the bastions of dignified care for the terminally ill cancer patient, they must be done well or not at all. Although physicians can now be reimbursed for this type of care, it is important to emphasize that economic factors should be the least important consideration in deciding whether or not to provide this type of care. The medical, nursing, and paramedical professions owe terminally ill and dying patients the benefit of their expertise in home care and must continue to improve, modify, supplement, and clarify the art, skill, and science of providing such care regardless of ability to pay, race, creed, religion, or country of origin. This is indeed the noblest thing we can do for our fellowmen, because one day many of us might be the recipients of this type of care.

References

1. Spiegel, A. D., *Home Health Care*, 2nd edition, National Health Publishing, Owing Mills, Maryland, 1987.
2. Puig, L., Health care comes home for saving, *Business Health,* 7:10–20, 1989.
3. Kübler-Ross, F., *On Death and Dying*, MacMillan, New York, 1974.
4. Paradis, I. F., *Hospice Handbook*, Aspen, Rockville, Maryland, 1985.
5. National Hospice Organization of the U.S.A., *Standards of a Hospice Program of Care*, Arlington, Virginia, 1981.
6. National Association for Home Care, Basic Statistics About Health Care—1991, NAHC Bulletin, 1991.
7. Rooks, J. P., Let's admit we ration health care—then set priorities, *Am. J. Nurs.,* 90(5):39–43, 1990.
8. Stair, J. and McNally, J., Home care, in *Cancer Nursing Principles and Practice*, 2nd edition, Groenwald, S. L., Fragge, M. H., Goodman, M., et al., Eds., James & Bartlett, Boston, 1990.
9. Steel, K., Gertmann, D. M., Crescenzi, C., and Anderson, J., Iatrogenic illness on a general medical service at a university hospital, *New Engl. J. Med.,* 304:638–642, 1981.
10. Daut, R. L. and Cleeland, C. S., The prevalence and severity of pain in cancer, *Cancer,* 50(9):1913–1918, 1982.
11. Clinical Practice Guideline, No. 9, *Management of Cancer Pain*, USDHHS, AHCPR Publication No. 94-0592, Rockville, Maryland, 1994.
12. Zimmerman, J. M., *Hospice: Complete Care for the Terminally Ill*, 2nd edition, Urban & Schwarzenberg, Baltimore, 1986.
13. Robinson, B., Validation of a care giver strain index, *J. Gerontol.,* 38:344–348, 1988.
14. Conkling, V. K., Continuity of care issues for cancer patients and families, *Cancer,* 64:290–294, 1989.
15. McNally, J. C., Home care, in *Cancer Nursing: Principles and Practice*, Groenwald, S. L., Frogge, M. H., Goodwin, M., and Yarbro, C. H., Eds., James & Bartlett, Boston, 1993.
16. Hoeman, S. P., Community-based rehabilitation, *Holistic Nurs. Pract.,* 6:32–41, 1992.
17. Watson, P. G., Postoperative counseling for cancer ostomy patients, *J. Enterost. Ther.,* 10:84–91, 1983.
18. Tack, S. A., Hospice, a concept of care in the final stage of life, *Comm. Med.,* 43:367, 1979.

19. Dobratz, M. C., Waade, R., Herbst, L., and Ryndes, T., Pain efficacy in home hospice patient: a longitudinal study, *Cancer Nurs.*, 14(1):20–26, 1991.

20. Slevin, A. D. and Roberts, A. S., Discharge planning: a tool for decision making, *Nurs. Manage.*, 18(12):47–50, 1987.

21. Elliot, K. and Foley, K. M., Neurologic pain syndrome in patients with cancer, *Neurol. Clin.*, 7(2):333–360, 1989.

22. McCafferey, M., Martin, L., and Farrell, B. R., Analgesic administration via rectum or stoma, *ET Nurs.*, 19(4):114–121, 1992.

23. Herbst, L. H. and Strause, L. G., Transdermal fentanyl use in hospice home-care patients with chronic cancer pain, *J. Pain Symptom Manage.*, 7(3 Suppl.):S54–S57, 1992.

24. Coyle, W., Cherny, N. I., and Portenoy, R. K., Subcutaneous opioid infusion at home, *Oncology*, 8(4):21–37, 1994.

25. Moulin, D. E., Kreeft, J. H., Murray, P. N., et al., Comparison of continuous subcutaneous infusion and intravenous hydromorphone infusion for the management of cancer pain, *Lancet*, 337(8739):465, 1991.

26. Hanks, G. W., Twycross, R. G., and Lloyd, J. W., Unexpected complication of successful nerve block. Morphine induced respiratory depression precipitated by removal of severe pain, *Anaesthesia*, 36(1):37–39, 1981.

27. May, G. and Lukacsko, P. K., A Guide to Parenteral Analgesia Using the CADD-PCA™ Infusion Pump, Med. Department, Hospital Products Division, Pharmacia, Inc., Piscataway, New Jersey, 1985.

28. Poplin, N. J., Intractable pain management with intravenous narcotic administration at home, *J. Intrav. Nurs.*, 12(4):228–232, 1989.

29. Cousins, M. J. and Bridenbaugh, P. O., Eds., *Neural Blockade in Clinical Anesthesia and Management of Pain*, 2nd edition, J.B. Lippincott, Philadelphia, 1987, p. 1171.

30. Obbens, E. A., Hill, C. S., Leaven, M. F., Ruthenbeck, S. S., and Otis, F., Intraventricular morphine administration for control of chronic cancer pain, *Pain*, 28(1):61–68, 1987.

31. Hester, N. O., Foster, R. L., and Beyer, L. F., Clinical judgment in assessing children's pain, in *Pain Management: Nursing Perspective*, Watt-Watson, J. H. and Donovan, M. I., Eds., Mosby-Yearbook, St. Louis, 1992, pp. 236–294.

32. Hester, N. O., Comforting the child in pain, in *Key Aspects of Comfort: Management of Pain, Fatigue, and Nausea*, Funk, S. G., Tornquist, E. M., Champagne, M. T., Copp, L. A., and Weise, R. A., Eds., Springer Publishing, New York, 1989, pp. 290–298.

33. Campos, R. G., Soothing pain-elicited distress in infants with swaddling and pacifiers, *Child. Dev.*, 60(4):781–792, 1989.

34. Gonda, T. A. and Ruark, J. E., *Dying Dignified, The Health Professionals Guide to Care*, Addison-Wesley, Menlo Park, California, 1984, pp. 179–192.

35. Portenoy, R., Pain management in the older cancer patient, *Oncology*, 6:86–98, 1992.

36. Singer, E. J., Zorilla, C., Fahy-Chandon, B., Chi, S., Syndullo, K., and Tourtellotte,

W. W., Painful symptoms reported by ambulatory HIV-infected men in a longitudinal study, *Pain*, 54(1):15–19, 1993.

37. Meyer, H., Medicare to pay for home care, *AMA News*, p. 24, January 9, 1995.
38. Twycross, R. G., Terminal care of the cancer patient: hospice home care, in *The Management of Pain*, Bonica, J. et al., Eds., Lea & Febiger, Philadelphia, 1990.
39. Stelzik K., Care giver demands during advanced cancer: the spouse's needs, *Cancer Nurs.*, 10:260–268, 1987.
40. Farrell, B. R., Grant, M. M., Rhiner, M., and Padilla, G. V., Home care: monitoring the quality of life for the patient and the family, *Oncology*, 6(2):136–149, 1992.
41. Twycross, R. G. and Lack, S. A., Symptom control in far advanced cancer, in *Pain Relief*, London, Pitman, 1983.

Home Parenteral and Enteral Nutrition

5

Paul Mangino, Pharm.D. and Paula Zelle, Pharm.D.

Characteristics of Home Nutrition Patients

Home parenteral and enteral nutrition (HEPN) is a rapidly growing segment of home care. This therapy offers patients a less costly alternative to care in a hospital with the opportunity to resume many normal functions.

The indications for home parenteral nutrition (HPN) have expanded over the past decade and have shifted from primarily gastrointestinal related to neoplasm related. The OASIS Registry began annual collection of data on HPN in 1984. In 1985, 15% of HPN patients were age 65 or older. The primary diagnosis for most patients was related to the gastrointestinal tract, with Crohn's disease and ischemic bowel disease accounting for the majority of patients; 21% of patients in the registry had neoplasms and only 2% had AIDS.[1]

A survey of 347 patients by Herfindal et al. in 1988 also found that most patients on HPN had either short bowel syndrome or a combination of gastrointestinal problems such as Crohn's disease, obstruction, or inflammatory bowel disease.[2]

The largest cohort of HPN patients was reported by the OASIS Registry in 1991 and included data from 2916 patients entered between 1984 and 1987. During this period, neoplasm accounted for the highest increase in new patients entered in the registry, while the gastrointestinal diseases remained fairly constant.[3] By 1991, the OASIS survey reported cancer as the leading indication for HPN, comprising 28.5% of all HPN patients.[4]

In 102 pediatric HPN patients studied at UCLA over 10 years, small bowel syndrome accounted for one-third of the reasons for HPN, Crohn's disease and small bowel obstruction for another one-third, and malignancy for 10%.[5] Table

Table 5.1 Most Common Indication for Home Nutrition Therapy

Gastrointestinal disorders	*Other causes*
Crohn's disease	Neoplasm
Short bowel syndrome	Radiation enteritis
Inflammatory bowel disease	Chronic renal failure
Congenital bowel disease	Hepatic failure
Motility disorders	Scleroderma
Chronic pancreatitis	Cellac sprue
Malabsorption syndrome	Anorexia nervosa

5.1 summarizes the common indications for HPN. Indications for home enteral nutrition are somewhat broader and may be considered in patients who are expected to be unable to eat for at least 3 weeks and who will be medically compromised by poor nutrition.

Long-term HPN patients average one hospitalization per year for complications directly related to the HPN. Herfindal found an average length of stay of 22.5 days for HPN-related adverse problems, with catheter complications the most common cause followed by electrolyte imbalances.[2] The OASIS Registry also reported 1.1 complications per year resulting in hospitalization, but rehospitalization was much lower in Crohn's patients than any other group. Cancer patients have been shown to have the same rate of hospitalization for HPN-related complications but a much higher rate of non-HPN-related admissions than Crohn's patients.[6,7] The 3-year survival rate for patients receiving home nutrition support for nonneoplastic diseases has been estimated at 60 to 80%.[8,9]

Elements of a Home Care Nutrition Support Service

The experience of the OASIS Registry and numerous other studies show that parenteral nutrition can safely be done in the home setting. However, HPN is not without risk, as inexperienced patients and family members take over catheter care and total parenteral nutrition (TPN) administration from the hospital setting where around-the-clock nursing care was available. Therefore, a well-planned organizational network which is available 24 hours a day is needed in order to successfully provide this therapy.

The home care provider must coordinate nurses, pharmacists, and ancillary personnel to work closely with the referring physician and patient or caregiver to provide and monitor HEPN service. In some models, all necessary personnel are in-house, while in other models, nursing service and pharmacy service are separate and must be coordinated by the discharge planner and all the providers.

The following key elements must be in place for a home care provider to provide nutrition services:

1. 24-hour availability of services
2. Written criteria for patient selection for HEPN
3. A staff of professionals with training and expertise in nutrition assessments, patient care plans, patient teaching, making home visits, compounding sterile solutions, and all other aspects of HEPN
4. A method for monitoring nutrition outcomes, including evaluating the number of home visits, physical assessment, laboratory studies, and communications with referring physician
5. Availability and familiarity with electronic infusion devices that are suitable for home use with TPN

Accepting a Patient for HEPN

A physician may make a referral for home TPN to the home care provider if he or she has identified that the patient cannot be maintained nutritionally by the oral route, has a reasonable life expectancy, has no major organ failure, and is willing to be a home patient. It then becomes the responsibility of the home care provider to decide whether or not to accept the patient based on the defined admission criteria. The home care provider should have written guidelines for assessing the patient's ability to comply with HEPN. The provider must verify that the patient has an understanding of the disease and need for HEPN and that the patient and family or caregiver are motivated and capable of training and are willing to accept their responsibilities. The provider must also verify that the patient's home environment is capable of supporting HEPN in terms of adequate electrical service, storage space, and cleanliness. Provisions for refrigerator storage, hospital beds, and other equipment and supplies may also need to be made. Patients who do not have a family member or caregiver to assist them and are not capable of performing all the necessary procedures alone may require skilled nursing home placement rather than HEPN. Finally, the provider should review the patient's financial resources and explain to the patient/family what sources and alternatives are available to them to meet their medical bills.

The home care provider can participate in the hospital discharge planning process. Ideally, prior to discharge from the hospital, the needs of the patient and family are assessed to determine their learning needs, abilities, and readiness. Any barriers such as cultural and religious practices, emotional state, physical or cognitive limitations, or language difficulties will need to be addressed by the home care provider before patient education begins.

The provider organization should work with the hospital staff to ensure that the patient and family have an understanding of the need for HEPN, including the psychological aspects, such as depression, and the need for compliance. The patient must also be taught how to care for the intravenous or enteral access site, how to use the infusion device, and how to attach the nutrition solution to the access port aseptically. The provider can also use this time to coordinate all the necessary supplies for HEPN administration and have them ready for home delivery. A hospital discharge planner may have already investigated the availability of insurance coverage before the home health provider becomes involved, but if not, this should be explained to the patient before proceeding.

All of the above discharge planning can be done directly by the physician and provider when the patient is not in a hospital setting.

Treatment Plan

A treatment plan is an individualized plan of care that states the goal of treatment, the expected duration, and the actual nutrition orders. The nutrition orders must describe the amount of each ingredient (dextrose, amino acids, electrolytes, etc.), the infusion time and rate, and an on and off tapering schedule for cyclic TPN. The treatment plan will also state the laboratory tests to be done, where the tests will be performed, who will draw the blood, and how the physician will be notified of test results. In addition, the plan should address such issues as when and how the patient may progress from intravenous to enteral feeding or from enteral to voluntary oral feeding and what physical limitations exist.

Some of these issues may not be fully determined at the onset of home therapy. However, the home nutrition provider should have a plan for recognizing that the optimal feeding method may change over time. The plan will need to be reviewed on a scheduled basis and updated with the participation of the patient's physician.

Teaching Plan

A teaching plan with written procedures should be developed for use by the home health nurse with the patient. Table 5.2 lists the elements needed in the plan. All training should be done by discussion and demonstration by the nurse or pharmacist, with return demonstration performed by the patient or caregiver or both. The goal of training is to make the patient as compliant and independent as possible.

The areas to be covered in the teaching plan include aseptic technique, accessing the infusion port, aseptically connecting to the infusion port, proper use of the pump, and, if necessary, heparin or saline flushing of the port, aseptic addition of drugs to TPN solution, the method for discarding needles and bio-

Table 5.2   Elements of a Nutrition Teaching Plan

Goals of therapy and possible side effects and how to identify them
Basic home safety
Hand washing
Catheter site care
Skin preparation
Aseptic technique and control of infection
Use, maintenance, cleaning, and storage of infusion pump
Heparin and saline flushing
Adding drugs to TPN bags
Reformulating enteral feeding products
Techniques for self-monitoring
Psychosocial needs and concerns including available community resources
Emergency procedures in case of complication of treatment or natural disaster
Handling and proper disposal of infectious or hazardous materials and waste
Other OBRA teaching requirements

logical waste, possible complications and side effects of therapy, and other information required by OBRA (Omnibus Budget Reconciliation Act) regulations, which vary from state to state.[10] The training process logically begins with catheter care and care of the skin around the catheter to prevent infection. If the type of catheter being used requires heparin flushing, the patient will need to demonstrate the ability to draw up the heparin in a syringe and actually flush the line aseptically.

All TPN solutions should be compounded aseptically by the pharmacy, which minimizes the need for the patient or caregiver to make final product additions prior to infusing the solution. Some formulations and organizational policies may require the patient to make a final product addition due to the stability of certain TPN additives. For example, some pharmacies choose to add multivitamins, cimetidine, vitamin K, insulin, etc. to all the solutions they compound. Other pharmacies elect to have the patient add these final products due to stability. Care should be exercised in deciding which method is appropriate for a specific patient, and addition of injectable products to the TPN solution by the patient should be kept to a minimum. In such cases, the patient must be taught how to draw and measure the correct amount of additive in a syringe and how to inject it into the TPN bag aseptically prior to infusing the solution. Since multiple days worth of solutions are generally mixed and delivered at one time, the patient will need to learn how to visually inspect the bags for precipitates. When lipid emulsion is added to the TPN solution (3 in 1 formulas), the patient will also have to recognize "oiling out" or the separation of the lipid and water layers. All patients must be told how to store the admixed TPN, and the provider may have to place a small refrigerator in the home temporarily.

Patients on enteral feeding will need instructions on how to reformulate the product if it is not a ready-to-feed formula and how to clean and reuse any nondisposable equipment. Patients on enteral feeding often get medication through the same catheter, and the patient should be given a schedule of medication administration times that avoids drug–nutrient interactions.

Next, the patient is taught how to monitor the nutrition program. A self-monitoring data form should be available for the patient to record daily weight, temperature, urine output, and the results of any urine or blood glucose measurements. These records are reviewed at each home visit. Part of monitoring teaching must include complication recognition. The patient should be able to detect catheter occlusion, fluid overload, and changes in urine color as well as signs of early catheter infection, such as fever, chills, or general malaise. Enteral nutrition patients should know how to treat diarrhea and when to report excessive diarrhea, vomiting, or signs of small bowel obstruction. All patients must know whom to contact in case of questions and pump malfunction or other complication on a 24-hour basis.

Finally, the initial patient teaching should include a discussion of the psychological aspects of HEPN. Depression is a common problem and can lead to noncompliance with the nutrition program. Sleep changes caused by nighttime infusions can further exacerbate depression or cause anxiety. Underlying family and financial problems may surface if the family is not prepared to cope with the patient's disease and their role as caregivers or if the patient was a primary wage earner. An early discussion of the common reactions to home care may minimize potential problems later for the family.

Patient education and teaching should be done in an interdisciplinary manner and coordinated among the staff members providing care to the patient in order to promote consistency and also to standardize the information the patient receives. This allows the patient to gain confidence earlier in the learning process. Many home health providers have the patient sign a form that outlines the procedures he or she has been taught and indicates the patient's understanding of the procedures and the patient's agreement to participate in his or her own care.[11] The form should also give the patient/caregiver the opportunity to request more instruction in a particular area if needed.

Nutrition Assessment

For most patients receiving HEPN, home therapy is a continuation of nutrition which was started in a hospital setting. Occasionally patients will initiate HEPN outside of an institutional setting or may require reevaluation of their protein, calorie, and electrolyte requirements. However, in all cases, the home care provider needs to make a baseline determination of the patient's nutritional status in order to evaluate the success of therapy over time.

The purpose of a nutritional assessment, then, is to evaluate the patient's current nutritional status and success of nutritional support. The assessment does not need to be a time-consuming or expensive process. A number of simple approaches have been developed that use readily available information from the patient's history and laboratory data. Nutrition assessment in the HEPN patient should also not be a one-time event done on admission to the home care program; rather, it should be repeated periodically to reassess the patient's progress with the current HEPN formula to allow for changes in therapy if necessary.

The first step in the nutritional assessment is to gather disease information, a brief history of the current course, and the patient's available physical and laboratory data. Disease information includes the patient's primary diagnosis (e.g., esophageal cancer) and any additional medical problems that would be indications for HEPN (e.g., radiation enteritis) as well as any underlying problems that may contribute to nutritional status (e.g., renal failure). A brief history of the current course includes amount of weight loss or gain, duration of current illness, amount of dietary intake (fluid and nutrition), and a performance score. Performance score, also called functional status, has been correlated with outcome for a variety of diseases. Several performance scales have been tested; the Karnofsky Scale (Table 5.3) is a good performance indicator for outpatient assessment and can be used over time to measure a patient's overall improvement or deterioration. The patient's physical data includes sex, height, usual

Table 5.3   Karnofsky Scale

Scale (%)	Description
100	Normal, no evidence of disease
90	Able to carry on normal activity, minor symptoms
80	Normal activity with effort, some symptoms of disease
70	Self-care consistent with age, unable to carry on normal activity
60	Needs occasional assistance but able to care for most needs
50	Requires considerable assistance and frequent medical care
40	Requires special care and assistance, disabled
30	Severely disabled but death not imminent
20	Hospitalized, active support treatment necessary
10	Fatal process progressing rapidly

weight, and current weight. The most recent laboratory data should be collected or a baseline chemistry profile should be obtained. This should include all the serum electrolytes, liver function tests, renal function tests, and protein, albumin, cholesterol or triglyceride, and magnesium levels. Most of these tests are available from any standard laboratory as a Chem-18 or SMA-18 test. Finally, the provider needs to know the type of parenteral or enteral access device to make an appropriate pump selection.

Other nutrition assessment tests can be performed, but their value in measuring nutritional outcomes is questionable. Anthropometric measurements (such as triceps skinfold to measure fat stores and arm muscle circumference to measure muscle mass) are difficult to obtain accurately, may vary from person to person doing the test, and have a wide range of normal values.

The second step in the initial assessment is to determine energy requirements. There are several methods for predicting energy needs. One is the Harris-Benedict equation, which was derived from indirect calorimetry and uses height, weight, gender, and age to calculate basal energy expenditure (BEE), the amount of energy consumed at complete rest:

For men
$$\text{BEE (kcal/day)} = 66 + (13.7 \times kg) + (5 \times cm) - (6.8 \times years)$$

For women
$$\text{BEE (kcal/day)} = 655 + (9.6 \times kg) + (1.8 \times cm) - (4.7 \times years)$$

Another method for estimating BEE in adults is based upon the assumption that most adults require 30 kcal/kg of body weight, which is 25% more than the BEE, so that:

$$\text{BEE (kcal/day)} = 30 \times (\text{weight in kg}) \times 0.75$$

The BEE must be multiplied by an activity factor to estimate the resting energy expenditure (REE). This determines the energy requirements of the patient's day-to-day living. A number of nomograms have been developed to determine the activity factor, but this remains a very subjective estimate. In general, an activity factor of 1.3 to 1.4 times the BEE is usually adequate for maintenance calories and a factor of 1.5 times the BEE usually achieves anabolism and weight gain. As a guideline, "usual" calorie requirements for maintenance using the enteral route are 25 to 30 kcal/kg and for the parenteral route are 30 to 35 kcal/kg.

In all the above calculations, an adjustment needs to be made for patients who are more than 130% of ideal body weight. The adjusted weight is one-half the difference between the actual weight and the ideal body weight:

Ideal weight (men) = 120 lb for the first 60 inches
+ 5 lb/inch over 60 inches

Ideal weight (women) = 100 lb for the first 60 inches
+ 5 lb/inch over 60 inches

Adj. weight = 0.5(actual weight − ideal weight) + ideal weight

The next step is to determine the daily fluid intake. Fluid requirements vary by age and diagnosis, but for most adult and pediatric patients 1500 ml/m^2/day is adequate to maintain tissue and renal perfusion. Patients with gastrointestinal fistulas, fever, or nasogastric tubes will need more and patients with renal insufficiency may need less. For very small children, normal fluid requirements are 100 ml/kg/day for the first 10 kg and an additional 50 ml/kg/day for the second 10 kg.

The fourth step uses the nutritional assessment to calculate protein and nitrogen requirements. For patients with no underlying organ failure, 1 to 2 g of protein per kilogram will prevent anabolism, with most patients needing 1.4 g/kg. Pediatric patients need 2 to 2.5 g/kg, and rarely will a patient need greater than 2.5 g/kg outside an acute intensive care setting. Adjustments in protein intake must be made for organ deficiency. Patients on chronic hemodialysis require 1 to 1.2 g/kg. If creatinine clearance is less than 30 ml/hour, protein load should not exceed 40 g/day.

As a double check to ensure that the nutrition supplement will deliver calories and protein in the optimal ratio, the calorie to nitrogen ratio can be calculated. Since amino acids are 16% nitrogen, the nitrogen content can be found by dividing the total protein by 6.25. The total daily nonprotein calories divided by the nitrogen content will provide the calorie:nitrogen ratio:

Total protein divided by 6.25 = nitrogen content

Total calories divided by nitrogen = nonprotein calories:
gram nitrogen ratio

Studies differ on the optimum calorie:nitrogen ratio, but a ratio of 150:1 should maintain a neutral nitrogen balance. A lower ratio formula may represent underfeeding and the risk that the patient will use protein as a calorie source rather than for tissue formation and wound healing. In addition, a lower ratio may lead to prerenal azotemia, while a higher ratio (overfeeding) may cause gluconeogenesis. Pediatric patients require more calories and a calorie:nitrogen ratio of 180:1 to 200:1 is reasonable. In adults, septic patients and patients with gastrointestinal fistulas or wounds to heal will require more nitrogen (lower ratio), while renal patients will require less nitrogen with normal calories (higher ratio).

The final step in the assessment is to decide how much of the total daily calories should be provided by carbohydrates and how much by fat. Protein should not be counted as a calorie source since the goal of nutrition is to provide adequate calories to utilize the protein for tissue building. Essential fatty acid deficiency (EFAD) can be prevented by providing 10% of the daily calories as linoleic acid or 500 ml of 10% commercially available lipid emulsion every 3 to 5 days. However, since fat is a more concentrated source of calories than dextrose, it is often advantageous to provide up to 30% of the daily calories as lipids. By comparison, dextrose delivers 3.4 kcal/g and lipids provide 10 kcal/g. Medicare currently limits the quantity of lipids that can be reimbursed each month and this may have to be taken into account in deciding the formula.

It is rarely necessary to provide more than 50% of daily calories as fat. Lipids should not exceed 2.5 g/kg or 60% of calories in adults. Patients with pulmonary disease may benefit from a higher fat content with less dextrose since fat is not metabolized to carbon dioxide, which may further compromise pulmonary function. In children, 0.5 g/kg/day of lipids will prevent EFAD and daily lipids should not exceed 3 g/kg/day. Lipids are contraindicated in patients with egg yolk allergy and patients with lipid metabolism disorders (e.g., hyperlipidemia, hypercholesterolemia, and hypertriglyceridemia).

TPN Formulas and Schedules

Formulating a TPN solution is an individual process. No standard formula is ideal for all patients and the same patient may require modifications in the TPN formula as changes in the medical condition evolve.

The initial formula is based upon the fluid volume, calories, protein, and fat requirements that were estimated in the nutritional assessment. To complete the formula, electrolytes, vitamins, trace elements, and other additives such as insulin must be determined.

Commercially available protein products consist of crystalline amino acids in various amounts. These products also contain small amounts of electrolytes. There are no current data to suggest that there is any clinical difference between any of the standard products listed in Table 5.4. Specialty amino acid products are also available but their use in HPN patients would be rare. The first are the branched-chain amino acid products which have been promoted in patients with severe liver failure or cirrhosis. Many patients with mild liver impairment will tolerate a reduced amount of standard amino acids, but there is evidence that in liver failure accompanied by hepatic encephalopathy there is benefit to using the branched-chain solutions which decrease aromatic amino acids. These products are listed in Table 5.5. The second specialty amino acid products, listed in Table 5.6, are formulated for patients with renal failure. Three of the four products contain only essential amino acids and the fourth contains some nonessential amino acids but in lower amounts than standard products. Intravenous dextrose

Table 5.4 Crystalline Amino Acid Products

Product	Aminosyn 5%	Aminosyn 7%	Aminosyn 8.5%	Aminosyn 10%	Aminosyn II 3.5%	Aminosyn II 5%
Manufacturer	*Abbott*	*Abbott*	*Abbott*	*Abbott*	*Abbott*	*Abbott*
Protein (g/100 ml)	5	7	8.5	10	3.5	5
Nitrogen (g/100 ml)	0.79	1.1	1.34	1.57	0.54	0.77
Sodium (meq/l)					16.3	19.3
Potassium (meq/l)	5.4	5.4	5.4	5.4		
Chloride (meq/l)			35			
Acetate (meq/l)	86	105	90	148	25.2	35.9

Product	Aminosyn II 7%	Aminosyn II 8.5%	Aminosyn II 10%	Aminosyn II 15%	Aminosyn PF 7%	Aminosyn PF 10%
Manufacturer	*Abbott*	*Abbott*	*Abbott*	*Abbott*	*Abbott*	*Abbott*
Protein (g/100 ml)	7	8.5	10	15	7	10
Nitrogen (g/100 ml)	1.07	1.3	1.53	2.3	1.07	1.52
Sodium (meq/l)	31.3	33.3	45.3	62.7	3.4	3.4
Potassium (meq/l)						
Chloride (meq/l)						
Acetate (meq/l)	50.3	61.1	71.8	107.6	32.5	46.3

Table 5.4 Crystalline Amino Acid Products (continued)

Product	Aminosyn (pH 6) 10%	Travasol 5.5%	Travasol 8.5%	Travasol 10%	Trophamine 6%	Trophamine 10%
Manufacturer	Abbott	Clintec	Clintec	Clintec	McGaw	McGaw
Protein (g/100 ml)	10	5.5	8.5	10	6	10
Nitrogen (g/100 ml)	1.57	0.925	1.43	1.65	0.93	1.55
Sodium (meq/l)	2.7				5	5
Potassium (meq/l)						
Chloride (meq/l)		22	34	40	<3	<3
Acetate (meq/l)	111	48	73	87	56	97

Product	Freamine III 8.5%	Freamine III 10%	Novamine	Novamine 15%
Manufacturer	McGaw	McGaw	Clintec	Clintec
Protein (g/100 ml)	8.5	10	11.4	15
Nitrogen (g/100 ml)	1.3	1.53	1.8	2.37
Sodium (meq/l)	10	10		
Potassium (meq/l)				
Chloride (meq/l)	<3	<3	114	151
Acetate (meq/l)	72	89		
Phosphate (meq/l)	10	10		

Table 5.5 Amino Acid Products for Hepatic Failure

Product	BranchAmin	Freamine HBC	Aminosyn HBC	Hepatamine
Manufacturer	Clintec	McGaw	Abbott	McGaw
Protein (g/100 ml)	4	6.9	7	8
Nitrogen (g/100 ml)	0.443	0.97	1.12	1.2
Sodium (meq/l)		10	7	10
Potassium (meq/l)		<3		<3
Acetate (meq/l)		57	72	62
Phosphate (mm/l)				10

is available in concentrations ranging from 5 to 70%, with the most concentrated solutions being the most economical to use. Fat emulsions are available in 10 and 20% solutions.

Since the total additives cannot exceed the amount of fluid per day, it is often easiest and most economical to use the most concentrated protein and dextrose product and add sterile water if necessary to complete the total volume. Substrates can be expressed as either a percent solution or in grams per day. Grams per day is the preferred method since it eliminates calculation mistakes in converting the nutritional assessment into the final working formula. For example, 90 g of protein per day would be 9% amino acids for a 1-liter TPN, 6% for a 1.5-liter solution, and 4.5% for a 2-liter formula.

Requirements for electrolytes can be divided into intracellular and extracellular ions. Extracellular electrolytes, sodium, chloride, and calcium are fairly

Table 5.6 Amino Acid Products for Renal Failure

Product	Aminosyn RF	Aminess	Nephramine	RenAmin
Manufacturer	Abbott	Clintec	McGaw	Clintec
Protein (g/100 ml)	5.2	5.5	5.4	6.5
Nitrogen (g/100 ml)	0.79	0.66	0.65	1
Sodium		5		
Potassium	5.4			
Chloride			<3	31
Acetate	105	50	44	60

constant regardless of disease type or nutritional status but may be affected by sudden dehydration or excess oral intake. Intracellular electrolytes, potassium, phosphorus, and magnesium are affected by nutritional status. As feeding takes place and new cells are formed, additional amounts of these electrolytes are mobilized intracellularly. Requirements may decrease as the patient enters into a maintenance nutritional state.

Sodium and potassium can be added to TPN formulas as chloride, acetate, or phosphate salts. In general, the chloride ion content should be equal to the sodium content. This means most or all of the phosphate will be added as potassium phosphate and the remaining potassium as potassium chloride. (4.4 meq potassium phosphate contains 3 mmol phosphate). The sodium content can then be calculated by adding the remaining chloride as sodium salt and the rest of the sodium as sodium acetate. Acetate salts should be avoided in patients with severe liver failure and reduced in patients with high serum carbon dioxide levels.

Calcium is added as the gluconate salt. The chloride salt is not as water soluble and should not be used in TPN solutions. A major incompatibility in TPN solutions is the reaction between calcium and phosphate. Formation of dibasic calcium phosphate precipitate depends upon the final pH of the solution, which is determined by the amino acid concentration. In TPN solutions with a low concentration of protein, the precipitate is more likely to occur. The interaction can be partially avoided by mixing all phosphate salts after the amino acids and adding the calcium last. Increased storage temperature can also cause precipitation. It is important during patient teaching to emphasize proper storage and administration temperature.

Fat-soluble and water-soluble vitamins must be given during parenteral nutrition. A multiple vitamin combination, MVI-12, which is based on the AMA-FDA recommended daily allowances,[12] is usually administered daily. Additional amounts of ascorbic acid, vitamin B_{12}, and folic acid are often supplemented as needed.

In 1979, the AMA published guidelines for six trace elements considered essential for parenteral use.[13] These are listed in Table 5.7 with their recommended daily allowances. A number of trace element mixtures are commercially available and single-element solutions are also available. Long-term HPN may result in iron deficiency anemia, which can be corrected with iron dextran added to the TPN formula if the patient is unable to take oral iron. Thiamine, selenium, and molybdenum may also need to be considered in patients receiving TPN for longer than 6 months.

Other additives that can be added to TPN formulas include insulin, heparin, and albumin. Normal glucose levels are necessary for optimal utilization of infused dextrose and to lower the risk of infection. Serum glucose concentra-

Table 5.7 Essential Trace Elements with Recommended Daily Allowances

Element	RDA
Zinc	2.5–4 mg
Manganese	0.15–0.8 mg
Chromium	10–15 µg
Selenium	40–120 µg
Iodine	1–2 µg/kg
Cobalt	2 µg

tions up to 150 mg/100 ml are acceptable during TPN infusion. Starting doses of insulin are based upon the serum glucose level. Levels between 150 and 200 mg/100 ml can be treated with 0.05 units/g of dextrose and 0.1 units/g of dextrose for levels greater than 200 mg/100 ml.

Heparin has been added to TPN to reduce the complication of blood catheter occlusion. The addition of 1000 units/liter has no anticoagulant effect and is compatible with all TPN formulas.

The addition of albumin to TPN is controversial. Since albumin is an important transport protein and helps maintain the oncotic pressure within the intravascular space, it may be desirable to provide albumin when serum albumin concentrations are 2.0 to 2.5 g/100 ml or lower. However, the amount of albumin required to raise the serum level is large, the effect lasts only 2 to 3 days as albumin equilibrates with the extracellular space, and the product is expensive and occasionally in short supply. Albumin is compatible in all TPN solutions but may clog in-line filters.

Scheduling of TPN for home use is done to maximize patient freedom. Patients who have been stabilized in the hospital may be ready for cyclic administration prior to discharge or on arrival home. Patients who are started on TPN at home should ideally begin with a 24-hour infusion and once carbohydrate, protein, and fat tolerance are established can begin receiving TPN over a shorter period each day.

One tapering method is to infuse the entire solution over 20 hours for the first day and then decrease the infusion time by 2 hours each day until the solution is being delivered over 12 hours, usually at night. Blood glucose should be checked on the first day 1 hour after the start of the infusion and 1 hour after the infusion ends. Intolerance to cyclic TPN manifests as hyperglycemia, glucosuria, excessive nighttime diuresis, shortness of breath, or muscle cramps. Some patients will have altered sleep secondary to the infusion and may wish to change the schedule to afternoon–evening.

Enteral feeding formulas contain protein, carbohydrates, fat, electrolytes, and vitamins mixed in fixed proportions that vary from product to product and are available in adult and infant formulas. The form of protein in the product is the major determinant of its use. Enteral formulas contain protein in three forms: intact protein, partially hydrolyzed protein, and crystalline amino acids. Intact proteins require a functioning gastrointestinal tract and pancreas. Partially hydrolyzed proteins are used in patients who have some but not all gastrointestinal functions, such as patients with short bowel syndrome and pancreatic insufficiency. The crystalline amino acid products require no digestion and are useful in patients with liver or kidney disease or patients who do not tolerate other formulas. For a complete discussion and comparison of available products, see *Enteral and Tube Feeding* by John L. Rombeau and Michael D. Caldwell (W.B. Saunders, Philadelphia).

Assessing HEPN Outcomes

Monitoring HEPN outcomes can be divided into three categories: laboratory data, clinical data, and patient self-monitoring data. All three categories should be included as part of the patient's home care record.

Laboratory monitoring can be done in the physician's office at scheduled visits, in a nearby hospital, or by the home care provider. All laboratory tests done outside the physician's office should be sent to the physician by the provider. The patient's clinical course, fluid, and renal status will dictate how often tests need to be done, but a reasonable schedule is for a complete blood count, electrolyte levels, blood urea nitrogen (BUN), and serum creatinine to be performed weekly for the first month, then every 2 weeks, then monthly as the patient stabilizes. Liver function tests, cholesterol, uric acid, and prothrombin time should be done at least monthly, although some of these tests are included in standard electrolyte panels. In long-term, stable HEPN patients, laboratory values can be measured every 3 months. Trace element and vitamin levels should be measured every 6 to 12 months.

The patient should be provided with a form to record pertinent self-monitoring data on a daily basis. Ideally, the patient should record daily weight, input, output (including fistula output), and an estimate of diarrhea and any blood or urine glucose levels. Urine glucose levels may be easier for patients to do as they do not require a finger stick, but diabetic patients and patients with unstable blood glucose level should be taught to use a glucometer. Patients must also record their daily temperature on the form.

This information is reviewed by the home care provider and the physician is contacted as needed. If urine output is 1000 to 1500 ml/day and the BUN and serum creatinine are stable, fluid intake is adequate. If a patient's urine output is less than 600 ml/day or if the patient notes ankle edema, the physician should be notified to discuss potential dehydration or fluid overload. The TPN volume may need to be decreased if the input is consistently greater than output by 500 ml or more.

In patients receiving high concentrations of dextrose, glucose intolerance can be monitored by checking urine glucose levels 1 hour after the TPN infusion is finished and again 6 to 8 hours later. If urine glucose is consistently 2+ or greater for 24 or 48 hours, the physician should be notified. Sudden onset of glucosuria may be a symptom of infection or hyperglycemia.

Fever greater than 100.4°F should be closely monitored, especially if accompanied by chills, sweats, or general malaise. Nausea, vomiting, and excessive diarrhea should also be closely monitored.

A record of the total enteral nutrition or TPN formula, requirement for additional fluids, weight gain or loss, and all laboratory tests should be included as the part of the patient's home health medical record. The physician should be notified if weight gain or loss is greater than 5 pounds in 1 week. Rapid weight gain can be a sign of fluid overload, especially if accompanied by low urine output or peripheral edema. Weight loss can be a symptom of dehydration. Rapid weight gain with adequate urine output and no peripheral edema may signal that a decrease is needed in the amount of calories being used.

A review of the patient's medical record should be done each time new laboratory values are recorded. The medication list should be updated and reviewed for drug–drug interactions and drug–nutrient incompatibilities. A nutritional assessment should also be calculated once a month. Laboratory values that are abnormally high or low should prompt a discussion with the physician, pharmacist, and nurse for possible fluid changes.

All hospitalizations should be closely monitored and recorded in the patient's home care record. Any changes in the formula while the patient is in the hospital will need to be communicated to the home provider prior to discharge.

Finally, psychosocial aspects of HEPN should be monitored during home nursing visits. There is little in the literature on monitoring coping strategies in long-term HEPN, although it is very important in compliance and recovery. Wolfe reported that 30% of complications during home TPN therapy were related to a nonsupportive home environment.[14] Herfindal used a list of possible complaints that affect everyday life as a method to assess quality of life. The most frequently cited complaints were frequent urination and lack of sleep, followed by hand and feet cramps. Greater than 20% of patients also complained of dry skin, weakness, depression, and joint pain. Patients were also asked to rate 14 daily activities on a five-point scale from very disruptive to very helpful and the impact that HPN had on each activity. Inability to travel, sleeping, going to the bathroom, and keeping a job were the activities most disruptive.[2] Lists such as these could be used to assess potential psychosocial problems.

Complications of HPN

Complications from HPN can be divided into catheter-related and noncatheter-related problems.[15] Catheter complications are the most widely reported and are directly related to the duration of use.[16]

Infection of the catheter is the most common HPN problem that requires rehospitalization, but the overall incidence is less than one admission per year.[16,17] Symptoms range from low-grade fever to sudden onset of hypotension and sepsis. Any fever in a patient with an indwelling central line catheter should be treated as serious. Treatment involves antibiotics and, occasionally, removal of the catheter.

Catheter occlusion, often caused by a blood clot or fibrin sheath at the tip of the catheter, is also a reported problem. This can be treated by instillation of 9000 units of urokinase into the catheter. If this fails to open the catheter, a dye study may be needed to examine the position of the catheter tip and the degree of clotting around the tip.

Thrombosis is a third catheter-related complication often detected by physical exam. Symptoms of subclavian vein thrombosis are arm, neck, or facial edema. Low-dose warfarin given orally or heparin added to the TPN solution is often used to prevent subclavian vein thrombosis. Swelling secondary to thrombosis in the superior vena cava is usually more dramatic, with bilateral swelling of the upper arms and neck. Treatment requires hospitalization and antifibrinolytic or anticoagulant therapy. Catheter-related thrombosis has been shown to be a risk factor for development of pulmonary embolus.[18]

The most common noncatheter-related complications are electrolyte imbalances, but with frequent laboratory monitoring these are easily treated with changes in the solution formula and are rarely a cause for hospitalization. Muscle weakness, lethargy, confusion, and nausea are the most common symptoms of electrolyte abnormalities and signal the need for more frequent laboratory monitoring. Long-term HPN patients may develop metabolic bone disease resulting in bone pain and early osteoporosis. The exact cause is unknown but may be related to vitamin D and calcium metabolism or lactic acidosis.[19–21]

Muscle cramps occur occasionally during parenteral nutrition infusions, usually within the first 1 to 2 hours. Cramps may be due to slow equilibration of electrolytes like calcium and magnesium from the extracellular to the intracellular space. Cramps usually resolve by tapering the TPN on slowly.

Psychosocial Considerations

With the advent of technologies which allow the administration of more therapies to patients in their homes come new psychosocial stresses for these same patients. This is especially true for the enteral and parenteral nutrition patients who suddenly are no longer able to consume food in the manner in which they have done so with family and friends since birth. Most individuals have eating preferences and established habits which have been reinforced over many years. Mealtime and food itself are integral parts of cultural, national, religious, and daily social celebrations. When this activity is restricted or totally removed, the adjustment to enteral or intravenous nutritional support is often a difficult one.[22,23]

The venous access device, catheter, intravenous line, and pump which are used to administer the parenteral solutions may be the cause of an altered body image which the patient cannot overcome. This can be a significant barrier in the patient's acceptance of the therapy long term. In addition, negative body image can have a profound effect on the sexual functioning of the home care patient or his or her significant other, which adds to the anxiety.

The infusion device can be a source of several potential problems. In the beginning, the patient may perceive the pump as a symbol of his or her illness and not appreciate the time and attention the pump and patient command by other caregivers or friends and visitors. Later on, it is possible that the patient may become very accustomed to the time and attention which the pump commands and thus may be hesitant to try another therapy, such as enteral feeding, which would not require the high-tech pump or additional staff instruction. The patient may fear a decrease in the amount of attention received if the device were no longer required. In addition, many patients simply fear that the pump will malfunction or break, causing major complications, and this anxiety may lead to compliance problems. Finally, the sound of the pump may keep some patients awake at night when they are cycling their TPN.

The above factors are important to consider when the initial assessment is done as well as for reassessments. The findings from these assessments should then be incorporated into the plan of care. Interventions and appropriate actions to be taken in achieving the stated goals need to be identified and monitored as well. It would be important to evaluate or consider the following strengths and weaknesses of a patient who is receiving long-term home TPN:[24,25]

1. Patient's coping skills and available social support system
2. Current mental health and past psychiatric history
3. Episodes of depression: frequency and severity

4. Past experience with the current disease and how the patient was able to cope previously
5. Concurrent stressful family or significant other
6. Willingness of caregiver or significant other
7. Changes in family dynamics and the patient's interpretation of the "sick role"
8. Financial situation
9. Knowledge of available community resources

Once these potential areas for problems have been identified, the interdisciplinary team together can initiate interventions which will help ease the identified problems as much as possible. Most long-term TPN patients cope very well and accept their nutrition therapy after a period of adjustment. A strong support system and a willing secondary caregiver are very beneficial.

Preparing for Accreditation

Many home care organizations that provide pharmaceutical services seek accreditation from the Joint Commission on Accreditation for Healthcare Organizations (JCAHO). In doing so, they must comply with the standards and requirements which have been developed in collaboration with selected home care organizations, professional associations, and societies. These include the American Society for Parenteral and Enteral Nutrition and the American Society of Health-System Pharmacists.[26]

There are specific standards relating to the provision of food and nutrient therapies in the 1995 Accreditation Manual for Home Care from the JCAHO. These standards are in addition to the standards required for all patients receiving services. A summary of these specific required standards follows.

There needs to be interdisciplinary nutrition care planning performed as part of the patient's care. The plan of care needs to include quantifiable goals which permit an evaluation of the patient's progress toward these goals. A time frame for implementation of the plan needs to be determined, as well as the process for assessing and reassessing the patient's response. A sample care plan is provided in Table 5.8.

An authorized individual needs to prescribe or order the food and nutrient therapies. These orders are verified by a nurse or pharmacist when required by state and federal law and regulation.

The organization must also define and assign responsibility for the safe and accurate preparation, storage, distribution, and administration of food and nutrition therapy.

Table 5.8   Sample Plan of Care for Nutrition[23–25,28,29]

PATIENT_____   DATE_____
RPh_____

1. **Problem:** Patient has weight loss of _____ lb/kg secondary to _____.

   Goal: Patient to maintain present weight or experience weight gain of _____ lb/kg over _____ days/weeks.

   Intervention: Pharmacist to determine/calculate the appropriate amount of kilocalories needed to maintain and/or increase the patient's weight using tables, equations, references, or nutrition consult.

   Monitoring: Patient's weight will be monitored and recorded every _____ days/weeks.

2. **Problem:** Patient may have/develop glucose intolerance.

   Goal: Patient's glucose will stabilize between _____ and _____ mg/dl.

   Intervention: Pharmacist to stabilize the serum glucose by:
   a. Tapering the TPN on and off with the following schedule:

      _____

   b. Addition of _____ units regular insulin to the TPN solution
   c. Substituting some of the glucose calories with lipid calories
   d. Adjusting the infusion time during the transition from continuous to cyclic infusions

   Monitoring: Patient's blood glucose will be monitored on a _____ basis via _____ initially, then on a _____ basis via _____.

3. **Problem:** Patient may have/develop fluid retention or dehydration.

   Goal: Patient to maintain adequate and appropriate fluid status.

   Intervention: Pharmacist to communicate with nurses providing care and monitor patient for fluid overload and dehydration.

   Monitoring: Pharmacist to monitor weight on a _____ basis. Review chart or interview patient every _____ days/weeks for signs and symptoms of fluid overload dehydration (i.e., weight gain or loss, difficulty breathing, increase or decrease in urination and thirst, sunken eyes, etc.).

4. **Problem:** Patient may have/develop hypophosphatemia.

   Goal: Patient's phosphate level will normalize between _____ and _____ meq/l.

   Intervention: Adjustment of abnormal electrolyte level by addition of necessary electrolyte.

   Monitoring: Patient's phosphate level will be obtained and monitored every _____ days/weeks. Suggest to limit the use of phosphate binders. Adjustments to formula made as per physician.

Table 5.8   Sample Plan of Care for Nutrition[23–25,28,29] (continued)

5. **Problem:** Patient may have/develop hypomagnesemia.

   Goal: Patient's magnesium level will normalize between _____ and _____ meq/l.

   Intervention: Adjustment of abnormal electrolyte level by addition of necessary electrolyte.

   Monitoring: Patient's magnesium level will be obtained and monitored every _____ days/weeks. Adjustments to formula made as needed per physician.

6. **Problem:** Patient may have/develop hypo- or hyperkalemia.

   Goal: Patient's potassium level will normalize between _____ and _____ meq/l.

   Intervention: Adjustment of abnormal electrolyte level by addition/reduction of necessary electrolyte.

   Monitoring: Patient's potassium level will be obtained and monitored every _____ days/weeks. Adjustments to formula made as needed per physician.

7. **Problem:** Patient may have/develop other electrolyte disturbances.

   Goal: Patient's _____ level(s) will normalize between _____ and _____ meq/l.

   Intervention: Adjustment of abnormal electrolyte level by addition/reduction of necessary electrolyte.

   Monitoring: Patient's _____ level will be obtained and monitored every _____ days/weeks. Adjustments made to formulas as needed per physician.

8. **Problem:** Patient may have/develop liver function test abnormalities.

   Goal: Patient's liver function tests normalize as per aspartate aminotransferase (AST) levels between _____ and _____ units/ml, alanine aminotransferase (ALT) levels between _____ and _____ units/ml, and alkaline phosphatase levels between _____ and _____.

   Intervention: Pharmacist to obtain and review liver enzyme tests and contact physician as necessary.

   Monitoring: Pharmacist to obtain and review liver enzyme tests every _____ days/weeks. Appropriate adjustments to formula are made per physician contact when elevated levels are reported for more than _____ days.

9. **Problem:** Patient may have/develop elevated BUN levels.

   Goal: Patient's BUN level will normalize between _____ and _____.

   Intervention: Pharmacist to obtain and review BUN levels and discuss with physician regarding decreasing protein load as appropriate.

   Monitoring: Pharmacist to obtain and review BUN levels every _____ days/weeks and adjust protein load in formula as per physician.

10. **Problem:** Knowledge deficit of self-administration of medication.

    Goal: Patient/caregiver knowledgeable regarding self-administration of medications.

Intervention: Pharmacist or nurse to provide education to the patient in the area of self-administration of medications.

Monitoring: Pharmacist verifies education or training has occurred as evidenced by documentation in the patient's chart (progress notes, patient education checklist, nursing reports). Follow-up of any adverse instances will occur with teaching being reinforced by the nurse or pharmacist.

11. **Problem:** Knowledge deficit of the infusion pump or ambulatory device.

    Goal: Patient/caregiver will be comfortable with the operation of the _____ infusion device. Patient/caregiver understands procedures to follow in the event of a pump malfunction to acquire a back-up pump.

    Intervention: Patient manual regarding instructions for pump to be reviewed and left in the home. Nurse or pharmacist available on-call to troubleshoot pump problems and to arrange for back-up equipment.

    Monitoring: Pharmacist verifies education or training has occurred as evidenced by documentation in the patient's chart (progress notes, patient education checklist, nursing reports). Follow-up of any adverse instances will occur with teaching being reinforced by the nurse or pharmacist.

12. **Problem:** Potential for infection of the central line.

    Goal: Patient will be comfortable with self-administration of parenteral nutrition and the access line will remain patent and free of infection.

    Intervention: Patient will be educated by the nurse regarding proper aseptic technique and will successfully give a return demonstration to the nurse regarding care and flushing of the line with heparin and saline. Patient and caregiver will be instructed to examine access site on a daily basis, checking for redness at site, tenderness, bruising, infiltration, and patency of the central line.

    Monitoring: Pharmacist to review documentation of patient education and to obtain feedback on the patient/caregiver's progress and ability.

As with all pharmaceuticals, the food and nutrition therapies need to be prepared and stored under proper conditions of sanitation, temperature, light, moisture, ventilation, safety, and security.

The food and nutrition therapies need to be distributed and administered in a safe, accurate, and timely manner to the patient.

There needs to be flexibility in the delivery and administration systems to accommodate the patient's changing needs which will continue to provide food and nutrient therapies when diet and diet schedules are altered.

Ongoing monitoring of the patient's response for the effectiveness and appropriateness of the nutrition therapy needs to occur to determine the extent to which the stated goals are being met.

A review of the medication profile is done to evaluate the appropriateness, duplication, and effectiveness of the current regimen.

The organization needs to ensure that the food or nutrition therapies are delivered in ways and times that will ensure drug stability and potency. For example, coolers with ice packs can be used to transport an appropriate supply of TPN to a patient's home.

The pharmaceutical services offered need to be available 24 hours a day, 7 days a week.

Patients who are moderate or high nutritional risk need to be identified from the data gathered on the initial assessment. These identified patients should receive a nutritional assessment by a qualified health care professional as defined by the organization. For example, criteria which would define a patient in the "at risk" category might include:[24,27]

1. Patients who are grossly overweight or underweight
2. Patients with open wounds
3. Patients who are on medically prescribed diets
4. Patients with actual or potential malnutrition such as geriatrics and pregnant or lactating women
5. Patients who have a limited family or social support system and are possibly dependent upon others for meal preparation
6. Patients who have had significant weight gain or loss within a certain time period as defined by the organization
7. Patients with altered metabolism due to their illness, complicating condition, treatment, or socioeconomic factors
8. Patients receiving medications which are antinutrient or catabolic (i.e., antibiotics, steroids, antineoplastic agents, etc.)

An example of a weight loss chart that could be used to identify and screen moderate-risk patients and severe- or high-risk patients is provided below:

Time	Moderate weight loss*	Severe weight loss*
1 week	1–2%	>2%
1 month	5%	>5%
3 months	7–5%	>7.5%
6 months	10%	>10%

* Percent weight loss based upon usual body weight.

The following is another example of a chart that may be used to identify patients at nutritional risk:

Weight*	Mild	Moderate	Severe
% IBW	80–90	70–80	<70
% usual weight	80–95	75–84	<75
Visceral protein stores			
Albumin (g/l)	2.8–3.5	2.1–2.7	<2.1
TIBC	150–200	100–150	<100

* IBW = ideal body weight; TIBC = total iron-binding capacity.

Examples of appropriate assessment tools may include a physical examination, medical history, and a nutritional history which would reveal any weight loss or weight gain and the number of days the patient has not had adequate oral intake. Including the patient's preferences for certain foods and any intolerances or allergies to foods or medications is appropriate. Laboratory tests such as serum albumin and total lymphocyte count and anthropometric measures can be used.

Communication with all health care professionals involved in the care of the patient needs to be maintained. This can be done with thorough documentation of conversations in the home care record or more completely by patient care conferences.

The pharmacist also needs to be involved in the selection process of the infusion device which is used to administer the parenteral solution.

The patient or caregiver should be thoroughly educated regarding the maintenance, cleaning, and storage of the infusion pump; flushing the intravenous line; storage of solutions and supplies; emergency procedures; basic home safety; hazardous waste; infection control; and self-monitoring techniques.

There are additional standards in the JCAHO manual which would be applicable as well to nutrition patients. For a complete detailed listing of all required standards, it is necessary to review the current Accreditation Manual for Home Care from the JCAHO.[24]

References

1. Orr, M. E., Nutritional support in home care, *Nurs. Clin. North Am.*, 24(2):437–445, 1989.
2. Herfindal, E. T., Bernstein, L. R., Kuzia, K., et al., Survey of home nutritional support patients, *J. Parenter. Enteral Nutr.*, 13(3):255–261, 1989.
3. Howard, L., Heaphey, L., Fleming, C. R., et al., Four years of North American Registry home parenteral nutrition outcome data and their implications for patient care, *J. Parenter. Enteral Nutr.*, 15(4):384–393, 1991.
4. Oley Foundation, OASIS Home Nutrition Support Patient Registry Annual Report,

American Society for Parenteral and Enteral Nutrition, Silver Spring, Maryland, 1991.

5. Vargas, J. H., Ament, M. E., and Berquist, W. E., Long term home parenteral nutrition in pediatrics: ten years experience on 102 patients, *J. Pediatr. Gastroenterol. Nutr.*, 6:24–32, 1987.

6. O'Keefe, S. J., Burnes, J. U., and Thompson, R. L., Recurrent sepsis in home parenteral nutrition patients: an analysis of risk factors, *J. Parenter. Enteral Nutr.*, 18(3):256–263, 1994.

7. Hurley, R. S., Campbell, S. M., Mirtallo, J. M., et al., Outcomes of cancer and noncancer patients on HPN, *Nutr. Clin. Pract.*, 5:59–62, 1990.

8. Meguid, M. M. and Muscaritoli, M., Current uses of parenteral nutrition, *Am. Fam. Phys.*, 47(2):383–394, 1993.

9. Sharp, J. W. and Roncagli, T., Home parenteral nutrition in advanced cancer, *Cancer Practice*, 1(2):119–124, 1993.

10. Varella, L. and Watkins, C. K., Training patients to administer total parenteral nutrition via subcutaneous infusion ports, *J. Intravenous Nurs.*, 13(1):51–54, 1990.

11. Cady, C. and Yoshioka, R. S., Using a learning contract to successfully discharge an infant on home total parenteral nutrition, *Pediatr. Home Care*, 17(1):67–74, 1991.

12. Parenteral multivitamin products, Notice of the FDA, *Federal Register*, 44(136):40933, 1979.

13. Expert Panel for Nutrition Advisory Group, AMA Department of Food and Nutrition: guidelines for essential trace element preparations for parenteral use, *JAMA*, 241:2052–2054, 1979.

14. Wolfe, B. M., Beer, W. H., and Hayashi, J. T., Experience with home parenteral nutrition, *Am. J. Surg.*, 146:7, 1983.

15. Koithan, M., Home total parenteral nutrition complications, *NITA*, 8:231–237, 1985.

16. Dudrick, S. J., O'Donnell, J. J., Deann, E. M., et al., 100 patient years of ambulatory home total parenteral nutrition, *Ann. Surg.*, 199(6):770–781, 1984.

17. Oley Foundation, OASIS Home Nutrition Support Patient Registry, Annual Report 1987, Albany, New York, American Society Parenteral and Enteral Nutrition, Silver Spring, Maryland, 1989.

18. Mailloux, R. J., DeLegge, M. H., and Kirby, D. F., Pulmonary embolism as a complication of long term total parenteral nutrition, *J. Parenter. Enteral Nutr.*, 17(6):578, 1993.

19. Seligman, J. V., Basi, S. S., and Deitel, M., Metabolic bone disease in a patient on long term total parenteral nutrition: a case report with review of the literature, *J. Parenter. Enteral Nutr.*, 8:722-727, 1984.

20. Karton, M. A., Rettmer, R., Lipkin, E. W., et al., D-Lactate and metabolic bone disease in patients receiving long term parenteral nutrition, *J. Parenter. Enteral Nutr.*, 13:132–135, 1989.

21. Larchet, M., Garabedian, M., Bourdeau, A., et al., Calcium metabolism in children during long term total parenteral nutrition: the influence of calcium, phosphorus and vitamin D intakes, *J. Pediatr. Gastroenterol. Nutr.*, 4:367–375, 1991.

22. Grant, J. A. and Kennedy-Caldwell, C., *Nutritional Support in Nursing*, Grune and Stratton, Philadelphia, 1988.

23. Caldwell, S. and Rombaeu, J., *Parenteral Nutrition*, W.B. Saunders, Philadelphia, 1990.

24. The Joint Commission 1995 Accreditation Manual for Home Care, Volume II: Scoring Guidelines, Joint Commission on Accreditation of Healthcare Organizations, Oakbrook Terrace, Illinois, 1994.

25. Catania, P. N. and Rosner, M. M., *Home Health Care Practice,* Health Markets Research, Palo Alto, California, 1994.

26. Kuhn, A. P., Latest JCAHO standards cover nutritional support for patients being treated at home, *Pharmacy Pract. News*, Oct.:22–23, 1994.

27. Finn, S. C., Nutrition screening, assessment and support, their crucial role in home care, *Caring*, July:16–22, 1989.

28. Plumer, A. L., *Principles and Practices of Intravenous Therapy*, Little, Brown, Boston, 1993

29. Traub, S. L., *Basic Skills in Interpreting Laboratory Data*, American Society of Hospital Pharmacists, Bethesda, Maryland, 1992.

Home Care Rehabilitation

6

David R. Watkins, M.D. and
Joanne Berryman, M.S.N.

Introduction

The purpose of this chapter is to introduce the reader to the concept of home care rehabilitation. Many people who have illness or injury require some restorative services to try to re-establish either an independent living existence or to establish a functionally adapted, independent living situation. Perhaps, however, they require services to establish an improved quality of existence even though a caregiver may be required. Often, these individuals are admitted to a rehabilitation facility where such training takes place in preparation for the third phase or community existence phase. Home care rehabilitation may be required to complete that phase of training in the home setting. In some instances, individuals may go directly from an acute care hospital to the home, but may still require restorative services which can be applied in the home setting. In either case, the home care team may be involved in the ongoing restorative phases that may be required to achieve the rehabilitation goals.

Many patients require a period of rehabilitation therapy following an injury or illness before they can return to their normal or adapted lifestyles. The home care rehabilitation program can be a cost-effective alternative to extended hospital stays. This program helps to return control of the patients' care to the patients, to the families, or to the support systems. The goal of rehabilitation then is to teach the patients (or in this instance, the home care clients) to maximize the use of their residual functional capabilities so they can perform the activities of daily living (ADL) as independently as possible within that home or dwelling setting.

We, as health care providers, must remember that we are dealing with a *whole person* and that the assessments we make must include not only the individuals, but their entire existence. This should include their educational levels, their living circumstances, and their support systems—be they family or other individuals. The goal of assessment in this instance is to define the functional capabilities and functional needs of the clients in question.

Home care services have included the use of rehabilitative therapeutics since the 1940s, when Martin Cherkasky organized one of the first home care teams. The team included a public health nurse, an internist, and a social worker. In the 1960s, due to the passage of the Medicare laws, the rehabilitative home care team was expanded to include physical, occupational, and speech therapists. Medical social workers and home health care aides were also added. Today, the expanded rehabilitative home care team is client centered, thus including the client and the family as team members and also including an insurance case manager, a psychologist, an attorney, and others as may be needed.[1]

Home health agencies have been formed to meet the needs of the home health care industry, and these agencies provide the services of nonphysician health care professionals such as therapists, nurses, home health aides, discharge planners, and case managers. Many home health agencies have formed alliances with other agencies to broaden their scope of services or to widen their geographic markets. This chapter presents simple, direct, informative, and basic principles and will be directed at the concept of home care rehabilitation intervention.

Rehabilitative therapeutic intervention is a four-step process: (1) the evaluation of the client's condition, (2) the identification of the necessary members of the support system, (3) the development and use of a goal-directed treatment plan, and (4) the measurement of the outcome of the therapy. This four-step process should be in a constant state of re-evaluation and evolution. The effect of this process should be to keep the plan of therapy dynamic and flexible to keep up with the changes seen in the client, the support system, or the environment.

Evaluation

General Guidelines

The evaluation of the client's condition, which should be directed by a physician, begins with the identification of medical and functional impairments that need to be treated. The physician first interviews and examines the client, takes a detailed history, and then performs a thorough examination. A list of conditions should be developed and any contraindications to any therapeutic interventions should be mentioned and discussed with the team. Likewise, the use of medications and their effects upon the client should be discussed and any precautions listed so that no confusion would exist in the treatment of the client in the home setting. A thorough physical examination should help to determine how the client's impairments impact personal independence and basic physiological functioning. Precautions and/or contraindications can be determined at the time of the thorough evaluation by the physician. These precautions and/or contraindications must later be discussed among the team members so as to provide the best and safest rehabilitative effort.

Once the physician has completed the evaluation, a prescription is then devised for the patient/client to be functionally evaluated by any combination of the other team members. Once their respective evaluations have been completed, the final step in the process is to decide whether or not a client is a good candidate for home care; if so, a team meeting is held to determine the courses of action. Fundamental criteria in making decisions for rehabilitation include:

1. The stability of the client's medical or injury condition
2. "Teachability" as it relates to the client's learning capacities as well as those abilities related to the support system itself
3. The definition of the constellation of the support system and the availability of that support system for home management and hands-on assistance
4. The availability of the home care team itself in the area where the home exists

One can see that if all of the above conditions are not met, successful home care rehabilitation is at risk.

Conditions that Benefit from Rehabilitative Home Care

Conditions that may benefit from rehabilitative home care can be generally classified as those that impede mobility and/or impede personal independent self-care. A partial list of conditions includes, but is not limited to, spinal cord injury, stroke, brain trauma, neuromuscular diseases, amputations, burns, cardiorespiratory diseases, various arthritides, joint replacements, acute and chronic pain syndromes, and deconditioned states, to mention a few. One must remember that the primary rehabilitation thought process centers around function. According to Kirby,[5] three factors help evaluate the effect of an impairment on the ADL:

1. Determination of the current and acquired level of function
2. Identification of the type of assistance required
3. Identification of other limiting factors

Functional Problems

Consider the following example of a functional problem. A client is referred to the home health care rehabilitation team because of poor nutritional status. If the evaluation reveals that nutritional status has been impaired because of the inability to swallow, possibly due to stroke, the team will then be obligated to assess the level of function required, the type of assistance required, and the identification of limiting factors which impact the poor nutrition. The client could have had problems with reflexes, speech or voice, management of secretions, poor supporting musculature, or perhaps even disorientation. Sample intervention techniques could easily include:[4]

1. Placing the client in an upright position
2. Stimulating a swallowing reflex (i.e., talking about food stimulates saliva flow; serving foods with different textures and temperatures stimulates chewing and swallowing reflexes)
3. Keeping the client oriented (i.e., attempt to minimize distractions by removing unnecessary items from the tray, serve the meal in a private place, minimize mealtime talk by limiting it to simple instructions, and separate liquids from solids)
4. Choosing the right foods (i.e., serve textured and aromatic foods and foods moistened with liquids such as gravy or sauces, avoid bland or untextured foods, and avoid sticky foods such as peanut butter or soft white bread)

Without a thorough functional assessment, one may simply miss the ultimate cause of the nutritional deficit and focus only upon trying to supply nutritional elements rather than correct swallowing dysfunction.

Another theoretical client could possibly suffer from the lack of knowledge of self-care procedures that are within his or her functional capacities and thereby inhibit the client's performance with simple ADL. Self-care knowledge can include such things as the timing and dosages of medications in addition to understanding the purposes and possible side effects of the medications. Clients could also be made aware of, and taught how to use, the various technologies currently available that promote self-care. Assistive technologies range from simple, low-technology self-care aids, such as long-handled combs, brushes, shoe horns, and the more sophisticated adaptive eating utensils, to the very high-technology and sophisticated environmental control devices which are computer assisted and the very sophisticated powered electric wheelchairs.[6] All of this information may be directed at the client as well as the support team, which is usually the family or a community of support individuals.

Support System

Types of Care Teams

Having a client referred to a home care team or system for evaluation and treatment demands that the team be available for such services. Several types of home care teams have been identified and include the multidisciplinary team, the interdisciplinary team, and the transdisciplinary team.[1]

The multidisciplinary team is most generally a trained, licensed group of health care professionals and other support people (such as case workers or attorneys) who work individually with the client to help achieve his or her optimal levels of functioning. The efforts of these team members are performed parallel to those of the other team members. Each team member focuses upon the problems associated with his or her particular specialty. This type of home care team has been the traditional home care team approach and many times lacks organization and efficiency.

The interdisciplinary home care team is a group of health care professionals from different disciplines who work toward a common goal. The members of this team need not only the skills of their specialty, but also the ability to contribute to a group effort. After team members evaluate a given client according to their own specialties, a team conference is held to communicate findings and determine an effective, comprehensive rehabilitation program for the client. This cooperative approach to therapy produces a better total outcome than each discipline could produce individually. The interdisciplinary home care team is probably the most common type of team approach used in rehabilitation therapy today, whether that be in a home care setting or in an institutional or facility setting. The team members work cooperatively. They report to each other on a regular basis and have a team leader to direct their discussions, which generally leads to a better outcome.

The transdisciplinary home care team can obtain an overlapping of treatment approaches because the members have, in addition to in-depth knowledge of their own specialties, an ever-expanding knowledge of other specialties on the team. In fact, some team members can perform some of the tasks of team members in other specialties. This kind of staff can blend its knowledge of multiple specialties into a specific functional activity that will benefit the client.

This approach ultimately shortens the length of rehabilitation therapy and maximizes functional outcomes. These teams are trained in rehabilitation philosophy, team techniques, and methods of treatment. They participate regularly in scheduled team conferences that include the client and his or her family or support system. They perform creative problem solving that is initiated by the team leader, who is often a physiatrist (a physician who specializes in physical medicine and rehabilitation). This team uses the talents and strengths of every team member, and each team member is trained in using the transdisciplinary approach. This type of team is an expansion of the interdisciplinary team concept and is an evolving process as a natural outgrowth of the team concept approach in rehabilitation medicine in general.

Members of the Care Team

The members of the rehabilitative home care team come from a variety of professions. The team is a group of health care professionals that is usually directed by a physician and almost always includes a rehabilitation nurse who assists in the coordination of activities and can also provide hands-on care and training as well. Equally important on the home care team are the physical therapist, the occupational therapist, the speech pathologist, the home health care aide, and the psychologist. Often included in the group are an insurance case manager, a social worker, and an attorney. The most important aspect, however, is the fact that the client and his or her family are also considered members of the team and the client should be the center of focus.

Generally, the physician who directs the team is a physiatrist. According to Ruskin,[8] physiatrists strive to restore measures of self-sufficiency to patients because often restoration of function is the only real and obtainable cure. He goes on to say that this physician especially bases his or her practice on six principles: (1) evaluation and management of the client's physical impairment is an integral aspect of medical care; (2) disability can be prevented or reduced through appropriate medical management; (3) the goals of management include improvements in physical, social, psychologic, and vocational functioning with or without basic disease process; (4) restoration, maintenance, or adaptation of the patient's functional abilities frequently demands efforts of many specialists, including nonmedical personnel and other specialized physicians, as well as physiatrists; (5) family and community resources are essential to the rehabilitative process and must be included in therapy efforts; and (6) planning for continuity of restorative care is a medical responsibility and should be oriented toward reintegrating the client into the social setting. Generally speaking, the physiatrist is a team leader.

A rehabilitation nurse specializes in the personal care of clients who are physically impaired. This nurse acts as a liaison between clients and the community and helps clients make the necessary adjustments when they return home from the hospital. The interdisciplinary home care team utilizes the skills of the rehabilitation nurse to coordinate services as necessary to enact its home treatment plan. The rehabilitation nurse is a clinical resource, a patient advocate, a care coordinator, a primary health care provider, an educator, and a definite team member.

The physical therapist helps the client restore or adapt functional capacities. This treatment may be accomplished through a series of exercises designed to increase strength, flexibility, coordination, and endurance. Treatment modalities may include heat or cold therapy, electrical stimulation, massage, traction, or other modalities as useful adjunctive treatment to try to restore strength and motion. The endpoint, however, is the restoration of, or adaption of, motion or function and not the modality itself.

The occupational therapist focuses upon the client's ability to perform ADL. Treatment is directed toward facilitating the client's independence through various adaptive measures. These measures may include training clients to perform necessary activities by simplifying tasks so as to minimize fatigue. The therapist may advise the use of adaptive equipment and assistive devices and then proceed to train the client in how to compensate for lost sensory, perceptual, or even cognitive skills.

The speech pathologist addresses speech/communication disorders, swallowing disorders, and/or cognitive disorders. Examples of associative disorders include those associated with laryngectomies, aphasia, dysarthria, dysphagia, and apraxia, as well as a host of other neuromuscular disorders that affect speech, swallowing, language, or cognition.

The psychologist generally helps prepare the client and the family or other support system for participation in the rehabilitation process. The psychologist generally identifies the client's personality profile, which will help determine how the client deals with stress and perhaps even problem solving. Many test tools can be used by the psychologist to aid the team in guiding the client through the rehabilitation program and to help support the client as the process continues and advances.

The social worker generally helps the client and family interact with the home care team and the community. Each member of the team assesses the client's total living situation, including lifestyle, family support system, finances, employment history, education level, and community resources available. The social worker helps to evaluate how the client's impairments will impact each of these areas.

The insurance case manager, who is often a rehabilitation nurse, strives to provide the best, yet most cost-effective, care for the client. This member of the home care team generally tries to facilitate the client's restoration of maximal function and minimize the back-to-work time span when applicable, while at the same time utilizing a cost-effective treatment plan.

The home health aide is literally a true helper who assists the client in ADL during rehabilitation. This team member has specialized rehabilitative training which allows him or her to encourage the client's self-care participation in the rehabilitation program and also helps to promote the client's dignity while at the same time understanding the deficits. The aide reports the client's daily progress or changes to the team for continued assessment and evaluation.

Treatment Plans

General Principles

After an initial evaluation by the physician and the various team members, a goal-directed plan is devised. The treatment plan will be based upon the functional problems identified. It is important to remember that sometimes the goals are to restore function and at other times to adapt to functional independence, even though normal function cannot be accomplished. The treatment plan becomes a coordinated set of functional goals designed to improve the client's quality of life by restoring the maximum level of function possible to impaired areas.

The plan is generally directed by the physiatrist or a physician, who writes the treatment plan with the input of the other health care disciplines that have been involved in the rehabilitation evaluation process. Each member of the home care team should identify goals specific to his or her own specialty area, with the responsibility of helping to evolve the plan. The plan is a dynamic document with the capability of changing as goals are met or as the needs of the client change or evolve. The fact that this plan is dynamic underscores the obvious purpose for having a team and frequent periodic team meetings to keep abreast of the patient's progress or the progress of the support system upon which the client may depend. Treatment plans always incorporate the family or the support group and their various preferences as well as their cultural practices and needs. Clients and families should be encouraged to share their problems and even their solutions to those problems because they tend to have unique insight into the situation, which the home care team may not yet have developed.

For clients with chronic disease, a return to previous lifestyle may not be possible. The treatment strategies for such patients would then be to prevent or correct additional disability to enhance unaffected body systems, to increase the function of affected body systems, to use adaptive equipment or resources to promote function, to modify the client's social and vocational environment, and to use psychological techniques to enhance the client's performance and perhaps advance educational and/or vocational skills.

When designing a treatment plan, the method of educating the client must match the client's particular learning skills or educational level to the needs that exist at that time so that treatment interventions can improve independence, self-care, and self-esteem. For example, if a client has problems performing a task, the task should be separated into a sequence of simple understandable steps which when applied separately can eventually be remolded into the more complex task or at least adapted to closely approximate the task so that the client can then perform satisfactorily.

Assistive Devices

Many types of assistive devices have been developed to help clients make their individual functioning in their own environments more plausible and to enhance their independence. These devices may also provide mechanisms by which the client can possibly compete in the work environment in an adapted fashion, enhance his or her independence, and certainly improve quality of life. Examples of these devices or adaptations can be divided in the following functional categories:[9]

1. **Aids for daily living**—Devices that assist with such activities as bathing, dressing, eating, cooking, toileting, and home maintenance.
2. **Augmentative communication devices**—Tools that provide a means of expressive and receptive communication for clients with limited speech or hearing abilities.
3. **Computer-assisted tools**—Input and output devices with modified or alternative keyboards or alternative access aids, which may be in the form of switches or special software, and other devices that assist clients with disabilities to use a computer.
4. **Environmental control systems**—Systems that enable immobilized clients to control appliances, emergency security systems, telephones, entertainment systems, and home heating and air conditioning systems, to mention a few.
5. **Home/work site modifications**—Structural adaptations such as ramps, lifts, bathroom changes, or other modifications that would remove or reduce physical barriers to impaired individuals.
6. **Prosthetics and orthotics/artificial limbs or braces**—Tools that replace, substitute for, or augment missing or malfunctioning body parts.
7. **Wheelchair/mobility aids**—These devices include manual and/or electric wheelchairs, adapted walkers or other hand tools, electric scooters

or other conveyances, and other utility vehicles used for increasing personal mobility.

8. **Seating and positioning adaptive devices**—Tools that usually fit a wheelchair or other seating system to provide greater stability for trunk or head support for upright posture and to reduce pressure on insensate or at-risk skin.

9. **Visual or hearing aid devices**—These include specialized magnifiers or glasses, speech and hearing devices, large-print screens, and possibly even computerized augmentative systems.

10. **Personal vehicle modifications**—These modifications include adapted driving aids, such as hand controls or special emergency systems, for personal independent driving and wheelchair lifts and modifications to allow independent entrance to and exit from a modified vehicle, thus allowing independent transportation or allowing the caregiver the ability to independently transport the client.

Specialty Items

Specialty items are available which may help increase independence and safety. Call-button emergency assistive devices enable clients with a variety of conditions to feel confident and safe within their home environments. A client who lives alone and has the capabilities can utilize such a device to obtain help in an emergency by simply pressing a button, thus improving the client's ability to maintain the lifestyle that he or she desires with peace of mind. For clients who have trouble remembering to take their medications on a regular schedule, online medication devices have been developed. These devices dispense medications and remind the client to take them by use of an audible alarm which sounds continuously until the medication is taken. If the medication is not taken, a signal can be transmitted over the telephone line to a service center, where an attendant will attempt to contact the client; if the client cannot be reached, a caregiver or family member is contacted. It is clear that specialty items do play a role in the rehabilitation of people with various impairments. These specialty items may raise the level of self-confidence and feelings of safety among people with various kinds of needs.

Outcome Measurement

General Principles

After proceeding through the evaluation measures and the rehabilitative measures that have been designed to re-establish independence or adapt functional capabilities for a better quality of life, and having helped the family or other caregivers proceed through the same process, measurement of outcome certainly becomes an important item to consider. The measurement of outcome of rehabilitative therapy is difficult and sometimes controversial. Three levels of measurement have been used to evaluate the outcome of therapy: the impairment level, the disability level, and the handicap level. These levels are general in nature and require some definition.

Impairment measures evaluate case severity as it relates to the disease or injury and aid in the development of short- and long-term plans and treatment objectives. Impairment measures deal primarily with a disease or injury process as it affects the body as a whole. Measurement of impairment may indicate whether or not a particular intervention could produce a significant improvement in a client's functioning.

Disability is a measurement of the evaluation of the client's ability to perform activities in the given situation and is therefore task dependent. One cannot define disability without having a defined task and a defined impairment that impacts that task.

Handicap is a term that is dependent upon the society or the situation in which a patient is placed. Measuring handicap may be a measurement of how the client's disabilities may have been reduced. Defining handicap incorporates the impairments, the disability, the environment, and the disadvantages to the client in terms of social norms or social expectations or even social barriers. For example, a truck driver who has had an amputation below the knee may still be able to drive a commercial vehicle. However, in spite of rehabilitation to independent ambulation and the use of a prosthesis, state law does not allow commercial driving if one or both lower limbs are artificial. Handicap in this sense is socially dictated. Accuracy in defining handicap is affected by family support, ethnicity, poverty, prior employment history, and environmental barriers, to name just a few.

These terms—impairment, disability, and handicap—and their measurements are pertinent to the overall goal of increasing the client's quality of life. Even though the level of physical impairment may not change dramatically, the level of function and the ability to perform ADL may improve.

Functional Measurement Tools

Functional measurement tools can be applied to the rehabilitation of any given individual, and these outcome measurement tools can display graphically that goals which have been established may well have been met. Improvement in percentage scores and final outcome scores should be used to provide the most complete evaluation of a given client's rehabilitative efforts. These tools can be applied periodically during rehabilitation (and certainly at the end of the reha-bilitation period) to help measure the outcome as it relates not only to the patient and the caregivers, but to the rehabilitation team itself so that the team can make critical assessments of its own efforts. These tools should help clients, their families, and/or their support systems see results in a more graphic manner and reinforce the positive aspects of the efforts of the rehabilitative team and the client, as well as the efforts of the support system. The tools may also be reapplied at a later date during follow-up to see if there have been changes, for better or worse, in the client's condition.

Many measurement tools have been developed to measure functional abili-ties, and these can be utilized by a rehabilitation team. It is recommended that the team choose a tool that it can apply consistently so that the tool becomes an aid in the development of rehabilitation programs and goals for clients. Some functional assessment tools under development are targeted to be used nation-ally so as to standardize functional outcome measurements. Two fairly simple and dependable tools are the Tinetti Assessment Tool and the Barthel Index.[10]

In 1986, the Tinetti Assessment Tool was developed by Mary Tinetti, M.D., to assess balance in gait. She devised ten areas of assessment, and each area was given a weight and score. The total score achieved with these balance and gait tests indicates a predictive value for assessing a client's risk of falling. The rehabilitative home care team can also use the results to assess its success or failure as it relates to a person's ambulation safety.

In 1965, Florence Mahoney, M.D., and Dorothea W. Barthel, P.T., devel-oped the Barthel Index. It has become a proven method of measuring a client's functional status and an aid in determining the need for assistance with ADL. This index uses a weighted scale that gives more points to more important activities. For example, it is considered more important to be able to move from a sitting to a standing position than it is to get in and out of the shower independently. The first section of the Barthel Index addresses personal care tasks such as drinking from a cup, eating, dressing the upper body, dressing the lower body, grooming, bathing, and controlling bowel and bladder evacuation activities. The second section addresses client mobility, such as getting in and out of a chair or getting on or off a toilet. This section also addresses use of a shower or tub, walking on a level surface, and using stairs. If walking is not possible, then the use of an adapted wheelchair becomes important, and in this section wheelchair usage is also assessed if it is the alternative method of mobility. It is clear that use of various tools for assessment can help the reha-bilitative team not only in assessing the patient's initial needs but in reassessing the client as he or she progresses through rehabilitative efforts. Such tools can also help the team to assess itself as it relates to the responses of the patient or the results that have been accomplished.

Follow-Up Care and Assessment

Once the client has regained the maximum levels of functional activities as defined by the initial evaluation and the ongoing evaluations made by the team (including the client and the support system), rehabilitation therapy is terminated. Usually the final duty of the home care team is to provide the client and his or her support system with a follow-up care plan to assist them in continuing the newly regained lifestyle in as functionally independent a manner as possible. This final care plan should incorporate suggestions for how the client can access the network of support which is available in the community. It should include a schedule of follow-up visits by the client to physicians or therapists if an outpatient setting can be utilized. It should also include in-home visits made by the team periodically to ensure continued best functional capacities.

It is important to remember that use of functional assessment tools not only aids in assessing client outcomes but also aids in assessing effectiveness of treatment protocols developed and applied during the home care rehabilitative process. Therefore, the treating team can use these tools to assess itself as well. These tools can also be useful when providing information to third-party payors who usually require justification of treatment.

Conclusion

The home care rehabilitation team can be successful in promoting functional restoration either back to a normal situation or to an adapted functional situation by coordinated, goal-directed efforts well conceived and consistently applied by an intelligent, caring, motivated group of individuals focused upon teamwork, with the client at the center of the focus. It is important to keep in mind that we as health care providers are here *because* of our clients, not in spite of them!

References

1. Jaffe, K. B. and Walsh, P. A., The development of the specialty rehabilitation home care team: supporting the creative thought process, *Holistic Nurse Pract.*, 7(4):36–41, 1993.
2. DeLisa, J. A. and Gans, B. M., Eds., *Rehabilitative Medicine: Principles and Practice*, 2nd edition, J.B. Lippincott, Philadelphia, 1993.
3. Theuerkauf, S. and Schuster, L. C., The changing role of the rehab nurse, *Caring*, July:48–52, 1994.
4. Loustau, A. and Lee, K. A., Dealing with the dangers of dysphagia, *Nursing 85*, Feb.:47–50, 1985.

5. Kirby, R. L., Clinical evaluation of the musculoskeletal system, in *Medical Rehabilitation*, Basmajian, J. V. and Kirby, R. L., Eds., Williams and Wilkins, Baltimore, 1984, pp. 33–43.
6. Portnow, J., Assistive technologies in the home, *Caring*, Sept.:58–61, 1994.
7. Hoeman, S. P., Community-based rehabilitation, *Holistic Nurse Pract.*, 6(2):32–41, 1992.
8. Ruskin, A. P., Ed., Psychosocial aspects: the physiatrist, physician to the disabled, in *Current Therapy in Physiatry, Physical Medicine and Rehabilitation*, W.B. Saunders, Philadelphia, 1984, pp. 567–568.
9. Enabling Technologies of Kentuckiana, Paper on Assistive Technology, Louisville Free Public Library, Louisville, Kentucky, 1995.
10. Moffa-Trotter, M. E. and Anemaet, W. K., Measuring up in home health, documenting objective, measureable progress in home care: two sample tools, *Advance/ Rehabilitation*, July/Aug.:23–27, 1995.
11. Sherry, D., Restorative nursing, *Home Healthcare Nurse*, 13(2):71–72, 1995.
12. Jaffe, K. B., Home health care and rehabilitation nursing, *Nurs. Clin. North Am.*, 24(1):171–178, 1989.
13. O'Toole, M. T., The interdisciplinary team: research and education, *Holistic Nurse Pract.*, 6(2):76–83, 1992.
14. McBride, S. M., Rehabilitation case managers: ahead of their time, *Holistic Nurse Pract.*, 6(2):67–75, 1992.
15. Wilson, A. A., Hartnett, M., and Ferrari, P., Outcome measurement from the functional status perspective, *Home Healthcare Nurse*, 10(3):32–46, 1992.

Home Care of Communicative Disorders

7

David R. Cunningham, Ph.D. and Barbara M. Baker, Ph.D.

Communicative Disorders Defined

A communicative disorder is an impairment in the ability to receive, send, process, or comprehend concepts or verbal, nonverbal, and/or graphic symbol systems. These disorders may be manifested in the processes of hearing, language, and/or speech production. They may range in severity from extremely mild and subtle to profound. A communicative disorder may be the primary disability, it may be secondary to other conditions, or it may be congenital, developmental, or acquired through disease processes or traumatic injury.[6] It is convenient to describe communicative disorders as problems associated with speech, language, hearing, or central nervous system processing. Each of these will be explained in greater detail, but it should be made clear that there is often significant functional overlap among these subtypes, and there are likely to be cause–effect relationships as well (e.g., early childhood hearing loss is causally related to delayed speech and language development).

A speech disorder is an impairment of the articulation of speech sounds. An articulation disorder is characterized by the atypical production of speech sounds. Abnormal articulation patterns may include the omission of certain speech sounds, the substitution of individual speech sounds or clusters of sounds for others, the addition or insertion of speech sounds, and/or distortions of speech sounds. These patterns interfere with the intelligibility of speech as heard by the listener.

A voice disorder is characterized by abnormal voice production to include the parameters of vocal quality, pitch, loudness, resonance, and/or voice duration which are inappropriate for an individual's age and gender. This would result in voice changes such as hoarseness, breathiness, weak volume, low or high tone, and/or too much or too little nasality.

A fluency disorder is an interruption in the flow of speech characterized by an abnormal rate or rhythm of speech. In layman's terms, this condition is known as stuttering. Speech production is characterized by the associated mannerisms of facial grimacing, excessive eye blinking, and a lack of eye contact with the listener.[6]

A language disorder is characterized by impaired comprehension and/or use of spoken, written, or other symbol systems. A language disorder may involve the "form" of language: a phonological disorder affects the sounds used to convey meaning, a morphological disorder affects the construction of word forms, and a syntactical disorder affects the combination of words to form sentences. A language disorder may involve the "content" of language: a semantic problem affects the meaning of words/phrases/sentences. Finally, a language disorder may involve the "function" of language: a pragmatic disorder affects the social appropriateness of language. Language disorders may affect children or adults. Adult language disorders generally result from traumatic head injury, cerebral vascular accident, or degenerative central nervous system dysfunction. Pediatric language disorders result from developmental delay, hearing loss, and traumatic head injury.[6]

A hearing disorder is the result of impaired auditory sensitivity, recognition, discrimination, comprehension, and/or perception of auditory information. A hearing disorder may limit the development, comprehension, production, and/or maintenance of speech and language. Hearing disorders may be classified by site of pathology (i.e., outer, middle, or inner ear; primary auditory neurons; brainstem; and/or other central nervous system manifestations). Hearing disorders are also classified by degree of impairment or hearing handicap (i.e., mild, moderate, severe, and profound hearing impairment).[6]

Central auditory processing disorders (CAPD) are deficits in information processing of audible signals *not* associated with peripheral hearing loss or cognitive impairment. A CAPD is characterized by problems in attending to, discriminating, filtering, sorting, storing, retrieving, organizing, decoding, or assigning meaning to auditory information.[6] This type of communicative disorders may share some of the same symptoms as those produced by head trauma, cerebrovascular accident, or space-occupying lesions. Nevertheless, CAPD is distinguished from these and is generally considered a disorder of central auditory "function" or "organization" rather than overt pathology or injury. (This distinction may prove to be arbitrary as new neurophysiologic and neuropathologic information unfolds in careful research.)

Causation and Prevalence of Communicative Disorders

Approximately 42 million Americans are affected personally by a communicative disorder of some type; 28 million suffer some measurable degree of hearing loss. About 73% of these are males. The most common causes of hearing loss are otitis media with effusion in children, presbycusis in the elderly, hereditary factors, and noise exposure. Hearing loss can also result from prematurity, neonatal anoxia, ototoxic chemicals, meningitis, otosclerosis, viral diseases, and head trauma. It can be associated with a very wide variety of genetic syndromes. At least 50% of congenital hearing loss is genetically based. Many cases of hearing loss with later onset in childhood have a genetic basis as well. There are 17 million Americans estimated to have permanent sensorineural hearing loss. Some 10 million Americans have noise-induced hearing loss. Approximately 2 million Americans are prelingually deaf. One child in 1000 has early onset hearing loss that impedes speech/language development. Approximately 30% of individuals 65 to 74 years of age have hearing loss secondary to presbycusis; at least 50% of people over 75 years of age have presbycusis. Hearing loss is clearly the single most common cause of communication difficulty in children and adults.

Speech and/or language disorders affect some 14 million Americans. These disorders are often associated with neurological impairments such as stroke, Parkinsonism, head trauma, brain tumors, spinal cord injuries, muscular dystrophy, multiple sclerosis, cerebral palsy, amyotrophic lateral sclerosis, Huntington's chorea, or dementias including Alzheimer's disease. Hearing loss is a significant causal factor for speech and language delay in children. Speech/language disorders are bimodally distributed in the general population: they are most common in preschool and school-aged children and older adults. Of individuals reporting chronic speech disorders, 45% are under 18 years of age. Stuttering affects some 2 million Americans. There are a number of specific disease entities associated with communicative disorders. The probability of having a communicative disorder in these subgroups is much higher than in the general population. These subgroups include:[8]

- 500,000 have Parkinson's disease.
- 300,000 have multiple sclerosis, about 25,000 have Huntington's chorea, and some 14,000 suffer from amyotrophic lateral sclerosis.
- Some 400,000 strokes (cerebrovascular accidents) occur each year in the United States; approximately 20% of these are related to aphasia.
- More than 1 million persons in the United States have some degree of aphasia.
- Alzheimer's disease afflicts 2.5 to 3.0 million Americans.

- Dementia affects 10% of the population over age 65 years and approximately 50% of those over age 85 years.
- Spasmodic dysphonia, a severely debilitating voice disorder characterized by a strained/strangled vocal quality, affects some 50,000 to 100,000 people.
- 6 to 8 million Americans have some type of language disorder.
- Language disorders affect approximately 2 to 5% of preschoolers and about 1% of the school-age population.
- Two-thirds of language disorders occur in boys. The most common causes of language disorders in children are mental retardation, brain injury, autism, and hearing loss.
- Dysphagia (swallowing disorders) affects some 15 million Americans.

Impact of Communicative Disorders

Communicative disorders have a significant negative impact on patients' lives. On the most fundamental level, communicative disorders cause normal interpersonal communication to be diminished. The sending, receiving, and/or interpreting of messages breaks down. The psychosocial impact of communicative disorders can be overwhelming. There will be loss of information, social intercourse is impoverished, and self-esteem and self-image are negatively affected. Social withdrawal, isolation, and depression are common symptoms. Family relations can be significantly strained. Vocational/occupational paths can be limited or interrupted altogether. This may lead to diminution or loss of personal/family income.

Communicative disorders affect the learning of new information. Children are normally voracious learners. Childhood communicative disorders challenge the educational process. Although professionals endeavor to educate children in the "least limiting environment," and this is usually construed to mean keeping children in the "mainstream" of the normal educational setting, children with communicative disorders often require special education, extended therapy, and/ or augmentative or alternative communication technologies. These strategies may be required whether the child is treated in the schools, as an outpatient, or in the home setting. Educators, therapists, and other caregivers have the dual responsibility of trying to remediate the primary communicative disorder while also imparting the content of the educational curriculum (math, social studies, science, language arts, etc.). It is important, therefore, that the communicative disorders therapist and the child's educators work in concert to realize the patient's maximum potential. The pediatric home care environment must accommodate not only the child's need for direct therapy, but also his or her educational requirements as soon as the child's general health status permits these interventions.[3]

Adults are also learners. Normal adults have mastered the fundamental communication processes (speech, language, listening skills, vocabulary, the subtleties of social discourse, etc.). These can be radically and catastrophically altered by a head trauma, stroke, or other disease process. The initial focus of the therapy may be reestablishing the basic communication infrastructure so that information that has already been learned and "stored" can be retrieved and used again. It is now accepted as dogma that early and continuing stimulation is essential in these cases. The adult's communicative disorder may also impede the learning of novel information. This includes not only the learning of new life skills (job-related information, hobbies, etc.), but also learning specific to the treatment plan (medications, exercises, new modalities to accomplish the activities of daily living, and so forth). The success of other treatments depends to a great extent upon the patient's ability to communicate his or her needs, symptoms, and concerns and to understand the instructions provided by caregivers. Unless and until the basic communication processes can be reestablished, the broader treatment plan and goals are jeopardized. Beyond stabilizing the patient medically, perhaps the next most important priority is establishing a communication system that links the patient to other communicators.[1,2,5,7]

The Home as a Treatment Environment

The patient's home is generally a natural environment for healing and relearning. It was "at home" that interpersonal communication was first mastered. Within earshot of his or her parents (or other caregivers), the infant child spends some 3000 hours listening to the spoken language of its particular culture before producing its first meaningful utterance. For most of us, there is a strong positive correlation between home life and ease of communication. Communication within the home is, hopefully, less threatening and less demanding than in an institution, in a formal treatment environment, or even within a "sheltered" workplace. The "flow" of conversation is likely to be less restrained in the home. There is more time to communicate, and the "audience" (parents, spouse, siblings, etc.) is generally more forgiving and nurturing. The home is a familiar place. The surroundings are laden with personal meaning and memories. These are natural stimuli and inducements for relaxed, casual communication. The therapist will have less need of contrived or artificial stimuli: the "real" objects, furnishings, clothing, food items, and facilities are readily available at home. Communications in the home are pragmatic, meaningful, and relevant. Communication retraining in the home can focus on tangible objectives. The timing and pace of treatment can be adjusted more readily than in other health care settings (i.e., clinics, hospitals, rehabilitation agencies, etc.). Because family members or friends are usually recruited into the home treatment program, the visiting clinician may have more information about the patient's lifestyle than what might be available in an institutional setting or outpatient clinic. This information will be valuable in custom-tailoring therapy to the individual's needs. There are more opportunities to observe the patient's problems and progress in the home setting. With family/friends involved on a more or less continuous basis in the rehabilitative process, the sheer numbers of "clinical" observations of patient behavior are increased dramatically over those seen in the typical "b.i.d." therapy sessions in an institution. Friends and family members are not only caregivers, they are "reporters." They are in a position to report to the visiting therapists on the patient's successes and failures, on his or her attitude, and to make observations or suggestions on other aspects of the treatment plan.

Interpersonal communication in the home environment takes on a "social" meaning and intent rather than the purely "functional" significance that would be typical of an acute treatment setting. The number of communication events generally is higher in the home, and retraining takes on an air of relevance that reinforces healing. The focus is diagnosis and system stabilization, not rehabilitation, in the acute care setting. Speech, language, and/or hearing "survival skills" are the priority in the hospital environment, where "length of stay" issues may mitigate against comprehensive treatment for communicative disorders. Extended-stay facilities (rehabilitation hospitals, intermediate care facilities, skilled nursing facilities, etc.) offer treatment for communicative disorders in an environment that is only a second-order approximation to the "home" setting. The focus is on "functional" communication skills: communicating basic needs and choices (feeding, toileting, reporting pain, and so forth). These activities are essential as stimulation and are absolutely necessary to the preservation of patient function, but it is within the home, however, that these exercises are elaborated and expanded to form the repertoire of self-expression, dialogue, and written and read symbolization. The home provides an infrastructure for communication that is natural, meaningful, realistic, and "reinforcing" (at least in terms of the number of communication events that are likely to occur). As long as the home environment is reasonably stable and not overtly dysfunctional or abusive, these benefits are likely to accrue to the patient who is treated in the home.[1,5]

The Communication Specialists

The professionals who provide home care for individuals with speech, language, and hearing disorders and/or dysphagia (feeding and swallowing disorders) are speech-language pathologists and audiologists. Speech-language pathologists and audiologists are certified in either discipline (or both) by the American Speech-Language-Hearing Association (ASHA). The certifying credential is known as the "Certificate of Clinical Competence" (CCC). The designations CCC/SLP and CCC/A denote professional certification in speech-language pathology or audiology, respectively. A clinician's certification status can be determined by contacting ASHA at 301-897-5700 or at 10801 Rockville Pike, Rockville, Maryland 20852. Certified members of ASHA have a master's degree or a doctoral degree in their discipline and hold a license to practice in most states.[2–4]

Although there are currently no specific credentialing requirements for practicing speech-language pathology or audiology in the home setting, the clinician should have experience and skills that relate to the unique aspects of home health care. Some of these experiences and skills may include:[1,4,5,7]

- Skill in the treatment of neurologically impaired children/adults
- Provision of services to patients with communicative disorders and/or oral-pharyngeal disorders resulting from trauma, severe illness, and/or surgery
- Knowledge of prespeech/language developmental skills in infants/ toddlers
- Skill in family intervention techniques
- Work experience in the home environment
- Knowledge of drugs/medication/illnesses and disabilities and their effects on communication
- Knowledge of infection control and universal precautions
- Knowledge of the roles, responsibilities, and contributions of other health care professionals
- Knowledge of documentation requirements specific to home care
- Knowledge of reimbursement and legislative issues that impact home service delivery

Qualified speech-language pathologists and audiologists can be located by contacting area clinics, hospitals, rehabilitation agencies, state speech/language/ hearing associations, or home health agencies.

Service Delivery

As described in a previous section of this chapter, the chief advantage of home-based treatment is having a more natural, familiar environment which may facilitate and maximize communication and rehabilitation. Speech-language pathology/audiology services provided in the home have some unique aspects, however. The home has some characteristics that differ from acute, intermediate, or skilled-level treatment facilities. These differences present a number of challenges to the speech-language pathologist or audiologist. Some of these unique aspects of home-based care include:[1,4,5,7]

- Increased pressure or risk from family members
- Working in an unknown environment
- Exposure to contagious diseases in less well-controlled environments
- Clinician travel; distance and time constraints
- Limitations in the type of specialized equipment available for home use
- Relative isolation of the clinician from other health care professionals
- Difficulties in coordinating multifaceted treatment components
- Relative disconnection from other health care facilities
- Less immediate oversight/help from supervisors

These factors must be considered when planning a home-based treatment protocol, as well as when selecting a knowledgeable speech-language pathologist or audiologist.

Guidelines for the Delivery of Speech-Language Pathology and Audiology Services in Home Care were developed by the ASHA Task Force on Home Care in November 1990.[5] Home care is rapidly expanding in today's health care industry. Factors contributing to this growth include: (a) the aging population, (b) a growing number of children identified as needing home care, (c) pressure on hospitals to decrease costs by reducing lengths of stay and limiting the number of beds, (d) government and private business efforts to contain costs, (e) technological advances, and (f) consumer need or preference for receiving services within the home.[5] Since the establishment of Medicare and Medicaid programs in 1965, home care has grown to include speech-language pathology and audiology services.

The Referral Process

The basic professional service components of speech-language pathology and audiology services in the home care setting include identification and referral, assessment, treatment, consultation, and education. The initial identification process may come from the physician, nursing, hospital discharge planner, discharging speech-language pathologist from various institutional settings, or other home care providers. The referral process may be initiated from an acute care hospital, a rehabilitation center, a long-term care facility, or from other home care providers already treating within the home. An individual patient can make a self-referral and can be seen without a physician order, if he or she wishes to pay privately for the services.

Referrals generally accompany an acute incident, medical necessity, progressive deterioration, or a decline in function. Maximum rehabilitation can be planned for a recent (within 6 months) onset of a disorder or a justifiable recent medical condition for a homebound individual. Continued therapy is dependent upon the patient's potential for progress and restoration of function. Maintenance therapy for progressive degenerative diseases or a recent decline in function is treated on a more limited basis.

Homebound infants and children with swallowing and medically based speech and language disorders can qualify for home health care services. These infants are usually discharged with sucking and feeding problems from the neonatal critical care nursery. These children are at risk for speech, language, oral-motor, and feeding disabilities or delays. Children in the birth to 36 months age range are not serviced by the public schools and may be followed by home health therapists for speech disturbance and language delay.[3] Some insurance companies will not cover developmental delay and will limit services to injury, traumatic brain injury, cleft lip and palate or craniofacial syndromes, seizure disorders, fetal alcohol syndrome, or neurological involvement.

Certain medical conditions affecting adults often trigger a referral. Typical etiologies are (1) transient ischemic attack and/or left cerebral vascular accident resulting in aphasia and/or speech dysarthria or apraxia; (2) right cerebral vascular accident resulting in perceptual dysfunction and neglect syndromes; (3) dementia or Alzheimer's disease which affects memory and judgment; (4) degenerative disease processes such as multiple sclerosis, amyotrophic lateral sclerosis, and Parkinsonism which affect speech, voice, and swallowing; (5) head injury resulting in confusion and judgment impairment; (6) head and neck cancer impairing speech, voice, and swallowing; (7) hoarseness resulting from benign vocal cord lesions; (8) hearing impairment; (9) dysphagia occurring from a multitude of medical and surgical interventions, necessitating nasogastric and gastric tube placement; and (10) respiratory and vocal dysfunction due to chronic obstructive pulmonary disease.

A physician order is needed for insurance reimbursement. The order is specific to the type of evaluation needed. If the patient exhibits a communication impairment, the physician should write the order in the following format: "Speech-language evaluation and treatment as indicated." Once the evaluation is completed, a specific frequency and duration is recommended by the speech-language pathologist. Orders for other specific evaluation and treatment plans would be issued for dysphagia and audiologic evaluation to rule out ear pathology.

Many times, a patient's deficits are noticed by family members or caregivers.

The family or nursing staff may have difficulty understanding the patient or in getting the individual to understand directions or to process information. The following signs/symptoms may trigger a referral:

- Aphasia/language impairment/developmental language delay
- Dysarthria/slurred speech/pediatric misarticulations
- Apraxia/motor programming problem
- Jargon
- Word retrieval problem
- Auditory comprehension impairment
- Reduced memory
- Impaired judgment
- Transient confusion
- Voice tremor, hoarseness
- Dysphagia: nasogastric, gastric tube, difficulty managing secretions, choking, aspiration pneumonia, difficulty with thin liquids, purees, or solid consistencies
- Hearing impairment
- Nonvocal secondary to tracheostomy and/or ventilator dependency

Assessment

Evaluation procedures typically focus on aphasia assessment, cognitive assessment for confusion or dementia, symbolic-perceptual assessment for right cerebral vascular accident, oral-motor measures to test for speech dysarthria, voice analysis, bedside dysphagia evaluation utilizing different food consistencies, and hearing assessment with a portable audiometer. A pediatric evaluation would include articulation assessment, language testing for language delay, and dysphagia assessment for sucking and swallowing impairment.

The overall assessment goals are to: (a) ascertain the patient's functional communication ability, (b) gather objective and informal data to devise or revise a treatment program, and (c) provide a baseline against which to document progress, regression, or a plateau.[5]

Background information is needed to compare the date of onset and/or exacerbation of the illness with the present communication or swallowing difficulty. A recent episode or a recent decline in function pinpoints the onset date. Patients with long-standing deficits and an old onset date may not be candidates for treatment (or insurance reimbursement), especially if rehabilitation has been instituted at an earlier time period. However, patients may be eligible for treatment if: (1) they had never received any services in the past or (2) previous rehabilitation efforts have been unsuccessful and a new therapeutic approach is warranted (i.e., an augmentative communicative device for a severe verbal apraxia).

The evaluation process takes various forms of data collection from standardized tests, direct observation of patient behaviors, nonstandardized tests, and consultations with family, physician, nursing staff, and caregivers. A complete case history would include a pertinent medical, educational, vocational, and psychosocial history. The medical diagnosis is correlated with the type of communication impairment. Assessment of previous treatment approaches and the outcome of those services are reviewed for the direction of further assessment. Formalized adult measures assess aphasia, cognition, auditory comprehension, visual comprehension, graphic skills, expressive speech production, vocal quality, and memory. Pediatric measures assess fluency, speech and language development, and vocal quality. Informal measures for children and adults include observation of social and communication interactions and oral-motor function and assessment of current swallowing and dietary considerations during mealtime. Interpretation of test scores and assessment data will determine rehabilitation potential, functional limitations regarding communication and swallowing outcome, and recommendations for intervention.

Treatment

Following assessment, a specific treatment plan is developed which denotes recommended frequency and duration of therapy, prognosis for improvement, and baseline data with measurable objective long- and short-term goals. Environmental factors such as opportunities for communication and level of stimulation are considered when developing the plan. The initial evaluation and plan must be certified by the physician responsible for the patient's overall care.

At the completion of 60 days of treatment, the plan of care is updated with the total amount of progress obtained for the certification period. The physician reviews the plan and recertifies the next month of treatment. Measurable and predictable progress will generally qualify a patient for continued services (see section on reimbursement). Discharge is made when goals have been met or a plateau occurs with no significant progress noted.

Treatment is based upon the medical history and diagnosis, the course of prior treatment, and the findings of the current assessment. Treatment aspires to help the patient become more communicative and functional within his or her environment. The needs of the patient and the caregiver are considered to make the patient functional within the context of the home environment. Long-term treatment goals are centered around achieving functional independence by: (a) increasing auditory comprehension, (b) increasing language skills to developmental age level, (c) improving speech intelligibility, (d) increasing visual and reading skills, (e) improving graphic productions, (f) improving oral-motor functioning, (g) increasing sucking and/or swallowing skills or upgrading diet levels, (h) prescribing assistive listening or augmentative communication devices, (i) initiating an aural rehabilitation program, or (j) recommending a hearing aid. Table 7.1 outlines preferred practice patterns as set forth by ASHA. Represented is the type of service, the professionals who perform the procedure, expected outcomes, the clinical process, and documentation standards.[7]

Reimbursement

Major sources of payment for home health services are Medicare and Medicaid. Some third-party insurers and health maintenance organizations (HMOs) include home health services in their policies as well.[5] Ancillary services are billed under the Medicare Part A program. Patients must qualify for the state-assisted Medicaid program. Each policy should be reviewed to determine the extent and method of coverage and the need for prior authorization of speech-language pathology and audiology services for persons who are confined to the home.

Speech-language pathology and audiology services are reimbursable under the Medicare home health benefit. Medicare publishes specific guidelines for these services. These must be followed by the treating therapist. Home health reimbursement per visit limits are published in the Federal Register for speech-language pathology and other professionals' services.[5] Medicare providers offering outpatient services in the home are rehabilitation agencies, Medicare certified home health agencies, and hospitals. Speech-language pathologists not affiliated with a certified Medicare provider are not eligible to become Medicare providers as independent practitioners but may have their practices recognized as rehabilitation agencies. Audiologists can obtain a Medicare provider number for diagnostic audiology services.

Home health services are a required benefit under the federal Medicaid plan.[5] Speech-language pathology and audiology services are optional services under the home health benefit. Direct speech-language pathology and audiology services are an optional benefit under the federal participation agreement. Before rendering services to Medicaid recipients, the speech-language pathologist and audiologist should review the state Medicaid plan to ascertain coverage of services in the home.[5]

Blue Cross and Blue Shield plans, commercial insurers, and HMOs may also offer home health services. However, each policy should be reviewed before initiating services to determine the extent of coverage and the need for prior authorization.

Reimbursement depends upon eligibility of the individual for coverage, homebound definition and determination, recordkeeping requirements of daily

Table 7.1 ASHA Preferred Practice Patterns

Type of service	Professionals who perform the procedure	Expected outcomes	Clinical process	Documentation
Speech screening	SLPs and audiologists	Identification of persons with speech disorders that interfere with education, health, development, or communication. Recommendations for comprehensive assessment.	Screening of oral-motor function, speech production skills: articulation, fluency, resonance, voice.	Statement of identifying information, results, recommendation, or referral.
Language screening	SLPs and audiologists	Identification of persons with language and/or cognitive communication disorders. Recommendation for comprehensive assessment.	Screening of comprehension and production of language and cognitive aspects of communications.	Same as above.
Swallowing screening	SLPs	Identification of persons with swallowing disorders that cause pulmonary aspiration, airway obstruction, inadequate nutrition, and/or hydration.	Observation of the patient during oral intake/feeding. Review of: medical/ pharmacologic history, cognitive/linguistic/behavior status, pulmonary/ respiration status, oropharyngeal swallowing dysfunction.	Same as above.
Hearing screening	Audiologists, SLPs (Pure Tone Air Conduction)	Identification of persons with auditory disorder that may interfere with education, healthy development, or communication. Recommendation for comprehensive assessment.	Screening of children with behavioral and/or electrophysiological procedures. Screening of adults with audiometry.	Same as above.

Table 7.1 ASHA Preferred Practice Patterns (continued)

Type of service	Professionals who perform the procedure	Expected outcomes	Clinical process	Documentation
Comprehensive speech-language pathology assessment	SLPs	Description of communication abilities of speech articulatory/phonology, voice, resonance and nasal airflow, fluency, spoken and written language, nonspoken language, cognitive-communication. Recommendations for treatment or follow-up.	Assessment includes: case history; interview; standardized and nonstandardized measures; analysis of associated medical, behavioral, environmental, educational, vocational, and social-emotional factors; patient counseling.	Includes background information, results and interpretation of formalized and nonformal tests, prognosis, and specific recommendations concerning treatment frequency, estimated duration, and type of service.
Spoken language assessment	SLPs	Identify and describe characteristics of spoken language skills. Diagnosis and clinical description of a disorder, recommendations for treatment, or referral. Recommendations for treatment or follow-up.	Assessment includes: case history, observation, standardized and nonstandardized methods to determine: comprehension/production of spoken language including phonology, morphology, syntax, semantics, and pragmatic.	Same as above.
Written language assessment	SLPs	Identify and describe patient's abilities to use written language as a functional mode of expression. Recommendations for treatment or follow-up.	Assessment includes: case history, standardized and nonstandardized methods to assess: orthography, morphology, syntax, semantics, pragmatic. Evaluation of the reading process.	Same as above.

Cognitive-communicative assessment	SLPs	Identify and describe strategies and deficiencies related to cognitive factors (attention, memory, and problem solving) and related language components (semantics and pragmatic). Recommendation for treatment or follow-up.	Assessment includes: case history, standardized measure to assess linguistic knowledge, spoken and nonspoken language comprehension and production, written language comprehension and production, and cognitive and pragmatic communication.	Same as above.
Articulation/ phonology assessment	SLPs	Description of the characteristics of speech sound production and to diagnose a communication disorder. Recommendations for treatment or follow-up.	Assessment includes: standardized and nonstandardized measures to assess developmental and acquired articulation disorders, oral-motor skills, phonological processes, and motor speech observation of voice, fluency, cognition, language.	Same as above.
Voice assessment	SLPs	To diagnose a voice disorder, describe perceptual phonatory characteristics, measure aspects of vocal function, examine phonatory behavior. Recommendations for treatment or follow-up.	Assessment includes: case history and vocal case history, perceptual aspects of voice production, acoustic paramedics of voice production, physiological aspects of phonatory behavior, psychological status, medical history, aerodynamic measures, electroglottography, imaging techniques such as endoscopy and stroboscopy.	Same as above.

Table 7.1   ASHA Preferred Practice Patterns (continued)

Type of service	Professionals who perform the procedure	Expected outcomes	Clinical process	Documentation
Resonance and nasal airflow assessment	SLPs	Diagnose normal and abnormal parameters of the swallowing system and other oral-pharyngeal functions. Recommendations for treatment and follow-up.	Assessment includes: case history; structural assessment of the head and neck; functional assessment of oral sensation, strength, tone, language and rate of structures, oral praxis, head-neck control, posture, suckling, suckling, developmental reflexes, and involuntary motion assessment of oral, pharyngeal, and upper esophageal structures needed during swallowing or feeding; observations of feeding, positing, food preference, swallowing, posture control, respiratory coordination. Assessment of relationship if intubation to oral-pharyngeal function. Observation of patient's coughing, choking, gurgling, reflux, and aspiration. Instrumentation used in interpretation is videofluoroscopy, ultrasound, manometry, endoscopy.	Same as above.

Augmentative and alternative communication (AAC) assessment	SLPs	Selection and obtainment of appropriate augmentative and/or alternative communication component to enhance communication. Recommendations for treatment and follow-up.	Assessment includes: observation of visual status, hearing status. Observation of posture, gross and fine motor coordination, and use of communicative boards and specialized equipment. Recommendation of devices, techniques, symbols, and/or strategies for the preferred AAC option.	Same as above.
Prosthetic/ adaptive device assessment	SLPs	Assessment to determine whether a patient is a candidate for a prosthetic/adaptive device such as palatal lifts, obturators, artificial larynges, tracheoesophageal fistulation prostheses, and speech prostheses. Correct use and maintenance of the device. Recommendations for treatment and follow-up.	Standardized and nonstandardized measures to determine appropriateness of prosthetic/adaptive devices to improve functional communication. Trial intervention with the device with rationale for the preferred option.	Same as above.
Basic audiological assessment	Audiologist	Quality and quantity by site of lesion, peripheral hearing loss on the basis of perceptual, physiologic, or electrophysiological responses to acoustic stimuli. Recommendation for further audiologic assessment, rehabilitation assessment, medical/educational referral, hearing aid/sensory assessment, aural rehabilitation.	Assessments: case history, aid and bone conduction, pure tone threshold measures with appropriate masking, speech recognition thresholds, word recognition (speech discrimination) measures, tympanometry, static immittance, acoustic reflex measures, auditory evoked potentials, evoked otoacoustic emissions.	Interpretation of test results and the type and severity of the hearing loss and associated condition.

Table 7.1   ASHA Preferred Practice Patterns (continued)

Type of service	Professionals who perform the procedure	Expected outcomes	Clinical process	Documentation
Comprehensive audiological assessment	Audiologists	Same as basic audiologic assessment.	Same as basic audiologic assessment. Procedures to assess cochlear versus retrocochlear (i.e., eighth cranial nerve, brainstem, or cortical auditory) disorders include: acoustic reflex threshold, acoustic reflex patterns, auditory-evoked potentials, performance intensity—phonetically balanced speech discrimination (PIPB), evoked otoacoustic emissions. Procedures to assess central auditory nervous system disorders include: auditory-evoked potentials, brief tone stimuli, distorted speech, dichotic stimuli, temporal ordering of stimuli, masking patterns, physiological measures of brain activity, including blood flow, metabolic rate, and electrical activity. Procedures for detecting or quantifying pseudohypacusis include: compiling pure tone averages and speech recognition thresholds, Bekesy audiometry, including lengthened off-time (LOT) and Bekesy Ascending Delayed auditory feedback, Stenger tests, acoustic reflex thresholds, auditory evoked potentials.	Same as above.

Pediatric audiological assessment	Audiologists	Same as basic audiologic assessment.	Assessment includes: case history, behavioral observation, visual reinforcement audiometry, play audiometry, tympanometry, static immittance and acoustic reflex measures, auditory evoked potentials, measurement of otoacoustic emissions.	Same as above.
Hearing aid assessment	Audiologists	To determine whether a patient is a candidate for amplification. Recommendation for hearing aid fitting/orientation, assistive listening system/device selection, product dispensing, sensory aids assessment, or aural rehabilitation assessment.	Frequency-specific measures of functional gain, work recognition. Real ear measurements. Electroacoustic evaluation of hearing aids, determination of ear mold characteristics and hearing aid configuration, administration of communication inventories or questionnaires, recommendation of hearing aids, referral for medical evaluation.	Same as above.
Aural rehabilitation assessment	Audiologists and SLPs	Evaluate and describe the communication skills of individuals with hearing loss. Recommendations for treatment and follow-up.	Assessment includes: evaluation of comprehension and production of language in oral, signed, or written modalities; speech and voice production; perception of speech and nonspeech stimuli in multiple modalities; listening skills; speech and reading; and communication strategies.	Pertinent background information, type of amplification system/sensory aid used, communication modality used, assessment results, prognosis, and specific recommendations.

Table 7.1 ASHA Preferred Practice Patterns (continued)

Type of service	Professionals who perform the procedure	Expected outcomes	Clinical process	Documentation
Speech-language pathology treatment	SLPs	Treatment is conducted to achieve improved, altered, augmented, or compensated speech, therapy, and cognitive communication behaviors and/or processes. Recommendations for reassessment or follow-up.	Short- and long-term functional goals and specific objectives are determined from assessment and represent the framework for treatment.	Pertinent background information, treatment goals, results, prognosis and specific recommendations.
Swallowing function treatment	SLPs	To improve the patient's oral-motor function, neuromuscular function and control, and coordination of respiratory function with swallowing activities for safe and efficient feeding and swallowing.	Treatment strategies include: no oral presentation of food or liquid, oral presentation of food or liquid, strategies that alter behavior (e.g., posture rate, learned airway protection measures, method of intake) modification of swallowing activity in coordination with respiratory or alteration of bolus characteristics. Short- and long-term functional swallow goals are determined from assessment and represent framework for treatment.	Same as above.
AAC system fitting/ orientation	SLPs	Use of individual AAC systems and components.	Fitting and orientation of the device. Counseling and training in system operation and maintenance.	Contains information about training provided to patient.

| Aural rehabilitation | Audiologists and SLPs | Facilitation of receptive and expressive communication of individuals with a hearing loss. | Treatment that focuses on comprehension and production of language in oral, signed, or written modalities; speech and voice production; auditory training; speech reading. Short- and long-term functional communication goals and specific objectives are determined from assessment and represent the framework of treatment. | Same as above. |
| Hearing aid fitting/ orientation | Audiologists | To achieve maximum understanding of and performance with the amplification system. Recommendation for aural rehabilitation assessment or treatment. | Fitting/orientation includes: a real-ear measurement, electroacoustic evaluation of hearing aids, earmold impression and modification, instrument dispensing, evaluation of hearing aid use with other listening devices. | Same as above. |

Note: SLP = speech-language pathologist.

Source: American Speech-Language-Hearing Association, Preferred practice patterns, *Asha*, 35(Suppl. 11):5–88, 1993.

or weekly progress notes, and documentation of functional improvement per goal per month. Physician recertification does not guarantee reimbursement. Some payor sources review claims retrospectively, which can cause a claim to be denied months after therapy has been discontinued. The burden of responsibility is on the practicing therapist to be familiar with qualifying reimbursement issues.

A determination is made concerning the need for skilled rehabilitation to restore function or a program designed to maintain function. A qualified licensed and certified professional is needed to initiate and carry out a skilled treatment program. The treatment plan must be within acceptable standards of the profession. Maximum reimbursement can be obtained for a recent (within 6 months) onset of a disorder. Justification of the patient's restorative rehabilitation potential with the expectation of reasonable and predictable progress is the criterion for continued treatment. A maintenance program can be designed by a skilled professional, followed by the training of the caregiver to conduct the program. Designing a program for maintenance therapy for progressive degenerative diseases or a decline in function is reimbursable, but on a more limited basis. The caregiver, not the skilled professional, is then expected to carry out the maintenance program without reimbursement from the third-party payor.

References

1. American Speech-Language-Hearing Association, The delivery of speech-language pathology and audiology services in home care, *Asha*, 30(3):77–79, 1988.
2. American Speech-Language-Hearing Association, Scope of practice, speech-language pathology and audiology, *Asha*, 32(Suppl. 2):1–2, 1990.
3. American Speech-Language-Hearing Association, The role of speech-language pathologists in service delivery to infants, toddlers, and their families, *Asha*, 32(Suppl. 2):4, 1990.
4. American Speech-Language-Hearing Association, Knowledge and skills needed by speech-language pathologists providing services to dysphagic patients/clients, *Asha*, 32(Suppl. 2):7–12, 1990.
5. American Speech-Language-Hearing Association, Guidelines for the delivery of speech-language pathology and audiology services in home care, *Asha*, 33(Suppl. 5):29–34, 1991.
6. American Speech-Language-Hearing Association, Definitions of communication disorders and variations, *Asha*, 35(Suppl. 10):40–41, 1993.
7. American Speech-Language-Hearing Association, Preferred practice patterns, *Asha*, 35(Suppl. 11):5–88, 1993.
8. Bello, J., Prevalence of Communication Disorders in the United States, American Speech-Language Hearing Association, Research Division, March 1994, pp. 1–12.

An Overview of Hospice Home Care

8

Barbara Head, R.N., C.R.N.H., A.C.S.W.

Hospice Philosophy

While affirming life, the hospice philosophy recognizes dying as a normal process and death as a natural part of the life cycle. Hospice care neither hastens nor postpones death. Quality of life rather than length of life is the focus of hospice care.

Hospice programs exist in the hope and belief that through supportive, palliative care and the provision of a caring community sensitive to their needs, terminally ill patients and their families may be free to attain an alert, pain-free life and a degree of emotional, mental, and spiritual preparation for death that is satisfactory to them.

History of the Hospice Movement

The word "hospice" comes from the Latin root "hospes," from which our words "hospital," "hospitality," "hostel," and both "host" and "guest" are derived. In medieval times, a hospice was a place of shelter and refuge for persons on a difficult journey—the outward journey undertaken as pilgrims sought to visit holy places or the inward journey faced by widows, orphans, lepers, and dying individuals.

The existence of hospices can be traced from that time until now. However, the modern hospice movement is generally considered to have begun in England in the 1960s with the establishment of St. Christopher's Hospice by Dame Cicely Saunders.

Educated at Oxford, Dame Saunders became a nurse, then a medical social worker, and finally, a physician. Deeply impressed by the death of a 40-year-old friend, she was moved into providing leadership for development of hospice care as it is now known. She combined the application of sound medical management utilizing the most modern medical treatment available with the goal of the medieval hospice, to provide spiritually inspired, loving care. Emphasis of this new approach was placed on caring for the patient, not the disease.

Dame Saunders toured the United States in the 1960s and inspired many through her contacts and lectures. This, plus the works of Elizabeth Kübler-Ross and others involved in terminal care, began to highlight this country's lack of satisfactory care for terminally ill persons and their families. These early pioneers shared the following ideas:

- Dying, the final stage of human existence, is normal and natural but is not an easy or simple process. It is a unique and important time in each person's life and can be an opportunity for growth and insight.
- Caring for dying persons and their families requires special skills and a different pace from other health care models. Primary emphasis should be placed upon physical comfort and emotional support.
- Dying patients should be informed about their medical condition and available treatment alternatives. The patient and family should have control over the decisions made regarding care.
- The medical system as it existed at that time did not deal with the unique needs of the dying.

Early leaders of the movement included concerned professionals, volunteers, family members, and friends of terminally ill patients who were allowed to die without appropriate care (including pain relief). Many gave countless hours of their time and boundless energy and enthusiasm to the cause.

Hospice care in the United States developed as a program or philosophy of care rather than a distinct physical setting, and it continues to emphasize caring for patients in their own residence while allowing short-term inpatient care for acute medical needs. The first hospice in the United States began serving patients in 1974 in New Haven, Connecticut; it was initially a home care and bereavement program but later (1979) an inpatient facility was opened. Subsequently, diverse hospice organizations developed in communities across the country; the need, available leadership, and resources for health care, social service, and spiritual care in each community shaped the design of each program.

Initially, hospice programs struggled financially to put together the resources necessary to provide adequate care for patients and families. Volunteer efforts and charitable contributions were the major resources available. Indeed, volunteers have always been the center of the hospice movement and continue to be a core component of hospice services. With the creation of the Medicare hospice benefit in 1983, hospice programs were able to realize some degree of financial stability. Many private and public health insurance providers now reimburse for hospice care. Donations and memorials, grants, support from religious organizations, and the United Way continue to enable hospices to serve all patients regardless of their ability to pay.

The hospice movement in the United States has realized significant advances in the research and knowledge base of palliative care as well as educating the public on the needs and special care of the terminally ill and their families. The National Hospice Organization, a nonprofit membership organization, based in Arlington, Virginia, has provided leadership and support to the various individual hospice programs in the United States which number over 2000 and now serve over 200,000 terminally ill patients and their families annually. Nationwide, 48 states have hospice organizations and over 3400 professionals work to provide hospice services.

Types of Hospice Programs

Hospices in the United States operate with a variety of affiliations and administrative models, depending upon the needs and resources of the communities in which they developed. Hospice programs may be hospital-owned and -administered, independently owned, community-based, or part of community-based comprehensive home health agencies. A smaller percentage are owned by skilled nursing or extended care facilities, county health departments, or psychiatric institutions. Inpatient care may be provided through contracts with acute or long-term care facilities and/or specialized units owned or managed by the hospice. There are a number of hospices which have developed their own independently managed "freestanding" inpatient hospice facilities. Of all hospices, 90% are not-for-profit organizations, while the rest are for-profit or government affiliated.

All hospices function to implement the hospice philosophy of care, and this goal can be realized within highly varied structures. Hospices certified by Medicare must meet all the specific conditions and standards of the Medicare hospice benefit and offer all required services. Due to a stronger financial base and higher census, larger hospice programs may be able to offer a wider menu of services to meet specialized patient needs, but even the smallest program will provide core hospice services.

Unique Features of Hospice Care

A number of key features differentiate hospice care from other health care programs and approaches:

* Hospice care is built upon the principles of palliative care rather than curative medicine. The focus is on aggressive symptom management to ensure patient comfort when efforts toward cure are futile or impossible.
* The patient, not the disease, is the focus of care.
* The patient and the entire family are considered to be the unit of care.
* An interdisciplinary team directs and provides care to each patient/family unit. Physical, psychosocial, emotional, and spiritual issues are all considered in developing the hospice plan of care.
* Volunteers are an essential component of each hospice organization and are utilized across all departments (administrative, development, patient care, bereavement services). Volunteers give more than 5 million hours annually to hospice programs across the nation. The Medicare hospice benefit requires each certified hospice program to annually match total staff hours in patient care with 5% volunteer hours.
* Care and support are readily available to the patient and family 24 hours a day, 7 days a week.
* Bereavement services are provided to the patient's family for at least one year after the patient's death.
* Hospice services are offered based on need rather than ability to pay.

Accessing Hospice Care

The National Hospice Organization (NHO) has as its goal universal access to hospice care for terminally ill individuals in the United States. With over 2000 programs now in existence, the majority of communities have hospice care as an available health care option for the terminally ill.

Most programs accept referrals from any source—patient, family, physicians and other health care providers, hospital discharge planners, clergy, friends, or neighbors. Once a referral is made, the hospice contacts the patient's doctor to assure that the physician agrees that hospice care is appropriate. Of course, the consent of the patient and family to hospice care is also essential prior to admission. Relevant demographic data are collected on the patient and a time for an admission visit is scheduled. Most hospices try to admit patients within 24 hours of referral unless the patient or family requests a later appointment.

In the past, many hospice programs required the patient to have a primary caregiver in the home at all times. More recently, hospices have allowed admission of patients who live alone as long as provisions are made to care for that patient as his or her condition deteriorates (i.e., nursing home placement, hired caregivers, or availability of friends or family to provide care at that time).

Although approximately 85% of those served by hospices are diagnosed as having some type of cancer, patients diagnosed with other end-stage diseases are also appropriate. Examples of such diagnoses include cardiovascular disease, pulmonary disease, cerebrovascular accident, Alzheimer's, amyotrophic lateral sclerosis, Parkinson's, multiple sclerosis, acquired immune deficiency syndrome (AIDS), renal disease, liver disease, and chronic debilitated state. In these cases, there needs to be documentable clinical progression of the disease, notable physical decline, progressive symptoms despite maximal medical therapy, and clinical evidence that the patient is in the end stage of the disease progress.

Age is not a factor in admission as long as other criteria are met. Hospices admit children, and many larger hospices have specialized pediatric teams. As might be expected, two-thirds of hospice patients are over 65 years of age, while only about 1% are under age 18.

The guiding principle in determining who should have access to hospice care is clearly stated in the NHO standards:

> Hospice offers palliative care to all terminally ill people and their families regardless of age, gender, nationality, race, creed, sexual orientation, disability, diagnosis, availability of a primary caregiver, or ability to pay.[5]

Upon admission, the patient and family begin receiving hospice services. Members of the interdisciplinary team begin their assessments and planning for care. The patient and family immediately have support available to them through their assigned team and on-call services.

Patient care extends through the patient's death. Hospice staff are available to be with the family at the time of death to assist with funeral arrangements and offer supportive care to grieving family members. Subsequent to death, hospice continues with bereavement care services for the family.

The scope of services available from most hospice programs is outlined in the next section.

Scope of Patient/Family Services

Nursing:
- Case management
- Nursing assessment
- Skilled care visits (including infusion therapy, wound care, ostomy care, patient/family teaching, etc.)

- Coordination with patient/family/physicians and other medical personnel
- Education of patient/caregivers
- Symptom control
- Emotional support
- Interdisciplinary team participation
- Supervision of home health aides
- Bereavement follow-up

Social Work:

- Psychosocial assessment
- Individual/family counseling
- Overview/assessment of family resources
- Emotional support
- Referral to community agencies
- Assistance with legal, financial issues
- Interdisciplinary team participation
- Client groups
- Bereavement follow-up

Pastoral Care:

- Spiritual assessment when indicated by the plan of care
- Spiritual support
- Coordination with patient/family denominational affiliations or assistance in establishing such support
- Funeral planning and participation
- Client groups
- Bereavement follow-up

Home Health Aides:

- Personal care: bath, shampoo, oral care
- Light housekeeping: changing bed linens, straightening immediate area around patient's bedside

Patient/Bereavement Care Volunteer:

- Respite
- Companionship
- Emotional support
- Assistance with personal care
- Hairdressing services
- Transportation/errands
- Recreational outings
- Interdisciplinary team participation
- Grief education

- Facilitation of expression of grief
- Assistance with gaining new skills during bereavement

Bereavement:
- Bereavement assessment/evaluation
- Grief counseling
- Emotional support
- Educational programs
- Support groups
- Ongoing correspondence/newsletters
- Memorial services
- Library resources
- Referral to community agencies

The Hospice Interdisciplinary Team

True interdisciplinary teamwork is the most essential element of hospice care. An interdisciplinary team of professionals and volunteers is the key to providing care which meets the varied and complex needs of the patient and family facing terminal illness. Communication and coordination of efforts are essential to the functioning of this team. Each team member brings unique skills and abilities to the problem-solving process of care planning and implementation.

Core services (those considered essential to each and every patient's care) include nursing, medical social services, physician services, and counseling services. The hospice program must directly provide these services through its own staff or volunteers who have received orientation, training, and education in terminal care. Bereavement services are also a required component of hospice care and are extended to the family for at least one year after the patient's death.

Most hospices also provide home health aide services through their own or contract staff. Various other therapies may be provided depending upon the patient's plan of care (i.e., physical, occupational, speech, or dietary therapy) and the therapists involved become members of that patient's team.

Volunteers are often assigned to specific patients and are an integral part of the interdisciplinary team. The hospice provides extensive training prior to any assignments to prepare the volunteer for involvement with patients and their families.

This interdisciplinary team meets regularly to develop and update care plans for the patients and families assigned to that team. The patient and family are also involved in care plan development, are viewed as team members, and are invited to attend team meetings.

In summary, the interdisciplinary team is fundamental to hospice care and its purposes are to:

- Provide a structure for interdisciplinary care planning, goal setting, and evaluation, which encourages patient/family participation
- Provide an interdisciplinary approach to case management issues and legal/regulatory requirements
- Provide a setting for problem solving and professional exchange which will enhance patient/family care with respect for confidentiality
- Provide a setting for individual and team self-reflection, accountability, mutual support, challenge, and nurture for the uniquely personal dimensions of hospice care[1]

The next section examines the roles of the individual team members.

The Hospice Physician

Each patient's medical care is coordinated by two physicians in most hospice programs: the hospice medical director and the attending or primary physician.

The **attending physician** orders hospice care for the patient and continues to follow the patient throughout the course of care. This physician is invited to attend team meetings, reviews and signs the initial plan of care, receives regular feedback and updates on the care plan, orders new treatments and/or medications, and has responsibility for continued medical care of that patient.

The **hospice medical director** oversees the medical aspects of the care of *all* patients served by the hospice. He or she must be an expert in symptom management and pain control in order to effectively direct the palliative, supportive medical care plans for the patients of the hospice. Often the medical director is called upon to make decisions or recommendations regarding the appropriateness of certain treatments, medications, or procedures. According to the standards of the NHO, the duties of the medical director include:

- Consulting with attending physicians regarding pain and symptom control
- Reviewing patient eligibility for hospice services
- Acting as a medical resource for the interdisciplinary team
- Acting as a liaison to physicians in the community
- Establishing guidelines and parameters for acceptable medical research[2]

In cases where patients do not have attending physicians, or in cases where the attending physician chooses to transfer the patient to the hospice medical director, the medical director may also serve as a patient's attending physician.

Some hospice programs also utilize their medical directors to make home visits to patients, provide on-call consultation as needed, make clinical rounds on the hospice patients receiving inpatient care, and help to market hospice services to community physicians.

The Hospice Nurse

An expert in palliative care, symptom management, and pain control, the hospice nurse provides direct patient care as well as education for patients and families regarding the disease process and terminal care. The nurse teaches the skills necessary to care for the patient in the home environment, thus enabling the family to manage the illness and dying process and empowering them to maximize the quality of life and death during the patient's final days. As a patient advocate, the nurse works with the attending physician, providers of inpatient care, and other systems to ensure that the patient's autonomy and choices are respected and that the hospice plan of care is realized.

The requirements of the Medicare hospice benefit state that the nurse will coordinate the interdisciplinary care plan. The hospice nurse must therefore be an effective communicator with patients and families as well as a liaison with other team members, including the attending physician with whom the nurse must initiate direct communication and offer suggestions for modifications in the plan of care. As a communicator, the nurse must be able to honestly address the issues surrounding death by inviting discussions of the truth and facilitating decision making.

The average caseload for a hospice nurse ranges from 8 to 12 patient/family units, with visits averaging between 18 and 25 per week.[3] The frequency of visits to each patient is determined by patient need and condition and may vary from once weekly to daily as the patient declines. The nurse provides hands-on patient care but also teaches the family to assume the responsibilities of daily care, including administration of medications and treatments, infusion therapy, dressing changes, and routine care of colostomies, tracheostomies, etc. The nurse supervises and coordinates home health aide services for the patient.

The Hospice Social Worker

Beginning with the psychosocial assessment of each patient, the social worker assumes responsibility for assisting the interdisciplinary team and the patient/family in addressing environmental, social, and financial needs and the stresses unique to terminal illness. The NHO's Standards of a Hospice Program of Care describes the social worker's role as providing "counseling and linkage to community services for the patient/family to assist them in:

- developing optimal coping strategies,
- accessing community resources,
- preparing for death, and
- making most effective use of the health-care system"[4]

The social worker must therefore be knowledgeable and skilled in finding formal and informal community resources; assisting with financial, legal, and insurance matters; providing supportive counseling; intervening in time of crisis; addressing the "unfinished business" of the patient (including financial concerns, wills, funeral plans, and advance directives, as well as unresolved emotional or familial issues and relationships); and mobilizing the coping skills of the patient and family. Like the hospice nurse, the hospice social worker must be comfortable in confronting illness and death, skilled in communication, capable of independent autonomous practice as well as teamwork, and creative in combining resources to meet the unique needs of each patient and family. The social worker leads the team in a nonjudgmental, sensitive response to the psychosocial needs of patients and their families.

The Hospice Chaplain

Spiritual care is a key component of hospice philosophy, and each hospice program assesses and attempts to address the spiritual needs of the patient/family unit. Most often this is accomplished by the hospice chaplain or spiritual care coordinator, who may be a volunteer or a paid staff member. In smaller hospices with fewer resources, other team members may be designated to assess the spiritual needs of the patient/family and mobilize existing community resources outside the hospice to meet those needs.

The hospice chaplain may provide direct spiritual counseling and religious services or rituals (i.e., prayer, sacraments, funeral services) consistent with the patient/family's beliefs. The chaplain's approach is nonsectarian, nondenominational, and nonthreatening. In cases where the patient and family are connected to a community of faith, the chaplain ensures that their spiritual needs are being met and coordinates support and involvement by that group.

In many instances, there may be a connection to a church or faith, but the patient or family has unmet needs or is more comfortable exploring spiritual issues with a trained hospice chaplain who is well versed in the concerns of the terminally ill. In all cases, patients and families are helped to define their spiritual needs and spiritual care is offered accordingly.

The hospice chaplain should have theological and clinical education and experience in pastoral care and must be able to respond to persons from various religious backgrounds and belief systems. Using a nonjudgmental approach, the chaplain addresses the questions and fears of dying people and their families while providing for open dialogue and spiritual companionship. Exploration of life's meaning and value and review of the patient's life story are also frequent components of the chaplain's interaction with the patient and family.

The Hospice Volunteer

Often a hospice volunteer is assigned to a particular patient/family unit and this volunteer becomes a member of the patient's interdisciplinary team. Services that a volunteer might provide include companionship and emotional support, short-term respite care to enable family members to have time away from the patient, running errands or picking up supplies, reading or writing letters for the patient, transporting patient or family to an appointment, helping with recreational outings, and providing special services related to the individual interests of the patient and his or her family (i.e., hobbies, music). Volunteers also work with family members in bereavement by providing grief education, allowing for healthy expressions of their grief and enabling them to develop new skills and relationships.

Often referred to as "the heart of hospice," volunteers freely donate their time to meet the needs of the terminally ill, and this commitment makes a clear statement to patients and families about the concern and dedication they bring to the relationships they build. The hospice volunteer often comes to know the patient and family on a very personal and meaningful level. As a result of this close bonding, the volunteer can offer significant insights to the interdisciplinary team.

The Hospice Home Health Aide

The hospice home health aide provides personal care to patients experiencing functional limitations as a result of illness. Supervised by the nurse, the aide may visit the patient from one to several times weekly, providing assistance with the activities of daily living such as bathing, hair care, shaving, skin care, changing bed linens, and helping to maintain a clean and safe environment. In some cases, the home health aide may do some light housekeeping, set up meals, or even run errands. As a member of the interdisciplinary team, the home health aide contributes a valued service which enables families to care for the patient at home. As one who works very closely with the patient on a regular basis, the home health aide offers observations and knowledge of the patient's needs that might otherwise be overlooked. Like other members of the team, the aide must be comfortable communicating with terminally ill patients and must have training and experience in providing comfort measures which meet the special needs of patients experiencing end-stage disease processes.

Other Team Members

If indicated by the hospice plan of care, various therapists may also be included as part of the interdisciplinary team. Some hospices are fortunate enough to have the funds to employ their own music or art therapists to meet the expressive needs of patients and their families. The use of art therapy is especially meaningful in working with children facing their own death or the loss of a loved one.

Physical, speech, and occupational therapy as well as dietary counseling may be included in the plan of care when specific symptoms interfere with quality of life. The hospice most often contracts with individuals or agencies to provide these specific services on an as-needed basis for patients. The hospice provides orientation and in-service education to contract personnel to ensure that they are knowledgeable about hospice philosophy and care.

The Hospice Patient and Family

A unique feature of hospice care is the emphasis on the patient and family as the unit of care; neither is assessed or treated in isolation from the other. The patient and family are integral in care planning and implementation of that plan of care. Hospice care focuses on empowering the patient/family unit to deal with the physical, psychosocial, and spiritual tasks necessary to facilitate quality of life during the terminal stage.

Generally, the requirements for hospice enrollment are as follows:

- The patient has been diagnosed with a terminal illness.
- The patient is seeking palliative care rather than treatment aimed at cure.
- The patient is in the advanced stages of terminal illness with a life expectancy of months rather than years. (Medicare requires that the referring physician estimate the patient's life expectancy to be 6 months or less.)
- The patient and family know the expected outcome of the disease.
- The physician, patient, and family agree to hospice services and consent to it in writing.
- Hospice care can be provided in a safe environment.

In hospice care, the family includes not only those who are legally related but also those united by the bonds of affection, caring, loyalty, and interdependence. The family is that group with which the patient shares a past and an emotional connectedness. Family members may or may not live together. Regardless of their location, the hospice team will make every effort to involve the patient's significant others in care planning and implementation.

While the majority of patients continue to reside in their homes, patients living in long-term nursing facilities are eligible for the same hospice services as those residing in their own homes. In such cases, the nursing home is viewed as the patient's residence and the nursing home staff as caregivers. The hospice interdisciplinary team assumes responsibility for medical management and implementation of a hospice plan of care.

Most patients enroll in a hospice program during the last 3 months of life (the current average length of stay being 64 days), but hospice programs would prefer earlier referrals to allow sufficient time for adequate palliation of symptoms and preparation for death (see Figure 8.1).

Timeline Phases of Terminal Care

All too often, referrals are made to a hospice at the very end of a terminal illness and the hospice team is unable to address all of the needs of the terminally ill and their families. In fact, the number one response from patients and families in a recent survey was "why didn't we know about hospice sooner?"

The timeline shown in Figure 8.1 illustrates progressive changes that commonly occur in the physical and psychosocial conditions of the patient over a 6-month period. It also describes how each member of the hospice team intervenes to provide comfort and support during the terminal phase and beyond death for family and loved ones. The earlier the hospice team intervenes, the more satisfaction is expressed by patients and families—time allows closure and resolution of many issues.

The timeline can assist physicians and other referring professionals in assessing and identifying patients' needs earlier so that patients and families have access to the full array of hospice services.

The Hospice Plan of Care

Following individual assessments of the patient and family, the interdisciplinary team members combine their knowledge, skills, and insights in the development of a coordinated plan of care with the ultimate goal of addressing the diverse needs and desires of that particular patient/family unit.

As stated previously, the medical component of the care plan will include care which is considered palliative in its focus. Each individual hospice program must decide what treatments can be included. Most programs allow for radiation and chemotherapy directed toward palliative symptom control, blood transfusions if they promote a better quality of life for the patient, and both high-tech

PROGRESSIVE CHANGES IN THE TERMINAL PHASE

| Progressive changes in physical and psychosocial condition vary with each patient | Generally patient is ambulatory, coherent, some side effects from curative measures/meds, initial stages of grief, anger, denial | Some weight loss, weakness, symptoms manifested, showing signs of stress, growing acceptance of terminal state of fear, depression | Continuing weight loss, decreasing appetite, physical manifestations, symptoms more pronounced. Grief work, planning, resolving |

HOSPICE PLAN OF CARE

HOSPICE TEAM	MONTH 6	MONTH 5	MONTH 4
Medical director (in collaboration with attending physician)	Initial examination of patient, certification for hospice care, develop plan of care, orders	Monitor/assess plan of care, IDT (Interdisciplinary Team) meeting, orders, evaluate symptoms, manage pain	Monitor/assess plan of care, IDT meeting, orders, evaluate symptoms, manage pain
RN case manager	Assessment for hospice conference w/family, confer w/physician, develop plan of care, order medications, order durable medical equipment, train/ instruct primary caregivers	Follow plan of care and direct team members. Provide direct care, report observations, establish rapport with patient and family	Monitor ongoing implementation of approved plan of care. Increased need for symptom management, pain control. Evaluate psychosocial needs of family/patient with other team members
Home health aides	Start personal care program, instruct primary caregiver	Establish supportive, loving, trusting relationship, provide personal care services as per plan of care	Assist w/personal care needs and identify and report special needs to Case Manager
Social services	Assess patient/family psychosocial/bereavement needs to develop plan of care. Establish trusting relationships with patient/ family	Monitor and implement approved plan of care— determine need for referral to other community resources. Identify dysfunctional patient/family problems, make recommendations	Continued monitoring of plan of care—ongoing assessment of patient/ family abilities to cope with terminal diagnosis and its impact on daily living
Chaplain	Spiritual assessment, confer with other team members for development of plan of care	Implement plan of care conference with patient/ family who desire spiritual support. Assess other needs requiring psychosocial intervention	Implement plan of care as appropriate, contact spiritual support person of denomination of patient/ family choice
Volunteers	Conference w/hospice team for direction, learn interest of patient, initial visitations	Establish supportive trusting relationship via ongoing visits and contact	Assist with letter writing, telephoning, reading, music, provide emotional support to patient and family—respite for family

Figure 8.1   Timeline phases of terminal care. Note: All care is coordinated and integrated with staff of skilled nursing facility if patient becomes resident of a skilled nursing facility anytime during this period. (Reprinted with permission from Community Hospice Care, Inc., Anaheim Hills, CA).

PROGRESSIVE CHANGES IN THE TERMINAL PHASE

Physical deterioration apparent, symptom- atology and pain increase, beginning of withdrawal, acceptance of terminal disease	Progressive physical deterioration, symptoms increase, pain management primary, may be bedridden, increasing withdrawal, resolution and closure	End-stage pronounced withdrawal, requires total care, intensive management of symptoms and pain, no appetite

HOSPICE PLAN OF CARE

MONTH 3	MONTH 2	FINAL MONTH	AFTER DEATH
Reassess for new bene- fit period, monitor/assess plan of care, IDT meet- ing, orders, evaluate symptoms, manage pain	Monitor/assess plan of care, IDT meeting, orders, evaluate symptoms, manage pain	Monitor/assess plan of care, IDT meeting, increased need for medication changes to manage symptoms and control pain, support family	May have further communication with family
Monitor ongoing imple- mentation of approved plan of care. Increasing need for order changes to manage symptoms and control pain. Con- tinued coordination— patient/family team	Monitor more closely, in- crease visits as needed, implementation of approved plan of care. Daily review of symptom management, pain control. Family support increased, coordination of psychosocial plan of care	Daily monitoring of end- state process, side effects of meds, symptoms mani- fested and pain management. Coordinate preparation for death with other team mem- bers, increasing support to both patient and family	Call and/or visit family, assess special bereave- ment needs, may attend funeral, complete dis- charge charting
Continue assistance w/personal care needs and identify special needs to Case Manager	Provide bathing, dressing, and other personal care needs as necessary. Provide comfort measures—report needs to Case Manager	Increase contact with patient and family for direct care, assure all personal care needs are met and provide comfort measures	May attend funeral
Evaluate patient/ family coping abilities & appropriateness of respite care, need for referral to other community resources	Continued monitoring of approved plan of care, assess patient/family for signs of dysfunctional grieving and provide appropriate intervention. Facilitate support systems	Continued monitoring of approved plan of care— assist patient/family in resolution and closure— ensure final arrangements. Facilitate support systems	Call and/or visit family. May attend funeral. Begin be- reavement follow- up, identify dys- functional grieving and initiate appro- priate intervention
Implement plan of care. Encourage family to continue observance and rituals that provide meaning and support to them	Implement plan of care. Provide spiritual support as appropriate to patient/family wishes, assist with final arrangements as requested	Implement plan of care. Provide support to patient/ family and hospice staff in preparing for separation	May visit family, in- struct family about bereavement groups and memorial ser- vice, provide grief/ bereavement support
Arrange for personal preferences of patient—food, visitation, special interests, respite for family	Provide respite periods for family, assist with visitation & personal needs	Provide respite periods for family, provide patient with emotional support	Provide bereavement support to family/sig- nificant others, main- tain regular contact for up to 12 months

and simpler methods of pain management as needed. Treatments often disallowed include dialysis (for end-stage renal disease), ventilator maintenance, and chemotherapy which is directed toward cure of the disease. Hospice services are not appropriate for patients or families who do not agree to a palliative approach.

Palliative care is just as aggressive and active as curative care but has a different goal—that goal being to provide relief from pain and other distressing symptoms while integrating physical, psychological, and spiritual aspects of care to enable the patient to live as actively as possible until death. Adequate pain control may require aggressive titration of medication dosages and use of a variety of pharmacological and nonpharmacological approaches. The efforts of the entire team may be necessary to mitigate or alleviate a symptom such as pain. For instance, the nurse may be securing physician's orders for titration of medication for pain relief while the social worker is teaching visual imagery or relaxation techniques and the chaplain is exploring with the patient the meaning of suffering.

The psychosocial and spiritual components of the plan of care are developed according to the coping abilities of the patient and family, their "unfinished" business, available resources for dealing with financial and caregiving demands, and their desires as they approach the patient's death.

The plan of care constantly evolves during the patient's course of care by the hospice and subsequent bereavement care for the family. The interdisciplinary team meets regularly to review the plan of care and to revise the strategy for obtaining desired treatment goals according to changes in the patient's condition and needs of the patient/family unit.

The hospice is responsible for ensuring continuity in the plan of care regardless of the patient's setting. This requires communication and coordination with the staffs of inpatient and skilled nursing facilities when patients are placed in residential care, as well as supervision and coordination when staffs of other agencies go into patients' homes to provide continuous care for a few days or respite caregiving over a period of time.

Bereavement Care Services

Every hospice has a planned program of support which is offered to surviving families for 12 or more months following the patient's death. Members of the patient's interdisciplinary team begin bereavement care with a visit to the family shortly after the patient's death. Subsequently, bereavement care staff and/or volunteers embark on a plan of regular contact with survivors to offer them opportunities for sharing and remembering, experiencing the grief process with support and encouragement, and completing the tasks of bereavement.

Bereavement care counselors or volunteers may provide phone contact, supportive counseling, and educational programs and may facilitate support or self-help groups. Newsletters and correspondence may be sent to the bereaved at defined intervals. Social events, as well as task-oriented seminars and programs on topics such as taxes, car maintenance, and social security, may be offered to assist the bereaved in assuming new roles and relationships. Family members experiencing complicated grief and in need of intensive counseling may be referred to other community resources.

Many hospices offer memorial services and invite staff and patient families to join together in a ritual of sharing and remembrance. This may be done annually at a community church or at the hospice office. Some hospices also have a lending library of books and resources relating to grief and bereavement issues from which family members can borrow.

Hospice bereavement services address the physical, emotional, social, and spiritual changes which follow the death of a loved one, with the goal of normalizing this process and helping the bereaved to cope effectively and adapt to the changes brought on by the loss. Some hospices make their bereavement care programs available to the wider community rather than limiting services to survivors of patients served by the program.

Reimbursement Sources and Hospice Costs

Three-quarters of all hospice revenues come from the coverage provided by the Medicare hospice benefit established in 1982 and state Medicaid programs modeled after that benefit (37 states now provide such coverage). The hospice program receives a per diem payment for Medicare/Medicaid patients electing the benefit and, in turn, provides the following:

- Professional services of the hospice interdisciplinary team, which includes visits by registered nurse, social worker, pastoral care coordinator, trained volunteers, home health aide, and bereavement staff or volunteers
- Prescriptions and over-the-counter medications for pain and symptom management related to the terminal illness
- Medical equipment and supplies
- Outpatient and emergency room services
- Lab work
- Consulting physician services
- Ambulance to and from a treatment or for a hospital admission
- Short-term inpatient care and respite care

- Ancillary services—physical therapy, speech therapy, occupational therapy, dietary counseling, etc.
- Continuous skilled nursing care during periods of medical crisis

In addition to these government-funded programs, many private insurance plans now cover hospice services. It is estimated that 80% of all employees of medium and large businesses have hospice coverage as an insurance benefit, and 82% of all managed care plans provide for hospice care. Hospices may also collect co-payments and other charges from patients and families as appropriate.

While health insurance coverage programs now pay for a large part of hospice costs, such payments rarely cover the entire expense of operating such an extensive program of care. Hospices often turn to fund raising, memorial contributions, community support, and grant resources for the revenue required to fully serve those needing services. Gifts to hospice programs enable them to continue to provide for patients without insurance benefits who are unable to pay.

Recent studies have found hospice to be a less costly approach to care of the terminally ill. The Hospice Benefit Program evaluation found that in 1988 Medicare was saving $1.26 for every dollar spent on hospice care. A more recent analysis (1991–1992) of the cost savings of the Medicare hospice benefit found that for every dollar Medicare spent on hospice patients, it saved $1.52 in Medical Part A and B expenditures.[7] Most of these savings occurred during the last months of life, when hospice programs were successfully able to substitute home care days for inpatient days. Traditional home care services were less successful in this substitution and were approximately 30% more expensive than hospice care during the last 24 weeks of life. The success of hospice in keeping terminally ill patients at home can be attributed in part to the interdisciplinary framework of hospice care, the 24 hours/7 days per week ready availability of support services, the special training and expertise of hospice staff and volunteers, and the motivation of those who choose hospice to remain in their home environment.

Education and Advocacy in Hospice

Since its beginnings in the early 1970s, the hospice movement in the United States has made great strides in educating the public about the special needs and issues confronting the terminally ill and their families. In addition to providing patient/family care and bereavement services, individual hospice programs spend a great amount of time and resources in education and advocacy efforts geared toward impacting the physical, mental, and spiritual care of all those facing terminal illness.

Through clinical experience and research, the hospice movement has contributed significantly to the development of palliative care protocols and methods of pain control which ensure patient comfort. By addressing the mental and spiritual pain of terminal illness, hospice has contributed to the establishment of a caring, supportive public community and has impacted health care systems nationwide.

As a major movement in health care, hospice has provided public information, become involved in legislative efforts which ensure humane care for the terminally ill, educated health care professionals and the general public, and addressed many ethical concerns related to terminal illness.

With the mission of enhancing quality of life for the terminally ill and their families, hospice programs have had immeasurable influence. From "micro" concerns such as assuring that a patient has a last visit with a favorite pet to "macro" concerns such as educating physicians on effective interventions for the end-stage AIDS patient, hospice is a real and present force in the current health care environment.

References

1. Hospice of Louisville Clinical Department Directors, memo of February 24, 1994.
2. National Hospice Organization, *Standards of a Hospice Program of Care Self-Assessment Tool*, Arlington, Virginia, 1994, p. 29.
3. National Hospice Organization, *Standards and Accreditation Committee, Hospice Services Guidelines and Definitions*, Arlington, Virginia, 1994, p. 3.
4. National Hospice Organization, *Standards of a Hospice Program of Care Self-Assessment Tool*, Arlington, Virginia, 1994, p. 35.
5. National Hospice Organization, *Standards of a Hospice Program of Care Self-Assessment Tool*, Arlington, Virginia, 1994, p. vi.
6. Manard, B. and Perrone, C., *Hospice Care: An Introduction and Review of the Evidence*, National Hospice Organization, Arlington, Virginia, 1994, p. ii.
7. National Hospice Organization, *An Analysis of the Cost Savings of the Medicare Hospice Benefit*, Press release, Arlington, Virginia, April 26, 1995.

General References

Amenta, Madalon O'Rawe and Bohnet, N. L., *Nursing Care of the Terminally Ill*, Little, Brown, Boston, 1986.

Beresford, L., *The Hospice Handbook*, Little, Brown, Boston, 1993.

Hospice of Louisville, *Careprovider's Manual*, Louisville, Kentucky, 1991.

Hospice of Louisville. *Caring for the Hospice Patient,* Louisville, Kentucky, 1993.

Manard, B. and Perrone, C., *Hospice Care: An Introduction and Review of the Evidence*, National Hospice Organization, Arlington, Virginia, 1994.

National Hospice Organization Task Force on Access to Hospice Care by Minorities, *Caring for Our Own with Respect, Dignity and Love the Hospice Way*, Arlington, Virginia, 1992.

National Hospice Organization, *Hospice Services Guidelines and Definitions*, Arlington, Virginia, 1994.

National Hospice Organization, *Standards of a Hospice Program of Care Self-Assessment Tool*, Arlington, Virginia, 1994.

National Hospice Organization, *The Basics of Hospice*, Arlington, Virginia, 1994.

Stoddard, S., *The Hospice Movement: A Better Way of Caring for the Dying*, Vintage Books, New York, 1978.

The Role of the Social Worker in Home Care

9

Bibhuti K. Sar, Ph.D. and Iris Phillips, M.S.S.W.

Introduction

Social workers have been involved in the delivery of home care—homemaker and home health services to meet the medical, physical, social, and emotional needs of persons homebound due to illness and injury—since the turn of this century. This tradition was certainly evident in the practice of "friendly visiting" during the early part of this century when members of the Charity Organization Movement visited the poor in order to "cure" them of their social ills and bring qualitative improvement to their lives. As the practice of home care took root, social workers' involvement first evolved as either directly developing, providing, or arranging for the delivery of *homemaker services*. For instance, in 1923, the first organized homemaker service was established by the Jewish Welfare Society in Philadelphia[1] to prevent unnecessary out-of-home placement of children. Women were placed to serve as housekeepers and provide child care in homes where the natural mother had taken ill.[1,2] During the Great Depression, health and welfare agencies used homemakers trained by the Housekeeper Aide Project, a federal program of the Works Progress Administration, to assist families in caring for their children, elderly family members, and chronically ill family members.[1,2] Such placement of homemakers was thought to allow welfare agencies and their caseworkers to more accurately diagnose the needs and problems of the client, prevent unnecessary institutional placement of the children, and ensure that the basic needs of the family, such as food and clothing, were provided.[3]

The involvement of social workers in the delivery of *home health services* came later in this century, even though social workers had been involved in delivery of health care services since 1905. At that time, Dr. Richard Cabot, a prominent physician and an early advocate of addressing social and environmental conditions contributing to illness and recovery, introduced the idea of hiring a social worker to assess the social and environmental factors influencing the delivery of health care at the outpatient medical clinic at Massachusetts General Hospital. However, social workers later came to be formally considered part of the home health care delivery system when Montefore Hospital in New York City offered medical, nursing, and social services to the chronically ill in their homes in 1947.[4,5] This was a late entrance for social workers as compared to physicians and nurses who had an established role in providing home care as early as the late 1700s. For example, in 1796 the Boston Dispensary created and administered the first hospital-based home care program through volunteers or trained doctors.[5] In 1877, the New York City Mission sent trained graduate nurses to care for the ill in their homes.[5] Soon after that, the Visiting Nurses Association was started in Boston and Philadelphia.[5]

The entrance of social workers into the home care field increased dramatically with the enactment of Medicare and Medicaid legislation in 1965. This legislation allowed primary skilled service providers to request social work services such as psychosocial assessments and short-term counseling to help clients manage their illnesses at home. The present role of social workers in home care continues to be defined in large part by Medicare and Medicaid legislative influence at both the federal and state level. The National Association of Social Workers continues to lobby Congress to legislate social work functions and tasks as reimbursable primary skilled services.

Despite present reimbursement limitations, social workers continue to be employed in home care agencies. It is likely that this trend will continue for several reasons. First, the intent of home care is consistent with the mission of social work. Home health care provides an alternative to hospitalization or skilled nursing facility care for patients with acute or chronic illness. Services provided to the patient in the home consist of education about prevention of disease and illness, promotion of a healthy lifestyle, restoration of health or rehabilitation, minimization of the effects of chronic illness, and maintenance of current levels of functioning. Today, social workers, as part of the home care team, play a major role in the delivery of home care services. By locating and linking resources with client needs, in addition to dealing with the psychosocial impact of illness on clients and their families, home care social workers promote faster recovery, increase the chances for longer stay at home, and strengthen family ties.[6]

Second, home care—based upon the principle of providing services to clients in their homes to maintain or improve their quality of life—has proven to be a more cost-effective alternative to institutional care. The majority of patients show a preference to remain in their homes when it is possible to receive home care. Advances in technology have made it possible for health services to include sophisticated in-home treatments and equipment. Complex services such as renal hemodialysis, ventilators, and infusion therapy are now available in a residential setting, providing an alternative to long hospitalization treatment.[7]

Third, involvement in home care allows social workers to serve vulnerable segments of the population. Current family demographics indicate that more families are living long distances from aging parents. In addition, greater numbers of women, who historically would assume the role of caregiver, are now in the workforce. Also, vaccinations, pasteurization, sanitation, and antibiotics have decreased sudden acute illness and have contributed significantly to an increasing life expectancy. With these changes has come a rise in the number of people suffering from chronic illnesses such as hypertension, diabetes, pulmonary disease, and cardiac disease. These types of illnesses develop over a long period of time and result in irreversible impairments of day-to-day life skills.[7] Clients suffering from chronic, degenerative illness drain family resources, both emotionally and financially. These forces have contributed to the increasing need for home health care services.

Home health care offers a variety of choices to meet a growing need for alternative nursing care. In a 1987 survey by the Agency for Health Care Policy and Research, approximately 2.5 million Americans, or 2.5% of the population, were utilizing some form of home health care. The over-65 age group accounted for approximately one-half of those using home health services. About 40% of those using home health services had at least one functional impairment in activities of daily living.[8] A 1992 study by the National Center for Health Statistics showed that 25% of clients receiving home health benefits had conditions related to the circulatory system. Diagnoses of stroke, chronic obstructive pulmonary disease, heart failure, major joint procedures, hip or femur procedures, and diabetes were frequent among patients discharged to home health services. Research indicates that women over 65 years old remain the primary users of home health care, although an increasing number of those under 65 are utilizing the services.[8]

On the other end of the spectrum, home care social workers have the opportunity to provide services to children with major health problems. By doing so, they make it possible for children to remain at home within the protective environment of the family. These children suffer from such illnesses as AIDS, hemophilia, cystic fibrosis, leukemia, severe kidney disease, and respiratory impairments, which require such services as home and school ventilator support, specialized feeding by intravenous tubes, and intravenous antibiotics over a prolonged period of time.

Therefore, this chapter addresses the role of the social worker in the delivery of home care services. Specifically, the roles of the social worker with the client, the client's family, and the home care team providing home care are examined. Medicare and Medicaid regulations and guidelines which govern eligibility and access to home care services are identified. First, however, the processes of referral, assessment, goal setting, intervention, and termination are outlined below.

The Social Worker's Role in Delivery of Home Care

Referral

The social worker's involvement in the delivery of home care services begins with a referral for social work services. The referral for social work services may come prior to the client's discharge from the hospital or after the client has been at home for some time. The referral may be initiated by a care provider, the client, or a family member. However, for social work services to be reimbursed by private insurance, Medicare, or Medicaid, an order for social work services must be written by the client's primary physician. The actual referral may be carried out by a medical social worker, who arranges for home care during the discharge planning process. A certified home health agency may provide for social work assessment and intervention as part of its package of services offered to home care clients and their families. More often, a client, his or her family, or a member of the home care team such as a physician or nurse may ask for social work assessment and intervention. Usually, this occurs during the treatment of the medical illness when health care providers initially begin to observe psychosocial issues negatively impacting the client's ability to manage, cope with, and adapt to the illness.

Assessment

When social work services are requested, the social worker is charged with conducting an assessment that includes obtaining a psychosocial history of the client, determining the availability of concrete and social support resources, evaluating the adequacy and safety of the home environment for home care, and appraising the client's competence and ability to comply with prescribed treatment. The social worker meets with the family to educate them about the role of the home care social worker, to gather information about the impact of the client's circumstances on the family, and to educate them regarding the services available to the client and family through social work involvement.

The ecological perspective is a useful framework for assessment of the needs of the home care recipient.[9] According to this perspective, all organisms (including human beings) strive toward a "goodness-of-fit" with their environments.[10] The extent to which this "goodness-of-fit" is achieved depends upon the interactions/exchanges of resources between the organism (in this case human beings) and the environment. The purpose of social work practice, then, is to "improve the transactions between people and their environments and to facilitate a better match—that is, a 'goodness-of-fit'—between human needs and environmental resources" (p. 630).[10] The ecological perspective suggests that problems faced by people are best understood as lack of resources in the environment, as problematic exchanges between systems, as coping strategies, or as delays in growth and development rather than problems located within the individual. Problems are viewed as a result of many factors rather than caused by a single factor. Problems experienced by one family member have an impact on all other family members.[11]

Given the limitations on when home care social work services can be requested in order to qualify as a reimbursable service, it is not uncommon for social work assessment to be requested by a skilled service provider only after the client has been receiving home health services for a period of time. Therefore, it is likely that the request for social work assessment may be precipitated by poor psychosocial adjustment to the illness and/or the home care by the client and/or the family. This, in turn, may threaten the progress of recuperation from the illness and/or the stability and continuity of receiving care in the home. Given these circumstances, a home care social worker will need to assess the situation from the perspective of the client, his or her family, and the home care team.

The following questions posed to the client and home care providers may help the home care worker during the assessment process to define and identify the problems experienced by the client receiving home care:[1,6,9–11,17–19]

- What is the client's current level of functioning in the home?
- What are the psychological, social, and emotional factors associated with the client's health problems?
- What has been the client's response to treatment?
- What has been the client's adjustment to care?
- What is the client's style of problem solving?
- What strengths and social supports are available to the client to cope with current circumstances?
- What are the psychological, social, and emotional barriers to the client's optimal functioning and recovery?
- What information does the client need to better cope with his or her present circumstances?

- What other services does the client require?
- What is the family's response to the client's disability?
- What are the barriers to service and how does the lack of service impact the client? The family?

In addition, during the assessment process, the home care social worker will need to ask the following questions of the family:[11–14,22,23]

- What is the family's reaction to the disability given the nature of its onset?
- How well does the family understand the reason for the family member's disability?
- How did the family view the client's capabilities prior to the onset of the illness?
- What meaning does the illness or disability hold for the family? Is this meaning influenced by their culture, ethnicity, or religion?
- What are the family's emotional responses to the illness?
- What was the family structure prior to the illness? How do family members envision it changing given the client's condition?
- What role did the patient have in the family system? Breadwinner? Homemaker? Caretaker?
- What was the relationship with extended family prior to the onset of the illness?
- How well connected was the family to the community prior to the onset of the illness?
- What roles do all the members play? What are their responsibilities?
- What cultural, religious, and language factors influence the family's health care practices, beliefs, and values?
- Who in the family will be providing care for the client?
- Which family member provides basic necessities?
- What are the usual family decision-making processes?

By asking these questions during the assessment process, the worker gathers information on the client's coping style, family interaction around the illness, living arrangements, and network of social support. The worker gathers information from the client on his or her lifestyle prior to the illness, past problem-solving style, attitudes, communication processes which may be blocking adaptation to the current life circumstances, and strengths available to cope and deal with current difficulties.[13]

After gathering information from the client and the family, the worker moves to categorize the information in terms of problems that are primarily due to lack of resources, poor communication and exchanges between the client system (client and family) and providers of home care, poor interactions between the client and family members, or problems with particular strategies used by the client to cope with present circumstances. Having formulated the nature and sources of the problems being experienced by the client, the worker is now in a position to develop a plan of care with specific goals and objectives.

Goal Setting and Plan of Care

After completion of the assessment, the social worker draws up a plan of care in consultation with the client and his or her family. The plan of care is a set of agreed-upon goals and objectives that are determined by the needs of the client and the family in order to maintain the client at home. The plan of care with the client may include objectives regarding supportive counseling to deal with issues such as depression, adjustment to and coping with physical illness, functional limitations, and death and dying issues. The plan of care with the family may include strategies for locating resources. The plan of care with the home care team may include maintaining open communication about the status of the client. This is crucial because the client is on home care and not all members of the home care team see and interact with the client on a daily basis, as may be the case with hospitalized clients.

Intervention

Once the plan of care has been devised, the home care worker proceeds to work toward fulfilling goals and objectives by working with the client, the family, and the home care team. The worker may engage in various functions including providing supportive counseling and linking the client and the family with community resources. In some cases, he or she may act as the case manager by arranging other services such as housekeeping and meal delivery. In other instances, he or she may act as the client care coordinator who oversees the delivery of all services in the plan of care. These tasks are performed in the context of the working relationship, which is characterized by concern, expression of empathy, and acceptance of the client. The home care social worker may play many different roles to carry out the plan of care. According to the literature, the primary roles of the home care social worker are brokering, advocacy, counseling, educating, mediating, and collaborating.[1,6,12,14-18] In taking on these roles, the home care social worker has the primary goal to "improve or maintain the social, emotional, functional, and physical health status of the patient; to enhance the capabilities and coping skills of the family and other caregiver systems; and to ensure that the patient's needs are being met in the home environment" (p. 241).[6] Each role is described briefly in the following sections.

Broker

Compton and Galaway[19] define the role of broker as "making connections between the client and the community to accomplish the objectives specified in the service contract" (p. 598). In taking on this role, the home care social worker informs clients, their families, and the home care team about the availability of resources in the community. These resources include financial (i.e., Supplemental Security Income [SSI], Medicaid, and Medicare), concrete (i.e., equipment), medical (i.e., specialists), and social supports (support group for family members).[6,16,18] Furthermore, he or she shares knowledge about eligibility guidelines and application procedures[14] for these resources. The home social worker not only links the client with the needed resources but assists the client in resolving problems with replacing resources.

Educator

As an educator, the social worker teaches or provides information to the client and the family about the client's medical condition.[14] The worker focuses on aiding the client in developing the necessary skills to use environmental supports necessary to continue to live at home independently.[16] The worker teaches clients and their families the skills necessary to interact with and respond to doctors and other health care personnel[13] to ensure that questions regarding the course of the illness and side effects of medications are addressed.

Social workers may become involved in the home training process of caregivers and may educate other home care staff about the interaction between the home care staff's responses to the patient, the medical management of the illness, and the client's long-term psychosocial adjustment to the illness. Social workers take on the role of educating other home care providers to understand their feelings toward the client and family, as well as offering insight into client and family interactions. Given their understanding of the client's behavior, they may offer suggestions regarding management of the client's psychosocial needs during a medical crisis and/or about interventions which might be successful.[14,20]

Counselor

Emotional difficulties and problems in family relationships become paramount concerns in the counseling process because they can directly undermine adjustment to the illness as well as the success of home care. A variety of psychosocial issues that have bearing on recovery arise in the course of the illness and its subsequent treatment. These include coping with illness and disability, dealing with loss of previous lifestyle, dealing with feelings of abandonment, being a burden to family, fearing death and dying, losing cognitive abilities, changing sexual capacities, grieving, and being depressed.[14] In the role of counselor, the home care social worker helps the client cope with these issues.[14,16]

In working with the client, the social worker first helps the client identify those factors that interfere with adjustment to illness and disability. These may include damaged body image due to disability, loss of function, and lowered social and economic status. Then, in a supportive manner, the worker helps the client discuss his or her feelings about these factors. At times, the worker aids the client to find ways to relieve tensions and counteracts feelings of helplessness and hopelessness. The worker's tasks with the client may also include encouraging communication with others, instilling confidence, and supporting strengths that promote social and emotional recovery.[13]

Regardless of the nature and course of the illness, some of the time spent with the client in counseling will need to focus on discussion of compliance with medical treatment.[16,18] For example, the worker will want to explore the client's feelings and attitudes about taking medication and the impact of the side effects of the medication on compliance.

In counseling the client and the family, the home care social worker brings a systems perspective to his or her work with the family. This means that the home care social worker views the family as a system composed of interdependent parts. A quick review of the systems perspective indicates that systems have boundaries or markers which make it possible to know what components are part of the system and which are outside of the system. Systems regulate the flow and exchange of resources (i.e., information, services) with other systems through their boundaries. System boundaries can vary from being fairly "open" to totally "closed" to environmental stimuli. Systems with "open" boundaries are said to be more flexible about exchanges with the environment, whereas "closed" systems are more rigid and regulatory. Systems are also characterized by their structure, organization, and feedback, or how components which make up a system relate back and forth to each other. Systems strive toward homeostasis or a balanced state in their functioning. When a system's homeostasis is disturbed, it can be said to experience stress. Through the mechanism of feedback, systems attempt to reorganize in order to achieve balance or equilibrium again. Sometimes, a substantial reorganization or change in the system takes place before equilibrium is achieved again. Whether minor or substantial, "a change in one part of the system may cause a change in many parts (subsystems) of the larger system and in the larger system itself" (p. 8).[21] Consequently, the whole system may be transformed in a way that is greater than the sum of its individual transformations.

A family is a system made up of members who influence and are influenced by every other member. Despite the diversity of the "family," all family systems have boundaries. All families have an internal structure which influences their organization, power and authority functions, and communication patterns, as well as assignment of functions, duties, and roles. Behavior in families is governed by rules and influenced by values, rituals, and culture. Behavior of family members can be need driven and influenced by the availability or lack of internal and external resources to meet family needs.

The primary functions of the family are to meet the physical, social, and emotional needs of its members. When the family is unable to meet one or more of these needs, and it lacks the necessary resources to meet those needs, the family homeostasis is disturbed. Consequently, the family experiences stress.[10,11] Therefore, any change affecting one family member, such as illness or disability, will impact and influence all other family members because a family system is "a dynamic order of *people* (along with their intellectual, emotional, and behavioral processes) standing in mutual interaction" (p. 7).[21]

Using this knowledge of families as systems, the home care social worker understands that the family equilibrium is disturbed when one family member is ill and is cared for in the home. Family roles change, relationships become strained, and less privacy becomes available to family members. Families must cope with a parade of health care providers coming in and out of their home. The family's concerns will most likely center around the impact of the illness on the client and family, the management of the client's illness, and the availability of resources to make home care successful. The challenge facing the worker is to help clients and their families deal with the changed home environment and make the changes to adapt to the client's illness while "preserving the vital function of the home as the nucleus of domestic serenity" (p. 528).[13]

In family counseling, the worker identifies and names for the family members the variety of burdens, emotions, feelings, and events that they are experiencing or may encounter. Some of these include increased daily care responsibilities and burdens, sense of loss of control over daily life, isolation from extended family and friends, disruption of sleep and social activities, depression, marital strain, reorganization and renovation of living space, lack of privacy, constant vigilance, restricted social life, and lack of time to meet personal and family needs.[22]

Initially, the worker listens and validates feelings and reactions of family members. For instance, Kohrman[23] notes that parents of children receiving home care experience a range of feelings from terror (that the child may die due to anxiety about their competence to care for a medically fragile child) to role confusion to exhaustion to the endlessness of caring for the child. Family members may feel the need to control their environment through controlling the illness. Christian,[24] in a study of families coping with a chronic illness in a child, reported that families used different strategies as means of coping with and controlling the illness. These strategies included minimizing the severity of the child's chronic illness or ignoring the problems, normalizing the illness as part of life, balancing the needs of the family and other family members by setting up a regular routine, and coordinating all of the care being provided.

The worker may need to educate the family about the nature of onset, the course, the outcome, and the degree of incapacitation brought on by the disease, as described by Rolland.[25] For instance, illnesses can have acute onset or gradual onset. The course of an illness can be characterized as progressive (disease progresses more severely over time), constant (disease progression is stable and predictable over time), or episodic (disease progression varies between stability and flare-up and exacerbation). In the last circumstance, the family and client's emotional status are enslaved by the unpredictability of disease progression. Families must be flexible enough to handle the "highs and lows" that accompany the episodic nature of certain illnesses. Lastly, knowing about the outcome of the illness (shortens life span or has no effect on life span) and the degree of incapacitation (degree of impairment) may give some predictability to family life as well as influence the specific adjustments family members make to attend to the needs of the ill person.

With life-threatening illnesses, the worker may have to help families begin to accept the possibility of death of the ill family member without feelings of abandonment. Rolland[25] suggests that "for both there exists an undercurrent of anticipatory grief and separation that permeates all phases of adaptation. Families are often caught between a desire for intimacy and a pull to let go, emotionally, of the ill member" (p. 436). When this happens, the client may be viewed as already deceased and the "end result can be the structural and emotional isolation of the ill person from family life" (p. 437).[25]

The home care social worker will need to facilitate families' discussion of their adjustment to home care. Feinberg[26] has identified three stages in the adjustment of families to home care of children. The first stage is the triumph of discharge from the hospital. In the second stage, which generally occurs between 6 weeks to 6 months later, exhaustion and frustration with health care providers and diminution of community support set in. In the third stage, families begin to integrate the technology-dependent child into daily family life. Families do expect occasional problems with insurance companies and health care providers, as well as medical crises and rehospitalization. Many families begin to understand their limitations in dealing with the child's condition in the home after the first year of illness.[22]

Families will need to hear that their ability to adapt to a member's disability does exist but may take some time. In addition, families may need encouragement to accept the benefits of home care to the well-being of the client and the recovery process without seeing it as a negative reflection on their capability to care for an ill family member. Families may benefit from hearing that, as Kohrman[23] has observed, home care promotes bio-psycho-social growth and development in children and lessens dependency in the elderly after discharge from the hospital. Also, family interactions and routines have a positive impact on the patient because home care offers the client the opportunity to be an integral part of family life.

Another task the worker can accomplish with the family is to create a supportive environment where the family can feel freed up to deal with some issues that are likely to factor into their caregiving and caretaking responsibilities. In particular, this includes dependence/independence issues[14] related to the client's disability. The worker encourages family members to achieve a realistic appraisal of the client's current level of functioning by addressing with the family their overreaction and/or underreaction to the difficulties experienced by the client. The worker may find that family members have to be reminded that they will have to divest emotional energy from other responsibilities in order to deal with the ill family member. The worker focuses on enabling family members to believe in their ability to care properly for the client.[14]

If the client needs long-term care, the home care social worker will be called upon to counsel the client and family on planning long-term care for the client. The focus of such counseling will be on assessment of the patient's need for long-term care, including evaluation of the home and family situation, requirements for enabling the patient and family to develop an in-home care plan, and arrangement for placement. If the client has an illness that is terminal, counseling will need to focus specifically on management of the terminal illness, reaction and adjustment to terminal illness, strengthening the family's support system, and the resolution of any conflicts related to the chronic and terminal nature of the illness.[6]

Advocate

As an advocate for the client, the social worker encourages the client to be more assertive in seeking and asking for services, intervenes directly with agencies on behalf of the client, removes barriers, and seeks out and develops new services in the client and family's geographic area. He or she also mobilizes and develops support groups for clients with the same medical condition[14] and interprets/explains needs and concerns of client to others, such as welfare and health care systems.[15,18]

Mediator

As a mediator/facilitator, the social worker interprets the client and family's situation to other members of the health care team.[14] Similarly, the worker explains to the family tasks and procedures performed or not performed by home care providers. The worker may find mediation may be necessary if the client and/or family become dissatisfied with care received, feel intruded upon, and want to control the comings and goings of home care providers or if roles played by family members and home care providers in caregiving become blurred.

Collaborator

Collaboration is a "cooperative process of exchange involving communication, planning, and action on the part of two or more disciplines" (p. 199).[27] The process of collaboration is carried out by the social worker through conferring (reciprocal exchange of views), cooperating (around a particular issue), and consulting (seeking advice from a knowledgeable provider).[27]

Specifically, the worker explains the psychosocial factors related to the illness to all service providers. In doing so, the worker helps the health care team understand and tolerate the client and family's direct and indirect display of emotional upheaval. The worker coordinates all treatment efforts in the home and monitors the process of collaboration among all service providers. The social worker facilitates communication at the interface of various disciplines and at the interface between the patient and the team members.[13,20] In order for the social worker to practice effective collaboration, he or she must understand the functions and tasks of the other home care service providers, such as home health aides, physical therapist, and nurses.

Termination

Ordinarily, the termination phase begins when there is agreement that the goals and objectives have been met to the satisfaction of the client and his or her family. The worker reviews both the initial plan of action agreed upon at time of assessment and the completed goals and objectives with the client and family.

The termination process is an opportunity for the home care social worker to review the working relationship established with the client, family, and home care team. If possible, the home care social worker should elicit direct feedback from the client, the family, and the home care team about their evaluation of services provided by the home care social worker. This information helps to guide the worker in a more effective fashion in future work with home care clients.

The termination of social work involvement may be forced due to client and family wishes, the worker leaving the agency, or further deterioration of the client's health status, resulting in rehospitalization, relocation to a skilled nursing facility, or death. When the last scenario occurs, under current billable services regulations, home care social workers are not able to provide supportive or grief counseling to families. A referral for grief counseling needs to be made for the family. Regardless of how termination occurred, a follow-up contact 3 to 6 weeks after end of service delivery should be made with the family. This is a another opportunity to solicit information about adequacy of services provided as well as to assess further needs of the home care recipient.

Reimbursement

As lifestyles, demographics, life expectancy, and types of illnesses have changed, so has the role of the social worker in the continuum of home health care. Social workers do play a pivotal role in the utilization of home health care services. Medical professionals recognize the importance of the social worker as part of an interdisciplinary team to provide quality care to home care clients. However, provision of social work services is directly affected by reimbursement of third-party payments, private pay, Medicaid, and Medicare. Currently, medical social work service is not considered a primary skilled service and is therefore not directly reimbursable under the present health care system. In this section, we will examine funding sources for the home health care services and the effect on social work service availability. The information presented on Medicare, Medicaid, hospice, and medical social work reimbursement guidelines is based on review of a number of different sources.[6, 28–38]

Medicare

Growth in the home care industry has been influenced by changes in Medicare reimbursement to hospitals and home health care agencies. Medicare is administered by the Health Care Financing Administration under the direction of the Social Security Administration. Individuals eligible for Medicare are those over 65 who have paid into the Social Security or Railroad Retirement system, individuals who have been disabled for longer than 24 months, individuals in the last stage of renal disease, spouses of recipients over 65, or dependent children of eligible participants. Medicare Title 18 is a federally funded amendment to the Social Security Act of 1965 which funds home health care. Medicare Title 18 has made home health services cost efficient and profitable. The capitalization of home health services has resulted in many new certified agencies and has increased availability of quality services.

In 1983, the introduction of the diagnostic-related group (DRG) system led to changes in Medicare payments to hospitals. Hospitals receive a specific amount of reimbursement based upon the diagnosis of the client, regardless of the number of diagnostic tests or length of hospitalization. As a result, this system of reimbursement encourages early discharge of more seriously ill individuals and intensifies the role of home health care.

Medicare Part A hospital insurance (HI) and Part B voluntary supplemental medical insurance (SMI) cover Home Health Agencies (HHA) services. To be eligible for HHA benefits under Medicare, each of the following criteria must be met:

- A client must be homebound. The client does not have to be confined to bed, but leaving his or her residence must require assistance or a significant effort.
- Services must be provided by certified agencies.
- Services are provided according to the care plan developed and reviewed at least every 60 days by the attending physician.
- The home health care client needs intermittent skilled nursing care. Skilled nursing care, as defined by Medicare, is services provided by a nurse, physical therapist, or speech therapist.
- Services must be reasonable and necessary.

In 1972, the Omnibus Reconciliation Act eliminated the 100 visits per year regulation for home health care recipients and the 3-day prior hospitalization period for receiving benefits under Medicare Part A. Once eligibility has been established, there are no limitations on use of services and prior hospitalization is not necessary. Medicare home health coverage does not include meals, home-delivered meals, homemaker services, drugs, blood transfusions, personal items, or round-the-clock nursing care.

Medicare does cover costs for intermittent skilled nursing care and home health aide services who provide for personal care of the recipient for a combined total of less than 35 hours per week. Skilled therapy such as physical therapy, speech therapy, and occupational therapy is covered if it is considered necessary to restore or maintain the patient's functional abilities affected by the illness. Medical supplies such as but not limited to surgical dressings, bandages, catheters, needles, syringes, irrigating solutions, and intravenous fluids are reimbursable. Durable medical equipment (equipment that has repeated use such as wheelchairs, beds, crutches, and canes that enable essential home health services to be provided) is 80% reimbursable. Under current provisions, medical social worker services are covered only when they facilitate recovery and/or maintain functional abilities outlined in the physician's care plan.

Medicaid

Medicaid Title XIX was enacted in 1965 as a means-tested entitlement program. Medicaid Title XIX is jointly financed by the federal government and each state.

States receive federally matched funds based upon the state's per capita income, with states having lower per capita income receiving the highest number of federal dollars. Medicaid regulations mandate that states cover the following individuals:

- Individuals receiving Aid to Families with Dependent Children (AFDC) and persons receiving SSI
- Low-income children
- Pregnant women
- Qualified Medicare beneficiaries and low-income Medicare recipients may receive assistance with co-payments, Medicare Part B premiums, deductibles, etc.

States may elect under Medicaid to cover:

- Medically needy individuals whose income is higher than allowable by the Medicaid program but whose medical expenses are so extraordinary they drain family resources
- Persons requiring long-term institutional care

States must provide home health services to eligible participants in the Medicaid program. Medicaid's home health regulations are structured much like Medicare, but the program is less restrictive. Federal Medicaid regulations do not require the recipient of home health services to be homebound. However, states design their individual programs and may apply limitations and restrictions to the number of visits and skilled services.

In 1975, Title XX to the Social Security Act added personal care and homemaker services to Medicaid provisions. Under this amendment, services such as assistance with personal hygiene, light housekeeping, shopping, and home-delivered meals may be provided by home health aides. Home health aides must be supervised by a medical professional following the treatment plan outlined by the attending physician. Restrictions to personal care services were again decreased by the Omnibus Budget Reconciliation Act of 1981, known as the "2176 waiver program." This act allows states to provide homemaker, personal care, and case management to the elderly, the mentally retarded, and the chronically ill. States must demonstrate that the cost of the waiver per recipient of home health services does not exceed the cost of institutionalized care under Medicare reimbursement regulations.

Hospice

Home health care under Medicare regulations makes the basic assumption that the client will regain health or maintain current functional abilities. However, the rise of more chronic and terminal illnesses necessitates residential care for the terminally ill clients. As an alternative to lengthy hospitalization for these clients, legislation was enacted by Congress in 1982 to create a Medicare hospice program. This legislation provides hospice benefits for Medicare recipients who have been certified as terminally ill by their attending physician and a hospice physician. Hospice provides services designed to control pain, to provide support and respite, and to allow the client to remain at home. Hospice services focus on the family support network and encourage active participation in treatment plans and care in order to maintain the patient in the home. Hospice provides comprehensive services including counseling for the family after the client has died.

Hospice services under Medicare are divided into four benefit periods—two 90-day periods, one 30-day period, and a lifetime period. Recipients must elect hospice care at each interval and be diagnosed with a terminal illness by both the attending and hospice physician. Medicare places a lifetime cap on hospice benefits which are adjusted each year. Benefits were capped at $12,846 per client as of July 1994. Medicare payments are based upon the following four categories:

1. **Routine home care**—Individuals receiving care at home. This service does not vary according to the level of care or intensity of services provided.
2. **Continuous home care**—Individuals who require skilled services for at least 8 hours a day for brief periods of time in order to allow the recipient to stay at home during a crisis.
3. **Inpatient respite care**—Care may be provided on an inpatient basis for no longer than 5 days at any one time.
4. **General inpatient care**—Service in a hospital, skilled nursing facility, or the inpatient unit of a hospice center.

Rates within these categories may vary according to the level of care required and allowable adjustments for area wages. Hospice care is optional under the Medicaid system. Currently, 36 states include hospice services under their Medicaid programs.

Medical Social Work Reimbursement Guidelines

Social work services are the most difficult for reimbursement regardless of the payment source. Medicare regulations are specific and restrictive, whereas Medicaid generally does not cover medical social work services at all. Social work services are considered a secondary service and may be provided only if the client is receiving a primary service such as nursing, physical therapy, or speech therapy. Under Medicare guidelines, medical social services may be provided by or under the supervision of a qualified medical social worker. Medicare defines a qualified medical social worker as an individual with a master's degree in social work from a Council on Social Work Education certified school and one year of experience in the health care field.

Medicare will reimburse for social work services if adequate documentation verifies that all of the following conditions are met:

- The client is homebound and receiving a primary service. The primary service must begin prior to social work services being initiated and social work services must be terminated prior to the end of the primary service.
- Medical social work services must be prescribed by the attending physician and outlined in the care plan.
- The patient care plan must document why medical social work services are needed. The care plan must demonstrate a specific link between the psychosocial needs of the patient and benefit to the medical recovery of the patient. The care plan must also document the necessity of the skills and knowledge of a qualified medical social worker.
- Social work services must be provided by or under the supervision of a qualified medical social worker.
- Medical social work services must be considered necessary to resolve emotional or social barriers to the client's speedy medical recovery.
- Medical social work services must be reasonable and in the physician's opinion must purposefully contribute to the treatment of the medical condition. The social work services must, in the judgment of the physician, contribute to the resolution of emotional and/or social problems impeding the patient's recovery. In the circumstance that for no known medical reason the patient fails to recover, the physician may suspect social or emotional difficulties and provide medical social work intervention.

Services reimbursable by Medicare and many third-party payors include:

- **Psychosocial assessments**—Assessment of the social and emotional influences relating to the recovery, adjustment, and treatment of the illness. This assessment may be conducted every 60 days in conjunction with the primary service provider to update the patient care plan.
- **Financial–environmental assessment**—Assessment of in-home services, treatment, the patient's financial ability to continue services, and available community resources.
- **Counseling**—Counseling services to assist the patient with adjustment to his or her medical condition and treatment.

- **Short-term planning**—Plans that incorporate specific goals toward a successful patient adjustment to terminal or chronic illness.
- **Community resource planning**—Assessing patient needs and providing referrals and linkages to available community resources.
- **Long-term planning**—Assessment of optimal care setting such as in-home with assistance, long-term placement, or available alternative care.

Documentation of the need and justification for medical social work services is key in receiving reimbursement. Medical social work services must assist the primary service provider in the maintenance of or recovery from the medical condition. Social work services dealing solely with concerns about the illness or treatment, services to minimize family and/or client problems in adjusting to the illness, or services to provide reassurance to the client or family are not covered under current Medicare and most third-party payors unless there is a direct medical benefit.

Conclusion

In this chapter, we have discussed the role of the social worker in the delivery of home care. Social workers are concerned with the negative impact of illness and disability on the client and his or her family. Social workers provide assessment of social and emotional factors related to the client's illness and seek out and deliver available resources to meet the needs of the home care client. Social workers work with the family to help them cope with and adjust to the illness of a family member. Social workers collaborate with other members of the home care team to coordinate and deliver services in a timely fashion to the client.

Overall, social workers play a pivotal role in the management of the client in the home. However, current Medicare and Medicaid regulations are impeding adequate delivery of social work services. For instance, Medicare participation in home care agencies mandates that social services be available to patients but does not require patients to be seen by social services or that social workers be involved in the care plan or assessment of the patient.[9] In some states, Medicaid regulations prohibit the involvement of home care social workers in the client's care on the grounds that the client already has a state-provided social worker in the Medicaid system.

Home care social work has not been defined as a skilled service, which makes reimbursement difficult. The number of individuals utilizing home care is increasing. In order to meet this growing need, the social work profession needs to be granted "skilled service" status under Medicare regulations. The services that a home care social worker provides, including assessment, supportive counseling, and case management, need to fall under "skilled services" and, therefore, be reimbursable. Physicians, nurses, and other "skilled service" providers involved in the delivery of home care should call on their respective professional organizations to join social workers and the National Association of Social Workers in calling for legislative changes to give "skilled status" to home care social workers. In the end, such advocacy can only result in better attention paid to the bio-psycho-social needs of the home care client.

References

1. Hart, E., Homemaker Services for Families and Individuals, Public Affairs Pamphlet No. 371, Public Affairs Committee, New York, 1965.
2. Council on Social Work Education and National Council for Homemaker Services, *A Unit of Learning about Homemaker–Home Health Aide Service,* Council on Social Work Education, New York, 1968.
3. Williams, J. U., The caseworker–homemaker team, in *A Unit of Learning about Homemaker–Home Health Aide Service,* Council on Social Work Education, New York, 1968, pp. 43–49.
4. Benjamin, A. E., An historical perspective on home care policy, *The Milbank Quarterly,* 71(1):129–166, 1993.
5. Jackson, B. N., Health care providers: functions and issues, in *Home Health and Rehabilitation,* May, B. J., Ed., F.A. Davis, Philadelphia, 1993, pp. 25–53.
6. National Association of Social Workers, *Social Work Speaks,* NASW Press, Washington, D.C., 1994.
7. Dieckmann, J. L., Home health administration: an overview, in *Handbook of Home Health Care Administration,* Harris, M., Ed., Aspen Publishers, Gaithersburg, Maryland, 1994, pp. 3–13.
8. National Association for Home Care, Basic Statistics about Home Care 1994, Washington, D.C., 1994.
9. Cox, C., Expanding social work's role in home care: an ecological perspective, *Social Work,* 37(2):179–183, 1992.
10. Germain, C. and Gitterman, A., The life model approach to practice revisited, in *Social Work Treatment,* 3rd edition, Turner, F. J., Ed., The Free Press, New York, 1986, pp. 618–643.
11. Hartman, A. and Laird, J., *Family-Centered Social Work Practice,* The Free Press, New York, 1983.
12. Keating, S. B. and Kelman, G. B., *Home Health Care Nursing,* J.B. Lippincott, Philadelphia, 1988.
13. Kirschner, C. and Rosengarten, L., The skilled social work role in home care, *Social Work,* 27(6):527–530, 1982.
14. Hart, M., Social services and community resources, in *Home Health and Rehabilitation,* May, B. J., Ed., F.A. Davis, Philadelphia, 1993, pp. 289–310.

15. Quire, E. and Stahl, I., The social worker, in *Home Health Care for the Aged,* Brickner, P. W., Ed., Appleton-Century-Crofts, New York, 1978, pp. 109–126.
16. Axelrod, T. B., Innovative roles for social workers in home-care programs, *Health and Social Work,* 3(3):48–66, 1978.
17. Oktay, J. S. and Sheppard, F., Home health care for elderly, *Health and Social Work,* 3(3):35–47, 1978.
18. Jacobs, P. E. and Lurie, A., A new look at home care and the hospital social worker, *J. Gerontol. Social Work,* 7(4):87–99, 1984.
19. Compton, B. R. and Galaway, B., *Social Work Processes,* Wadsworth Publishing, Belmont, California, 1989.
20. Peterson, K. J., Integration of medical and psychosocial needs of the home hemodialysis patient: implications for the nephrology social worker, *Social Work in Health Care,* 9(4):33–44, 1984.
21. Okun, B. F. and Rappaport, L. J., *Working with Families: An Introduction to Family Therapy,* Duxbury Press, North Scituate, Massachusetts, 1980.
22. Perrin, J. M., Shyne, M. W., and Bloom, S. H., *Home and Community Care for Chronically Ill Children,* Oxford University Press, New York, 1993.
23. Kohrman, A. H., Psychological issues, in *Delivering High Technology Home Care,* Mehlman, M. J. and Youngner, S. J., Eds., Springer Publishing, New York, 1991, pp. 160–178.
24. Christian, B. J., Quality of life and family relationships in families coping with their child's chronic illness, in *Key Aspects of Caring for the Chronically Ill,* Funk, S. G., Tornquist, E. M., Champagne, M. T., and Wiese, R. A., Eds., Springer Publishing, New York, 1993, pp. 304–312.
25. Rolland, J., Chronic illness and the family, in *The Changing Family Life Cycle*, 2nd edition, Carter, B. and McGoldrick, M., Eds., Gardner Press, New York, 1988, pp. 433–456.
26. Feinberg, E. A., Family stress in pediatric home care, *Caring,* 4(5):38–44, 1985.
27. Germain, C., *Social Work Practice in Health Care,* The Free Press, New York, 1984.
28. Silverman, H. A., Use of Medicare-covered home health agency services, 1988, *Health Care Financing Rev.,* 12(2):113–126, 1990.
29. Ruther, M. and Helbing, C., Use and cost of home health agency services under Medicare, *Health Care Financing Rev.,* 10(1):105–108, 1988.
30. Helbing, C., Sangl, J. A., and Silverman, H. A., Home health agency benefits, *Health Care Financing Rev.,* Annual Supplement:125–148, 1992.
31. Milone-Nuzzo, P. F., Third-party reimbursement for home care of clients with diabetes, *The Diabetes Educator,* 19(6):513–516, 1993.
32. Hospice Association of America, Hospice Facts and Statistics, Washington, D.C., 1994.
33. Coughlin, T. A., Ku, L., and Holahan, J., *Medicaid Since 1980,* The Urban Institute Press, Washington, D.C., 1994.
34. Visiting Nurses Association of Kentucky, Personal communication, January 1995.
35. Department of Health and Human Services, Health Care Financing Administration,

42 CFR Part 484, Medicare program: Home health agencies: Conditions of participation, *Federal Register,* 56:32967–32975, July 1991.

36. Samuel, F. E., High technology home care: an overview, in *Delivering High Technology Home Care*, Mehlman, M. J. and Youngner, S. J., Eds., Springer Publishing, New York, 1991, pp. 1–22.

37. Spiegel, A. D., The economics of high technology home care: doing right for the wrong reason, in *Delivering High Technology Home Care,* Mehlman M. J. and Youngner, S. J., Eds., Springer Publishing, New York, 1991, pp. 23–66.

38. Webb, P. R., Medicare conditions of participation, in *Handbook of Home Health Care Administration,* Aspen Publishers, Gaithersburg, Maryland, 1994, pp. 23–55.

Legal Aspects of Home Health Care

10

Brian K. Brake, Esq.

Introduction

Home care in the United States is a diverse and rapidly growing service industry. About 15,000 providers deliver home care services to some 7 million individuals who require such services because of acute illness, long-term health conditions, permanent disability, or terminal illness. Annual expenditures for home health care are expected to have exceeded $27 billion in 1995.[1]

With the growth of the home care industry and the increase in the elderly population requiring home health care, liability for medical malpractice in the home health care field is likely to expand in the coming years. This chapter serves as an overview to familiarize the home health care provider with (1) the legal elements required to establish a medical malpractice claim, (2) other areas of potential liability for the home health care provider, and (3) a broad overview of federal regulations for Medicare reimbursement.

Medical malpractice is a civil tort or wrong arising from the breach of a duty owed by a health care provider to a patient. Depending upon the circumstances, such claims may be governed by federal or state law or by a combination of both. There is wide variation among the different states on such crucial issues as statute of limitations (i.e., how long after the injury a patient has to bring a lawsuit), presuit mediation procedures, limitation of damage awards, availability of punitive damages, and insurance coverage, to name only a few. A comprehensive review of these issues on a state-by-state basis is beyond the scope of this chapter. Specific questions should be referred to competent counsel in the appropriate state.

Elements of a Medical Malpractice Claim

The injured patient, known as the "plaintiff," must prove four basic elements in order to recover against a defendant health care provider for medical malpractice:

1. That the health care provider owed a **duty** to the patient arising out of a provider/patient relationship
2. That the health care provider **breached that duty**
3. That the breach of the duty was **the proximate cause** of injury to the patient
4. That ascertainable **damages** resulted

Each of these four elements must be proved by the plaintiff to a reasonable certainty by the greater weight of the evidence. This is sometimes referred to as the "preponderance of the evidence" and is the lowest burden of proof imposed upon litigants. This burden of proof is sometimes referred to as a "more likely than not" standard, meaning that the plaintiff need only establish a greater than 50% probability that each element is true. By contrast, criminal cases must be proven beyond a reasonable doubt. The plaintiff has the burden of proving each of the four elements by the greater weight of the evidence; a failure to prove any one means the plaintiff cannot recover. For example, even if the plaintiff is able to prove that the health care provider owed a duty and the health care provider breached that duty, the plaintiff would be precluded from recovering if he or she is unable to establish that the breach of that duty caused injury. Likewise, the simple fact that a plaintiff was injured does not itself entitle him or her to recover unless it is established that the health care provider failed to comply with the standard of care required and that this caused the injuries.

Duty/Standard of Care

In the absence of a particular state or federal law, a health care provider has no legal obligation to accept as a patient everyone who seeks his or her services.[2] A health care provider's duty arises only upon the creation of a provider/patient relationship; that relationship arises from a consensual transaction, a contract, expressed or implied, general or special. Whether a health care provider/patient relationship is created is a question of fact, turning upon a determination of whether the patient entrusted his or her treatment to the health care provider and if the health care provider accepted the case. For example, a plaintiff's allegation that she "had an appointment with the defendant" would be insufficient to establish a physician/patient relationship for it is not implied that the health care provider had agreed to see him or her. But if the health care provider had granted an appointment at a designated time and place for the performance of a specific medical service, this would be sufficient to establish a consensual transaction giving rise to a health care provider/patient relationship and a duty to perform the services contemplated.[3]

Unless the services to be rendered are conditioned or limited, the health care provider/patient relationship continues until the services are no longer needed. However, the relationship may be terminated earlier by mutual consent or by the unilateral action of the patient. Under certain circumstances, the health care provider has a right to withdraw from a case, provided the patient is afforded a reasonable opportunity to acquire the services he or she needs from another health care provider. In the case of a physician, the doctor/patient relationship does not terminate simply because a patient's care is provided in his or her home rather than in a hospital. Unless the doctor/patient relationship has been formally terminated by one of the methods listed above, a physician retains the duty of care when the patient is discharged into a home health care setting.

As a practical matter, plaintiffs usually have no difficulty establishing that the health care provider owed them a duty arising out of a relationship. This is generally established if any health care is provided.

Once a duty is created, the health care provider will be found to have committed medical malpractice if he or she fails to exercise that degree of skill and diligence practiced by a "reasonably prudent" practitioner in his or her field of practice or specialty. This is generally referred to as the "standard of care" required. For instance, a home health care nurse will be held to the standard of care required to be practiced by a reasonably prudent nurse, while a physician will be held to the standard of care of a reasonably prudent physician under the circumstances of the case. In order to recover, a plaintiff must prove that the health care provider breached the applicable standard of care.

The specific duties encompassed by the "standard of care" are established on a case-by-case basis through the testimony of expert witnesses and in some instances through texts and learned treatises. It is the job of the finder-of-fact in each case, usually the jury, to determine what the standard of care is and whether it was met by the defendant.

Because the standard of care varies according to the qualifications of the health care provider and the circumstances of each case, it is difficult to generalize what the standard of care requires. However, the mere fact that a health care provider has failed to effect a cure or that his or her diagnosis and treatment have been detrimental to the patient's health does not in and of itself establish a breach of the standard of care.[4] Nor is a health care provider held to the highest degree of care known in his or her profession. Rather, the standard of care only requires the health care provider to have done what a reasonably prudent or "average" health care provider would have done under the circumstances.

Case History No. 1

Plaintiff alleged that a home health care aide was careless in the care provided. The home health care aide removed a footrest from the plaintiff's wheelchair, causing plaintiff to develop decubitus ulcers on his heels. Plaintiff underwent left and right lumbar sympathectomy to improve poor blood supply to the heels. Plaintiff had prior peripheral vascular disease resulting in poor blood supply to the lower extremities. Complications resulting from these decubitus ulcers were a contributing cause of plaintiff's death. The case was settled for $75,000. To establish breach of the standard of care, the plaintiff relied upon two home health care registered nurses, a physician practicing in general surgery, and a physician practicing in family practice. *Seaton v. Beebe*, Docket No. 92-807-CA-09G (Florida, 1992).

In the above case history, it was necessary for the plaintiff to establish through home health care registered nurses that the defendant home health care aide did not comply with the standard of care in treating the decubitus ulcers. It is likely that the plaintiff employed a general surgeon and a family practitioner to establish that the complications from the decubitus ulcers resulted in the plaintiff's death.

As stated, the standard of care required will depend upon the facts and circumstances of each case. However, courts have determined as a general matter that the standard of care requires a health care provider to perform the following duties:

1. To take a complete history from a patient
2. To perform follow-up examinations in an appropriate period of time
3. That the examination be geared to the specific complaint of the patient
4. To advise the patient to consult with a specialist if necessary

The above are general duties that have been recognized by some courts; this list is not intended to be exhaustive. The actual standard of care in any given case depends upon the particular facts and circumstances of the case. The standard of care to be applied is determined at the time the treatment was rendered to the patient, not at the time of trial.

Establishing the Standard of Care: Expert Testimony

Expert testimony is generally required to establish the standard of care and the health care provider's departure from that standard. This is because the standard of care against which the conduct of a health care provider is measured is a matter particularly within the knowledge of experts and beyond the scope of lay persons. In most cases, this testimony comes from expert witnesses not connected with the plaintiff's care who are hired by the parties to review the case and render opinions about the appropriateness of the defendant's care. Expert testimony may also come from the defendant or other treating doctors and experts. A malpractice action will usually be dismissed if the plaintiff does not present expert testimony that a violation of the applicable standard of care occurred.

Case History No. 2

> Plaintiff, a high school senior, was referred to a physician to have a blood sample taken. The sample was taken by a student technician while plaintiff was seated. When the technician turned to place the tube on a table, plaintiff stood up, fainted, fell, and was injured. Plaintiff asserted that the doctor and his staff were negligent in not telling him to remain seated for some moments after the sample was taken. The plaintiff failed to offer expert testimony as to the standard of care for taking blood samples. The court dismissed the action for failure to present expert testimony on the standard of care. *Carroll v. Richardson*, 201 Va. 157, 110 S.E.2d 193 (1959).

The expert witness must establish familiarity with the methods of customary and proper medical diagnosis and treatment in the community. A specialist may testify to the standard of care of a general practitioner or a different specialist as long as the witness is knowledgeable about the standard of care. Expert testimony is not necessarily limited to expert physicians. Qualified nonphysician experts may also be permitted to testify in certain circumstances. The question of whether a witness qualifies as an expert is a discretionary matter for the trial judge.

Evidence as to the applicable standard of care may often be provided by the defendant's own testimony. It is generally accepted that the testimony of the defendant may serve to prove the standard of care by which the defendant's treatment is to be judged. In a few jurisdictions, evidence as to the applicable standard of care may be provided through the introduction of medical treatises.

Although the general rule is that expert testimony is necessary to establish the standard of care, some courts have held that where the negligence is sufficiently obvious as to lie within the common knowledge of a lay person, expert testimony is not required. The so-called "common knowledge exception" applies where the evidence suggests to people of ordinary intelligence the proper standard of care. A typical situation is where a foreign object such as a sponge or needle is left within the body of a patient. Another well-established application of the common knowledge exception is where the physician has disregarded the directions of the manufacturer in administering or prescribing a drug. An exception has also been applied to establish that a doctor's delay in taking tests, or in submitting them to a laboratory for analysis, constituted negligence. Expert testimony may also be unnecessary where the physician willfully abandons the patient.

Case History No. 3

> Patient was diagnosed as having Alzheimer's disease and was placed in a nursing home. Members of patient's family had informed the nursing home that she was unable to eat without assistance and had previously choked on her food. On December 17, 1989, an employee of the nursing home delivered a dinner tray to the patient. No one assisted the patient with her food. The patient was found sitting up in her chair with her head turned sideways and was reportedly dead at the time. At trial, the plaintiff did not present any expert testimony as to the standard of care required in feeding patients. The court held that in this particular case, expert testimony was unnecessary because the alleged negligence was within the range of the jury's common knowledge and experience. *Beverly v. Nichols*, 247 Va. 264, 441 S.E.2d 1 (1994).

The standard of care may also be established by a statute or regulation. Some courts have found that compliance with federal and state regulations may satisfy the legal standard of care. In at least one case, the court held that the requirement of the Nursing Home Care Reform Act to provide adequate general supervision did *not* raise a rebuttable presumption in favor of plaintiff who had fallen that the defendant had failed to provide adequate care.[5]

The current Medicare regulations for home health care agencies set forth standards of physician supervision of home health care services. The regulations require a plan of treatment, physician review of the plan of treatment, and nurse's conformance with the physician's orders. Arguably, a violation of these federal regulations could be introduced as evidence of a breach of the standard of care.

Causation

It is not enough for a plaintiff to prove that the health care provider breached the standard of care. To recover damages in a malpractice action, the patient must prove that the breach of the standard of care proximately caused injuries. Causation is contested in most malpractice cases. Many malpractice plaintiffs lose their cases because they fail to prove causation, even though they successfully establish that the defendant violated the applicable standard of care. To establish causation, the patient need not prove that the defendant's negligence was the only cause of the injury suffered. In most jurisdictions, the patient must merely prove that the health care provider's conduct was "a cause" of or "a substantial factor" resulting in the injury suffered. Causation is a special problem in malpractice cases because health care providers treat people who already have illnesses or injuries. In each case, therefore, there is a question whether the negative result complained of was the normal and expected result from the disease or whether the patient's condition was made worse by the health care provider's negligence.

Most courts require the plaintiff to prove causation to a reasonable degree of probability. Courts have used various standards such as "the preponderance of the evidence," "substantial factor," and "reasonable medical certainty," but the essence of the standard is that the plaintiff must prove that it is more likely than not that the health care provider's negligence was a cause of the harm complained of by the patient.

"Vicarious" Liability

Under the doctrine of vicarious liability, an employer is liable for injuries caused by the negligent acts or omissions of its employee committed within the scope of employment. To the extent that a hospital discharges a patient into a home health care program and its staff physician fails to supervise the treatment, the hospital and the physician may be jointly responsible for any injuries the patient incurs.

Once a home health care provider undertakes the care of a patient, the provider is under a duty to perform that care in a reasonable manner. By negligently performing a treatment ordered by the supervising physician or by negligently training nonmedical personnel to perform the services themselves, a home health care provider may breach this duty. A physician may be held liable for these negligent acts and omissions to the extent he or she has control or a right of control over the provider's actions. Hospitals also risk liability for the negligence of hospital-based home health care providers under the theories of respondeat superior and apparent agency and for the negligence of nonhospital-based providers under theory of negligence in the selection of the provider.

Other Areas of Potential Liability

Negligent Hiring

A home health care agency may be liable for negligently hiring employees who assault or otherwise harm patients in the home health care setting. Some states have enacted legislation prohibiting home health care agencies from hiring persons who have been convicted of felonies or other serious crimes.[6] Some statutes require that the home health care agency perform a background check of the potential employee's criminal record before hiring. Regardless of whether the state in which the home health care agency is licensed is required to perform a background check, liability may be imposed for the negligent failure to do so.

Case History No. 4

Plaintiff, a 60-year-old female, was assaulted, tied up, and robbed in her home by two former employees of the home health care agency. Plaintiff claimed that the assailants had gained access to her file through their employment and acting upon this information gained access to the plaintiff's home. Plaintiff claimed that the home health care agency was negligent in hiring the two assailants without testing, references, or other guidelines. The assailants had been convicted of robbery, manslaughter, and other crimes prior to their employment with the home health care agency. The home health care agency contended that it had dismissed the two assailants four months prior to the subject incident and at the time of the incident they were neither in the course or scope of their employment with the home health care agency. A jury returned a verdict for $90,000 in favor of the plaintiff. *Morett v. Kimberly Services*, Case No. 127068 (California, 1990).

Case History No. 5

Plaintiffs Ms. Rue, a 55-year-old actress, and Wright, a 93-year-old retired teacher, asked for in-home care from defendant Action Health Care Services. The attendant, Pamela Reese, worked for Rue from November 1989 to July 1990. During that time, Reese stole several hundred thousand dollars through unauthorized credit card charges, unauthorized automatic teller withdrawals, and forged checks. Rue fired Reese in July 1990. Reese returned to Action Health Care Services under a different name, unknown to Action Health Care. She was then sent out to plaintiff Wright, where she was arrested and pled guilty to grand theft.

Plaintiff claimed negligent referral, vicarious liability, and ratification. Plaintiff also alleged violation of the Elder Abuse and Dependent Adult Act, as well as breach of fiduciary duty, and that Action Health failed to check on Reese and aided and abetted her by not cooperating sooner with the police. Defendant argued that the references, if checked, would check out clear, and there was no criminal background available to Action Health. Defendant also argued that the statute requiring a background check was not applicable because it became effective after the events occurred. The jury returned a verdict for $162,800, $125,000 against Reese and $37,800 against Action Health. *Rue and Wright v. Reese and Action Health Care Services*, Case No. SC011687 (California, 1993).

Abuse Reporting Statutes

Some states require health care providers who suspect that a child or adult has been abused or neglected to report the matter immediately to the local department of social services in which the person resides or in which the abuse or neglect is believed to have occurred.[7] These statutes normally direct that the health care provider shall disclose all information which is the basis for the suspicion of abuse or neglect and upon request to make available to the local department investigating the reported case of child abuse or neglect any records or reports which document the basis for the report.

It is possible that if a home health care agency is aware of such abuse and fails to report it, thus allowing continued abuse, this could give rise to an action for civil damages for failure to make the reporting. (*See* Case History No. 5 above.)

Antitrust Violations

Antitrust problems may arise if a hospital refers all of its patients to one home health care subsidiary. For example, serious antitrust allegations may be raised by competitors who are excluded from exclusive referral arrangements. In a case against Radford Community, Twin County Community, and Giles Memorial Hospitals,[8] a durable medical equipment (DME) supplier contended that the hospitals violated Virginia and federal antitrust laws under the following theories:

1. Unreasonable restraint of trade in violation of the Sherman Act, Section 1
2. Monopolization, attempted monopolization, conspiracy to monopolize, and monopoly leveraging in violation of Sherman Act, Section 2
3. Exclusive dealing in violation of the Clayton Act, Section 3
4. Tortious interference with business relationships under Virginia common law

The U.S. Court of Appeals found that the DME supplier stated a cause of action and the matter was remanded to the district court for trial on the facts. The case centered on allegations that the hospitals directed their discharge staff to refer all DME business to a subsidiary and to deny competitors any access to their patients. Further, the plaintiffs in the case claimed that the marketing presentations made by the hospital discharge planners were biased in favor of the hospitals' subsidiary in that they did not inform discharge patients about other potential suppliers of DME. The suit also alleged that, on occasion, the discharge planners ordered DME from the subsidiary without first consulting the patients.

This case was followed by *M & M Medical Supplies and Services, Inc. v. Pleasant Valley Hospitals, Inc.*, 981 F.2d 160 (4th Cir. 1992), where the appeals court again reversed a district court and held that a DME supplier stated a cause of action when a hospital steered all of its patients to a hospital's DME subsidiary. This situation is also discussed in the same conclusion reached in the widely cited decision of the U.S. Court, in *Key Enterprises of Delaware, Inc. v. Venice Hospital*, 919 F.2d 1550 (11th Cir. 1990).[9]

By analogy from a DME supplier to a home health care agency, a hospital is clearly at risk for litigation from competitors that are not given access to the hospital's patients. Whether the competitor would win such a lawsuit is subject to the facts of each case and is difficult to determine in the abstract. However, factors the court will consider in deciding whether an antitrust violation has occurred include:

1. Whether there is a specific intent to monopolize the relevant market
2. Predatory or anticompetitive acts in furtherance of the intent, and a dangerous possibility of success
3. Liability may also be imposed if the court finds that the hospital used monopoly power in a market to foreclose competition, to gain a competitive advantage, or to destroy a competitor in another distinct market

Because antitrust law is very complex, questions regarding possible antitrust violations should be directed to a competent attorney.

Advance Directives

A person may take legal steps while still mentally capable to anticipate and prepare for eventual incapacity by directing future medical treatment and/or voluntarily delegating future medical decision-making power. It is imperative that the home health care provider have a system in place to assure that these directives are followed.

Living Will

A living will is a document that allows a person to give specific advance directions concerning medical treatment in the event of subsequent mental incapacity. Most states have enacted statutes specifically authorizing the execution of a living will document.[10] In addition, courts in several states without living will statutes have ruled that the written directive of a competent person concerning future medical treatment is entitled to be given legal standing after the person becomes incompetent. In addition to providing a mechanism for expressing future treatment preferences, the living will under many state statutes may also be used by people to designate another individual as their representative and substitute decision maker in the event of future incapacity.

Durable Power of Attorney

A durable power of attorney is a legal document in which an individual may direct, through the appointment of an agent, the making of medical decisions in the event of future incapacity. Every state has a durable power of attorney statute. Even in states without such specific statutes, there appears to be no reason to prevent the general durable power of attorney from applying to medical decisions.

Under the Patient's Self-Determination Act, home care agencies must have policies and procedures for determining whether a client has executed a living will or durable power of attorney. The home care agency must develop and maintain a close working relationship with the substitute decision maker, if any, to whom a client has delegated decision-making authority. The home care agency should obtain a copy of any purported advanced planning document executed by a client, should verify the document's authenticity, and should place that copy in the client's permanent file. The agency must also have policies and procedures for communicating a client's advanced directives status to relevant staff, in a manner that is effective and assures that the client's wishes are respected but that also protects the client's right to confidentiality.

"Do Not" Orders

"Do not" orders may only be written by the client's physician. These orders are predicated on perspectively made decisions, ideally resulting from full discussion between the physician, other members of the health care team, and the client or client's substitute decision maker, to withdraw or withhold certain types of medical interventions from specified clients. Most attention has been devoted to "do not resuscitate" orders, or instructions by the physician to refrain from attempts at CPR in the event of a cardiac arrest. However, other kinds of "do not" orders also are important, especially in the home care environment, such as "do not hospitalize" and "do not treat" orders.

Under the Patient's Self-Determination Act and Joint Commission for the Accreditation of Health Care Organizations standards, home care agencies should develop policies and procedures regarding the entry of "do not" orders for clients. Provisions must be included regarding the decision-making involvement of authorized substitute decision makers, family and friends without formal legal authorization but who function and practice as substitute decision makers, the competent client, and members of the health care team. The agency's policies and procedures also must spell out the relationship of the home care agency and the client's attending physician concerning "do not" orders, expectations of the physician in this regard, and means of monitoring the physician's satisfaction of those expectations and of correcting communication or documentation problems. It should be emphasized that only a licensed physician, and not the home care agency acting independently, may enter a valid "do not" order. Agency staff should receive in-service training regarding the implementation of "do not" orders.

Medicare/Medicaid Reimbursement

Although over 7,000 of the 17,561 home health agencies (HHAs) in the United States remain uncertified for Medicare reimbursement, most HHAs that provide skilled nursing care or that wish to expand their client base beyond "private-pay patients" seek to participate in Medicare.[1] The incentive for participation is the opportunity to share in serving Medicare recipients.

In addition, Medicare certification is a prerequisite for certification for Medicaid and other state-administered programs. In some states, no additional licensing or certification is required once federal certification has been achieved. In other states, there are additional licensing or certification requirements.

In order to become and remain certified, an HHA must be prepared to fulfill the conditions of participation detailed in 42 Code of Federal Regulations 484 and the Home Health Agency Guidelines promulgated by the Health Care Financing Administration (HCFA). Although there are many conditions of participation, they may be grouped in the following categories for a summary overview of the scope of the regulations.

42 CFR Description

484.10 Residents' Rights—Each HHA must "conscientiously try" to inform *each* resident of his or her rights in writing and orally in a language that the resident understands. These rights include a right to: (1) be treated with respect,

(2) voice grievances, (3) have complaints investigated, (4) participate in planning care in advance of the delivery of treatment, (5) have records remain confidential, (6) be informed as to all charges not covered by Medicare or Medicaid, and (7) be informed of the toll-free home health agency hotline in that state.

484.12 Compliance with Statutes, Regulations and Professional Principles—Each HHA must comply with all certification standards and disclosures, and all professional staff must comply with relevant professional standards.

484.14 Organization, Services and Administration—Each HHA must have an established administrative structure and monitor and control all services provided by subunits or subcontractors. The guidelines stress that an HHA may not delegate supervisory administrative responsibilities to a full-time employee of another legal entity.

484.14(a) strictly limits services to "part-time or intermittent skilled nursing services and at least one other therapeutic service...in a place of residence used as a patient's home."

Each HHA must have a governing body with legal authority and responsibility for the operation. The regulations and guidelines prescribe specific qualifications and tasks for the administrator and for the supervising physician or registered nurse who must be available at "all times and at all hours."

Personnel policies must be written, and hourly or per-visit contracts must be written and provide for ongoing supervision by the HHA. All personnel are required to coordinate their efforts and prepare a summary report on each patient every 62 days. Each HHA must prepare institutional plans for annual budgets and capital expenditures.

484.16 Group of Professional Personnel—Each HHA must maintain such a body to establish and review policies.

484.18 Patients—Each HHA must anticipate meeting every patient's needs and formulate and follow a plan of care written by a physician. Each plan must be reviewed by that physician every 62 days.

494.30-38 Staff and Services—The regulations describe the required qualifications of staff and the specific care to be delivered for skilled nursing; physical, occupational, and speech therapy; medical social services; and home health aid services. The regulations include requirements for in-house service training and supervision of home health aides.

484.48-50 Records—Each HHA must maintain, in confidence, patient records for a period of five years.

Although Medicare is the largest single payer of home health services, its regulations provide few details on which services are covered and which are not. The regulations do require that an HHA *must* provide part-time or intermittent skilled nursing services and *at least one other therapeutic service* from a list including physical, speech, and occupational therapies; medical social services; and home health aid services.[11]

Even a certified HHA that has fulfilled these regulatory requirements may find that the HCFA denies payment due to the patient's physical situation or care needs. The reason for this is that Medicare restricts coverage to beneficiaries in certain situations and will only pay for care for those who:

- Are confined to their homes or in an institution that is not a hospital or nursing facility
- Are under a physician's direct care
- Require only "intermittent care"[12]

While the first two restrictions are relatively straightforward, the requirement that care be given only on an "intermittent" basis has raised significant problems. In brief, the HCFA will deny as "not intermittent" any skilled nursing care in excess of 4 days per week, although it will allow reasonable and necessary skilled nursing care for up to 7 days per week for a period of 2 to 3 weeks.[13]

Medicaid will become an increasingly important source of HHA revenue in the 1990s, as long-term care and other institutional costs continue to rise and budget-conscious state Medicaid programs begin to move more recipients into home care settings.[14] Federal regulations require that Medicaid programs utilize only Medicare-certified HHAs. The regulations mandate that a state provide part-time or intermittent skilled nursing, home health aid, and medical supply services. States have the *option* to provide physical, occupational, or speech therapy; speech pathology; or audiology services.[15]

Because of these options, there is wide variation in services covered and in reimbursement issues from state to state. These problems include: (1) denials for "nonintermittent" services, (2) delayed or denied payment due to prior authorization programs, and (3) state limitations on the scope of services.[16]

An HHA affiliated with a nursing facility must be a separate entity. As the guidelines note in regard to the 42 CFR 484.14 requirements of an independent administrative staff, an HHA may not use a full-time employee of another legal entity such as a hospital. If a nursing facility were to organize an affiliated HHA, it would need to establish a completely separate legal entity with a complete separate administrative staff. The guidelines, however, do acknowledge that an HHA may be affiliated with an institute such as a nursing facility. They recognize, in discussing the Group of Professional Persons, that such group need not create wholly new policies if the HHA is "part of a larger organization (e.g. state, county, hospital, etc.)."

References

1. Basic Statistics about Home Care 1995, National Association for Home Care, Washington, D.C.
2. An example of a law requiring a health care provider to accept a patient is the Emergency Medical Treatment and Active Labor Act. This federal law requires a hospital emergency room to accept the patient and perform an appropriate medical screening to determine if the patient is suffering from an emergency medical condition.
3. *Lyons v. Grether*, 218 Va. 630, 239 S.E.2d 103 (1977).
4. *Brown v. Koulizakis*, 229 Va. 524, 331 S.E.2d 440 (1985).
5. *Flinn v. Four Fountains, Inc.*, 536 N.E.2d 89 (5th Dist. Ill. 1989).
6. *See* for example Va. Code Ann. § 32.1-162.9:1.
7. *See* for example Va. Code Ann. § 63.1-248.3 and Va. Code Ann. § 63.1-53-3.
8. *Advanced Health Care Services, Inc. v. Radford Community Hospital*, 910 F.2d 139 (4th Cir. 1990).
9. The Key decision was vacated (*see* 797 F.2d 806 [1992]) after the parties reached a settlement of the case.
10. Much of the information in this section is taken from Haddad, A. M. and Cap, M. B., Withholding and withdrawing medical treatment, *Caring,* 10(9), 1991.
11. 42 CFR 484.14(a); 42 CFR 409.40.
12. 42 CFR 409.42(b).
13. Home Health Agency Manual (HCFA) Publ. 11 § 205.1.C.
14. *See* Dombi, W. A., Medicaid: Home Care, materials from the *Medicare Home Health Conference* (Center for Health Care Law), May 1–3, 1992, pp. 81, 82.
15. 42 CFR 440.70.
16. Dombi, W. A., Medicaid: Home Care, materials from the *Medicare Home Health Conference* (Center for Health Care Law), May 1–3, 1992, p. 83.

Additional References

1. *A Provider's Guide to a Medicare Home Health Certification Process,* National Association for Home Care, Washington, D.C., 1994.
2. Medicare "Cost Containment" and Home Health Care: Potential Liability for Physicians and Hospitals, 21 Ga.L.Rev. 9010 (1987).
3. Home Health Care and Long Term Care: Joint Opportunities, National Health Lawyers Association, Goldberg, Allen S., Esquire.
4. National Association for Home Care, 519 C Street, N.E., Stanton Park, Washington, D.C. 20002-5809, (202) 547-7424.

Total Quality Management in Home Health Care

11

Vanita Bellen, B.S., B.Comm., M.H.S.

Introduction

Total Quality Management (TQM) is a strategy of self-assessment that relies on scientific management principles to proactively make improvements in service so that customers' needs and expectations are met. TQM is a lifelong goal that places an obligation on an organization and all its constituents to do the right thing, all the time. In order for TQM to be successful, it is highly dependent upon management's sincere conviction to uphold ethical practices, its commitment to meeting the needs of the customer, and its respect for and support of its employees' decisions.

Those organizations that have followed these tenets are currently leaders in today's fiercely competitive markets. Those that have not are long forgotten or are perhaps relegated to serve as examples of poor managers of quality in TQM texts. Home health care, being a relatively young field, is in a tremendously advantageous position to learn from others' experiences and consequently avoid pitfalls that manufacturing and service industries have typically encountered.

The Joint Commission on Accreditation of Healthcare Organizations (JCAHO) has been a strong proponent of these principles as evidenced by the evolution of home care standards over the last few years, to a point where the JCAHO now firmly embraces the objectives of TQM. Specifically, the JCAHO views the 1995 home care standards as completing "the transition of home care standards from those that focus on capability to those that focus on actual performance of those functions and processes—both clinical and organizational—that most significantly impact patient care."[1]

©GR/St. Lucie Press CCC 1-884015-93-X 1/97/$100/$.50

The revised standards recognize that processes tend to cross departmental boundaries and, consequently, are organized by function (e.g., leadership, assessment, education) rather than by type of service as in past years (e.g., personal care and support service, pharmaceutical services, equipment management). This, then, allows organizations to be portrayed as they truly are—a wholly integrated system—rather than composed of distinct units that function independently.

The revised standards further support the principles of TQM by not being prescriptive in nature. Instead, as long as the intent of the standard is met, organizations are encouraged to develop innovative strategies to improve quality. In addition, by linking the standards across all functions necessary to home health care, the implication is that the management of quality is the responsibility of *all* individuals and departments within the organization.

Finally, the JCAHO stresses the use of scientifically based methodologies for improving performance. The general framework proposed by the JCAHO is (1) *design* processes to meet customers' needs, (2) *measure* the performance of these processes, (3) *assess* the performance data and identify opportunities for improvement, and (4) *implement* the improvement and *redesign* the process, as necessary. Whether an organization follows the JCAHO's framework—the Shewhart cycle (Plan-Do-Check-Act)—or some other model, it is crucial that the methodology selected is scientifically based and applied consistently.

Undoubtedly, ten different home care agencies surveyed across the country would provide ten different descriptions of their respective quality management programs. Nevertheless, there are some fundamental components of any quality management program, including clinical and nonclinical indicator measurement, customer satisfaction, risk management, staff development, infection control, and utilization review. In addition, the concepts of benchmarking and reengineering have recently become techniques that are integral to improving quality. The remainder of this chapter will address each of these components, their importance to home health care, and the methods by which they can be employed.

Indicator Measurement

An indicator is a quantitative measure that can be used to assess and improve the performance of important functions affecting patient outcomes.[2] The basic types of indicators are structural, process, or outcome based and sentinel events. Structural indicators refer primarily to the rules and regulations under which care is provided. Examples of organizational structure are policies, procedures, resources, and equipment. Process indicators assess those activities that are necessary to deliver home health care.[3] According to the JCAHO, the most beneficial process indicators are those that identify processes which, when conducted effectively, increase the probability of attaining positive patient outcomes. Process indicators can monitor activities that are related to the direct provision of care or those activities that support the patient care function. Outcome indicators assess what occurs after a process is carried out or interventions have been implemented.[3] Finally, sentinel event indicators identify a serious or rare patient care event. All sentinel events warrant in-depth investigations.

Whichever indicators a home care agency selects, it is absolutely crucial that they be reflective of the organization's patient population and target those aspects that have significant impact on the delivery of home health care and health outcomes. When in doubt as to the relevance of selected indicators, it is beneficial to compare them to the JCAHO's focus on activities or elements of care that (1) pose significant risk, (2) affect a large volume of the agency's patient population, and (3) have a tendency to be problem prone.

It is also advisable when selecting indicators that the agency identify each of its key processes and then develop indicators to measure their effectiveness. Elaine R. Davis, in her text *Total Quality Management for Home Care*, suggests that there are approximately 14 distinct functions in the average home care agency:[4]

1. Intake
2. Insurance verification
3. Data entry
4. Scheduling
5. Service delivery
6. Quality assurance/utilization review
7. Medical records
8. Recruitment
9. Staff development
10. Payroll
11. Billing
12. Collections
13. Accounts payable
14. Sales and marketing

An organization that has developed indicators for each of these functions has in all likelihood a comprehensive indicator measurement system.

Data collection or indicator monitoring does not necessarily have to be conducted on a routine basis. It is the agency's decision to prioritize the indicators and decide which ones would yield the greatest value for the patient and the organization if monitored routinely. If an organization uses sampling as a data collection strategy, statistical principles must be followed. Arbitrary data collection methods can yield results that are neither valid nor reliable, and in a time of limited health care dollars, this is an inefficient use of resources. It behooves the organization, then, to carefully select indicators and data collection strategies.

The assessment of indicators can be initiated in various ways. One approach is to define thresholds or acceptable levels for each indicator which, once exceeded, signal the need for investigation into the root cause and the potential or actual effect on the quality of care or service. Second, particular trends observed in indicator data may also signal the need for investigation into the cause of the trend or pattern. The establishment of thresholds and acceptable levels is discussed more fully in the section on benchmarking.

Problem identification and problem solving methods are used extensively during the assessment phase. Although specific problem identification and solving techniques are discussed in this section, these techniques are entirely appropriate for use when quality issues are identified through any of the other components of a quality management program. Also, a significant amount of literature is currently available on problem identification and solving methods. It is the objective in this chapter to describe only a few of these tools and to encourage the reader to investigate other methodologies as well as to develop his or her own techniques.

Brainstorming (sometimes called mind mapping) is best utilized in situations where a large number of creative ideas need to be generated in a short time.[5] Brainstorming can be in either written or oral form.

The *cause-and-effect* (or fishbone) diagram has become one of the most widely used tools in assessing data and conducting root cause analysis. The essence of this method is that the desired outcome of a process is affected by specific types of causes: materials, methods, equipment, and people. Used in conjunction with brainstorming or Pareto charts, the cause-and-effect diagram can further assist in identifying the actions necessary to improve performance once a problem and its cause has been identified.[6]

The *problem selection* matrix is a useful tool for "checking on the need to actually do what you are about to do"[7] (Figure 11.1). This method requires evaluating alternatives or solutions for the identified problem by calculating numerical scores. The criteria by which they are evaluated include the feasibility of acting on the problem, the timeliness with which the problem can be acted upon, potential cost savings, and general importance of the issue. The alternative(s) with the highest score would probably be the solution of choice.

There are several other ways of prioritizing issues and weighting alternatives. Kepner and Tregoe,[8] for example, suggest evaluation using the criteria of

Problems	Variable	Variable	Total

Figure 11.1 Problem selection matrix. (From Forsha, H. I., *Show Me: Storyboard Workbook and Template*, ASQC Quality Press, Milwaukee, Wisconsin, 1995.)

"seriousness, urgency, and growth." In addition, simple scales that rate problems or alternatives as being of high, medium, or low importance can be utilized.

"A flowchart is simply a graphical description of the flow of activities in a system, process or organization."[9] A flowchart is most beneficial when there is a need to know exactly what and who is involved in a process. It is an excellent tool to gain a common understanding of a process and is highly effective because often areas for improvement will be obvious even after simply delineating the process in use.

The *tree diagram* (also known as a *steam and leaf display*) is a useful tool for breaking down a solution into its component parts.[10] This methodology begins with the identification of the root cause and continues by asking at each level why the problem occurred. In this way, branches representing all the possible faulty processes or possible solutions to the problem are identified. (See Figure 11.2 for a general outline of a tree diagram.) Taken a step further, by estimating the probability of each branch, it becomes possible to understand the relationship of one action to another and the relative value of individual actions. This approach is not new and has traditionally been used in making business decisions.

Forsha[11] believes it is unlikely that any improvement activity can be documented without the use of a *Pareto chart*. The Pareto principle, or the 80/20 rule, states that a few activities or items are likely to contribute the most to a problem or an opportunity.[12] When using a Pareto chart, data are categorized and graphed in decreasing order using a bar chart. If a steep decline in bar height is evident, the Pareto principle is in effect and it would be to the organization's advantage to act on the vital few items or activities (see Figure 11.3). If the slope is slight, then an overriding opportunity for improvement has not been identified.

A *run chart* is essentially a line graph that indicates time on the horizontal

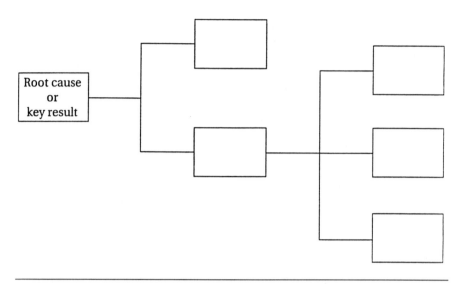

Figure 11.2   Tree diagram. (From Forsha, H. I., *Show Me: Storyboard Workbook and Template*, ASQC Quality Press, Milwaukee, Wisconsin, 1995.)

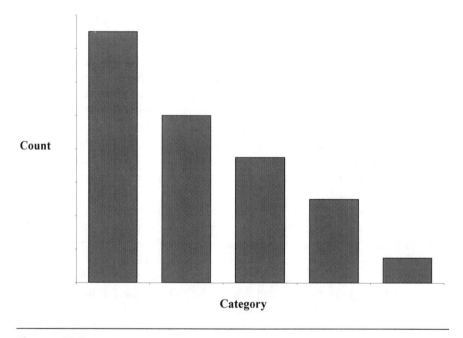

Figure 11.3   Pareto chart.

(x) axis and actual performance data on the vertical (y) axis.[13] Run charts are of most significance in depicting trends and in making comparisons over time. It is recommended that when comparing one period of time to another, the general conditions affecting the organization should be similar. As an example, Davis[14] cites that comparing total visits performed each month in a year of slow growth to the same month in a year with rapid growth would likely yield unreliable assumptions. At a minimum, however, the run chart can be used to determine the average and observe the variation around the average. An example of a run chart is provided in Figure 11.4.

Control charts take the run chart to the next level and portray "the variability of the process characteristic being measured as time passes."[15] Using statistical formulae, control limits can be determined from the performance data collected.

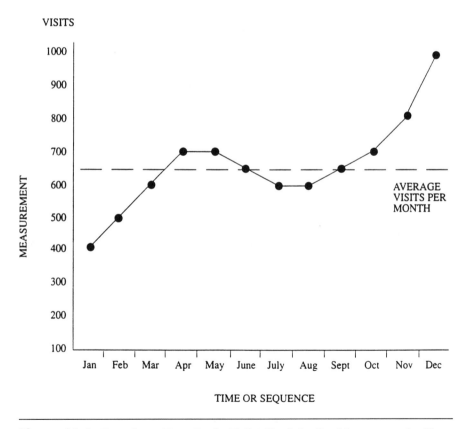

Figure 11.4 Run chart. (From Davis, E. R., *Total Quality Management for Home Care*, Aspen Publishers, Gaithersburg, Maryland, 1994.)

These upper and lower control limits show the range of normal variation that occurs in a particular process. However, "normal" does not necessarily imply acceptable. When a process is in control, then it behaves in a normal way and performance data commonly fall within the upper and lower control limits. A process that is in control can be used to predict future performance.

When a process is out of control, variations that are not normal to that particular process are present. This does not imply that the process is behaving in an unacceptable manner. A process that is out of control simply indicates that a special cause is present and should be removed. As long as abnormal variation is present, then the process cannot be used as a predictor and must be brought into control before improvement efforts can have a reliable effect.

As a point of reference, Davis[15] cites that W. Edwards Deming believed "that over ninety four percent of all problems with processes are common cause occurrences or normal variation and that the remaining six percent are special cause or abnormal variation and, furthermore, that common causes of problems can be attributed to problems with organizational policies, procedures and systems, whereas special causes are a result of individual action." See Figure 11.5 for an illustration of a control chart.

Obviously, the performance improvement tools described do not constitute an exhaustive list. However, it is important to recognize that the power of

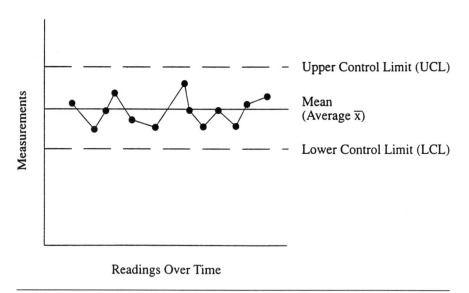

Figure 11.5   Control chart. (From Davis, E. R., *Total Quality Management for Home Care*, Aspen Publishers, Gaithersburg, Maryland, 1994.)

problem-solving tools increases tremendously when they are used in concert. Therefore, an organization that trains all its staff in even a few tools and actually uses them is likely to demonstrate more effective management of quality than an organization that invests heavily in data collection instead of data assessment and implementation. Furthermore, quality improvement tools used in conjunction with "creative thinking, critical thinking and reflective thinking" in a balanced way will increase the likelihood of achieving the best possible result.[16]

The final steps in the JCAHO performance improvement framework require implementation of actions plans and redesigning processes if necessary. Once this stage is reached, the need for data collection, however, is not over. Instead, it is best to view the framework as an ongoing cycle of events that inherently promote continuous or ongoing improvement. Therefore, new designs must be continually monitored in order to yield positive health outcomes.

Outcomes Measurement

Recently, the emphasis by managed care organizations, accrediting bodies, and regulatory agencies has been on the measurement and management of health outcomes. In response to this, many home care agencies have begun to turn to the use of practice guidelines. The goal of these tools is to ensure "that specific patient outcomes can be achieved within fiscally responsible time frames (lengths of stay) while utilizing resources appropriate (in amount and sequence) to the specific case type and the individual patient."[17] This is accomplished through the development of a "multidisciplinary plan [of care] that focuses on the processes of care in relation to outcomes." The descriptors of quality outlined in the tool can be "considered standards of patient care, because they define what the patient can expect and what goals should be achieved by the patient."[17]

Used correctly, these tools become even more powerful because not only do they "set standards but they also provide a framework for the evaluation of these standards."[17] Evaluation occurs by examining variances from the established guidelines or plan. Variances may be positive or negative and, regardless of their status, should be systematically reviewed as they serve as pointers to improving the care provided.

A distinct advantage to these tools is that they allow patient and family involvement in the plan of care and outline patient/family and agency responsibilities as well as the expected outcomes and time frames involved. Furthermore, they put "cost and quality in balance."[17] Most importantly, inherent in the use of practice guidelines are the key components of the quality improvement process: assessment, evaluation, problem solving and implementation, and ongoing follow-up.

A great opportunity exists for home care agencies to develop practice guidelines in collaboration with other health care providers in the community, thereby achieving a seamless care plan that optimizes the concept of continuity of care. Where this may not be feasible, agencies should at minimum work in conjunction with physicians in the community. In any event, it is probably most cost effective to develop guidelines for those diagnoses that have the greatest variation in lengths of stay, visits, frequencies and patterns, cost, and resource consumption. High-cost and high-tech diagnoses should also be examined.

Currently, much research is being done throughout the country in the measurement of outcomes in home health care. For example, the Center for Health Policy and Services Research at the University of Colorado is involved in a number of projects, including the development of a universal outcomes-based assessment tool, revision of the Functional Assessment Instrument for use by home health care surveyors, and comparisons of outcomes in rural and urban settings.[18] The National League for Nursing has obtained consumer opinions to define quality of outcomes. The result has been the development of a scorecard to measure one agency's performance against similar home care organizations.[18] An additional example of research being conducted is Brandeis University's work in developing measures of the adequacy of care being provided by paraprofessionals in home health care.[18]

These tools are readily available and, even if an agency is not involved in their testing, should be sought out and utilized to measure outcomes. This can be done relatively simplistically, by focusing, for example, on changes in functional status (activities of daily living and independent activities of daily living) between admission and discharge. Another issue to review may be readmissions to the acute care setting. Of additional benefit may be to compare the findings among the various insurers in the agency's mix and identifying trends in practice patterns and resource use. The message however is clear: home care agencies must in some way, however simplistic, begin to focus on the outcome of the care and service they provide.

Customer Satisfaction

In TQM, the key to an organization's success is the satisfaction of its internal and external customers. The literature consistently stresses that the initial step in meeting customers' needs and expectations is to first define who the customer actually is.

In the home health care environment, external customers include payors, governmental and other regulatory bodies, physicians, referral sources, and patients and their families. Internal customers include all employees of the agency, both as individuals and as representatives of a function or department.

Davidow and Uttal,[19] in their book *Total Customer Service, The Ultimate Weapon*, suggest that customers' expectations are shaped by the way an organization has treated them in the past. New customers or infrequent users have their expectations shaped primarily by word of mouth.[19] Negative word of mouth can be detrimental to an organization, whether it is cited by external or internal customers. Depending upon the industry and the nature of the negative experience, the unhappy customer will complain to between 10 and 20 individuals.[20] In comparison, positive experiences are likely to be shared with only a third as many individuals.[20] With odds such as these, the only reasonable action an organization can take is to know what its customers need and want and then offer a level of service that satisfies every customer.

In keeping with the JCAHO framework for performance improvement, a crucial element in meeting customers' needs is the assessment of customers' satisfaction levels. Traditionally, customer satisfaction has been viewed as a "soft" indicator of quality.[21] It is "soft" because the focus is on perceptions and attitudes rather than objective criteria. This is not to say that perceptions and attitudes cannot be measured at all. To do so effectively, however, the measurement tools selected should be well constructed and scientifically based. If not, the viability of an organization may be at risk, particularly because the data will be used as the basis of some strategic planning decisions.

Complaints are an invaluable source of information because they are often filed immediately after a negative incident has occurred, when details are clear and can be readily analyzed. In addition, because the incident may have occurred in the recent past, the organization may still have the power to rectify the situation even to a small degree and perhaps not lose a valued customer. Monitoring complaints is also cost effective because most governmental and regulatory bodies require that the home care agency have a system of tracking and following up on customer complaints. Therefore, there is no need for the duplication of resources.

Assessing complaint data is most effectively done by observing trends in the nature of complaints. Because each complaint will have its own particular circumstances, it may be useful to identify several categories of complaints and define the elements that constitute these types of complaint. See Figure 11.6 for examples of complaint categories. When analyzing complaint data, it is useful to look for trends in complaint types in relation to other elements, such as specific departments, teams, branch offices, patient demographics, etc. The objective in doing this is not to focus on individual performance but to work with the appropriate departments in determining the root causes of the incidents and then deploy resources to minimize the frequency and severity of that type of complaint.

- Communication and Behavior

- Practice/Duties

- Provision of Service

- Alleged Theft

- Timeliness of Service

Figure 11.6 Sample complaint categories.

A rating system can be beneficial in complaint analysis. The scale may be simple, such as one that rates a complaint as being of high, medium, or low severity. However, it is best not to rely solely on severity data because of the subjectivity in evaluating the complaint. Also, a high frequency of minor complaints could be more detrimental than an infrequently occurring type of incident that has a high severity rating. This type of information can be beneficial in awareness campaigns as the agency tries to communicate to staff the types of complaints and their effects. Another analytical approach to examining customer satisfaction data, while accounting for the growth in an agency, is the frequency of complaints relative to the volume of patients served or relative to the number of patient days. The organization can then establish a threshold or acceptable level which when exceeded warrants additional analysis and action.

Satisfaction questionnaires can be one of the easiest methods to gather data that accurately represent customers' needs and expectations and can be administered to internal and external customers. When developing a questionnaire, Hays recommends first defining dimensions of quality that the organization believes to be important in satisfying customers.[21] Examples of quality dimensions that are particularly applicable to service industries are availability, responsiveness, convenience, and timeliness.[22] Questions can be developed for each dimension as well as for determining overall satisfaction with the agency, and scores can be tabulated using a scale such as the Likert scale. Furthermore, through regression analysis, the impact of each dimension on overall satisfaction can be ascertained. This then allows for a systematic deployment of resources that target those needs on which the customer places the highest value. See Figure 11.7 for an example of a patient satisfaction survey.

Organizations that cannot invest heavily in a 100% review of all customers via questionnaires should consider the use of sampling methods and focus groups to gain satisfaction data. It is crucial, however, that this data be collected in one way or another because the long-term viability of any organization depends upon satisfying its customers' needs.

Please indicate the extent to which you agree or disagree with the following statements about the service you received from Genesee Region Home Care.

Genesee Region Home Care staff:

	STRONGLY AGREE	AGREE	NEITHER AGREE NOR DISAGREE	DISAGREE	STRONGLY DISAGREE
1. Were organized and well prepared.	☐	☐	☐	☐	☐
2. Answered my questions in a thorough and knowledgeable manner.	☐	☐	☐	☐	☐
3. Provided services to me in a timely manner.	☐	☐	☐	☐	☐
4. Handled my telephone inquiries promptly and politely.	☐	☐	☐	☐	☐
5. Treated me and my belongings with respect.	☐	☐	☐	☐	☐
6. Included me and/or my family in planning my care.	☐	☐	☐	☐	☐
7. Were neatly dressed and well groomed.	☐	☐	☐	☐	☐

Overall:

8. Genesee Region Home Care's staff and service met my expectations.	☐	☐	☐	☐	☐
9. If I ever needed home care again, I would request Genesee Region Home Care.	☐	☐	☐	☐	☐
10. I would recommend Genesee Region Home Care to others.	☐	☐	☐	☐	☐

How do you feel about the following services and the people who served you?

	VERY SATISFIED	SATISFIED	DISSATISFIED	VERY DISSATISFIED	DID NOT RECEIVE SERVICE
• Home Care Coordination (in hospital)	☐	☐	☐	☐	☐
• Community Health Nursing	☐	☐	☐	☐	☐
• Home Health Aide	☐	☐	☐	☐	☐
• Social Work	☐	☐	☐	☐	☐
• Physical Therapy	☐	☐	☐	☐	☐
• Occupational Therapy	☐	☐	☐	☐	☐
• Speech Therapy	☐	☐	☐	☐	☐
• Equipment and Supplies	☐	☐	☐	☐	☐
• Oxygen Services/Respiratory	☐	☐	☐	☐	☐

How did you first hear about Genesee Region Home Care?

☐ Physician   ☐ Discharge Planner   ☐ Social Worker   ☐ Family/Friend   ☐ Other _____ (please specify)

If we would like further details, may we call you?   ☐ Yes   ☐ No

Comments: _____

_____

Optional:

Patient's Name: _____   Name of Survey Respondent: _____

Address: _____   (Relationship to Patient): _____

Phone Number: _____

Figure 11.7   Genesee Region Home Care client satisfaction survey. (Reprinted with permission of Genesee Region Home Care, Inc., Rochester, New York.)

Employee satisfaction data should be given serious consideration because it can be a predictor of the views of the external customers. If conducting a staff satisfaction survey, the organization must be prepared to respond to the comments and suggestions in a timely manner. If an organization is unable to respond to staff needs, it is better to defer the exercise until such a time when a response will be timely and complete. Otherwise, the impression left with employees is that the exercise may have been conducted to appease them and that the organization does not place a high value on their opinions and suggestions. See Figure 11.8 for an example of a questionnaire that can be used to evaluate employee satisfaction with internally provided services.

Communicating patient satisfaction data to the members of the organization is just as important in promoting continuous improvement as is the collection and assessment of the satisfaction data. Since the employees are the emissaries of the agency, their comprehension of customer needs directly affects the degree to which these needs can be met. Their efforts can be supported by management through the provision of complete information and acknowledgment of their significance to the overall success and viability of the organization.

Staff Development

The education of agency staff is a key element in promoting and sustaining high-quality services. The 1995 JCAHO standards require that the home care agency have a well-defined educational plan aimed at improving the outcomes of care.[1] Any educational plan should begin with a thorough employee orientation. It is during this time that the agency's mission and philosophy should be conveyed and the groundwork set to assure staff of their value to the agency and the agency's continuing support in improving their knowledge base. It is also imperative that new staff are made aware of the functions performed by all departments in the agency, as this promotes not only a common understanding of the organization's objectives but stimulates communication and coordination among disciplines in the long run.

The testing and demonstration of competence is another component of staff development that receives considerable attention in the home care standards. Organizations are responsible for deciding which competencies must be maintained by a particular employee group. In addition, all employees should be able to demonstrate competence in concepts such as emergency/disaster preparedness, and clinical specialists must have continuously updated information that proves their competence in their area of specialty, as must those who provide education to other staff members.

Directions: **When completing this questionnaire, keep in mind that as an internal customer** **you or your department depend on other departments within GRHC to provide a service(s)** **to you. Please indicate the extent to which you agree or disagree with the following statements.**

Overall at GRHC, most departments	STRONGLY AGREE	AGREE	NEITHER AGREE NOR DISAGREE	DISAGREE	STRONGLY DISAGREE
1. Are available when help is needed.	☐	☐	☐	☐	☐
2. Are quick to respond to requests.	☐	☐	☐	☐	☐
3. Complete jobs/tasks within the agreed time frame.	☐	☐	☐	☐	☐
4. Complete all phases of the job agreed upon.	☐	☐	☐	☐	☐
5. Conduct themselves in a professional manner.	☐	☐	☐	☐	☐
6. Listen to their internal customers.	☐	☐	☐	☐	☐
7. Treat their internal customers in a considerate manner.	☐	☐	☐	☐	☐
8. Provide high quality results/response.	☐	☐	☐	☐	☐
9. Generally meet expectations.	☐	☐	☐	☐	☐

Which departments provide you with high quality service?

_____

Specifically, what characteristics do you believe contribute to this high quality service:

_____
_____
_____

Which departments do NOT provide you with high quality service?

_____

Specifically, what characteristics do you believe contribute to this lower quality service:

_____
_____
_____

Ideas/suggestions for improving the quality of service GRHC departments provide **to their internal customers:**

_____
_____
_____
_____

Comments:

_____
_____
_____
_____
_____

(Please use back of sheet for additional comments and suggestions)

Figure 11.8 Genesee Region Home Care staff satisfaction survey. (Reprinted with permission of Genesee Region Home Care, Inc., Rochester, New York.)

Areas for demonstrating competency may be altered depending upon the changing patient population and the strategic objectives of the organization; therefore, they should be reviewed periodically. Demonstration of competencies should not be limited to clinical personnel either, because all individuals and departments indirectly or directly contribute to the facilitation of a process to

	Satisfactory	Unsatisfactory	Comments
1. Selects a suitable work space for bag (adequate size, as convenient as possible to handwashing facility, using moisture-resistant furniture if possible).			
2. Protects furniture and nursing bag (uses newspaper under bag, or acceptable substitute).			
3. Washes hands without contaminating inside of bag, removes at least 3 towels and soap-permeated towelette. Closes bag. Removes jewelry and frees arms to elbows. Washes thoroughly, using friction, starting at forearms and working toward fingertips. Rinses under running water. Dries thoroughly. Uses appropriate water supply, bathroom if possible.			
4. Puts on apron.			
5. Removes extra towels for later handwashing.			
6. Anticipates and removes needed equipment for visit. (For taking rectal temperature in this case.)			
7. Closes bag and does not re-enter without washing hands.			
8. Uses thermometer with proper technique.			
9. Disposes of waste adequately and safely (all liquid waste in toilet, rather than sink).			
10. Cleans or wraps used equipment appropriately before placing in bag.			

Figure 11.9 Genesee Region Home Care checklist for performance of nursing bag technique. (Reprinted with permission of Genesee Region Home Care, Inc., Rochester, New York.)

meet the patient's health care needs. Figure 11.9 provides a sample of a post-test required to determine new clinical staff's competence in bag technique.

An organization's commitment to staff development must be demonstrable to the JCAHO surveyor. One way to obtain this information is through staff interviews. Needless to say, no elaborately written educational plan will be of assistance to the organization if staff do not believe that management supports and provides for their educational needs. Management, in turn, may want to consider setting aside a number of hours annually, quarterly, or monthly for staff education and present topics that are appropriate to the agency's patient mix.

Agencies with limited resources for establishing educational programs should consider linking up with other agencies and investing in interactive (educational) software and audio and video cassettes, as well as self-study courses. Any home care agency that wishes to remain competitive must acknowledge the connection between staff development and improved quality of care and service and act accordingly.

Risk Management

Incident Reporting

Although issues pertaining to the management of risk in the home health care environment have been touched upon in preceding sections, the subject warrants some additional discussion. The objective of any risk management program is to identify risks and prevent them from occurring. The most effective method of identifying risks is to have this done by those who come into contact with them on a daily basis, whether these risks are in a client's home, on the way to a visit, or in the administrative office. Staff participation, therefore, in the identification of risks is an integral factor in either preventing or minimizing those risks.

Incident reports are fundamental to the gathering of risk information and determining organizational trends. In order to be truly useful, however, reporting must occur in a timely manner (for example within 24 hours); otherwise, the ability to minimize or prevent loss is diminished. Because they are such valuable tools, incident reports should be formulated in such a way that information can be readily extracted. It may be helpful, therefore, to set up reports that provide triggers or locators for completion, rather than having entirely narrative explanations. This does not, however, discount the necessity for narrative explanation.

The type of data that can provide clues to agency practices and trends includes not only the type of incident but also the location of the occurrence, the time of day, patient/employee demographics, and psychosocial factors. With this specific information about the agency's client and employee incidents, resources can be allocated in the most efficient manner.

Once incident data are collected, they should definitely be related back to employees. Awareness at this level is a crucial factor in minimizing risk, as these individuals are on the front line. See Figure 11.10 for a sample report.

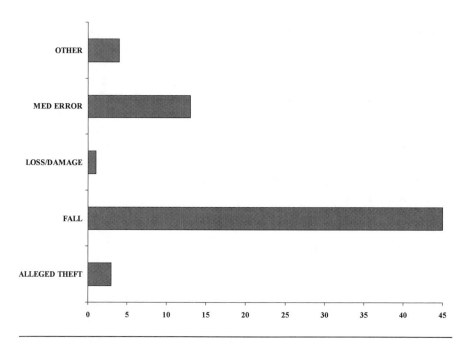

Figure 11.10   Sample incident reporting (fictitious data). (Reprinted with permission of Genesee Region Home Care, Inc., Rochester, New York.)

Focused monitoring of particular incident types is also encouraged. Some of these are important due to their relevance to the home care environment while others are high-risk or high-liability issues. For a sample of incident types, see Figure 11.11. It should be mentioned that JCAHO standards specifically require examination of medication errors and adverse drug reactions. If not already being monitored, these two items should be added to an agency's incident report.

In keeping with the JCAHO performance improvement framework, once incidents are identified, actions should be taken to prevent future occurrences. The formulation of an action plan can include the individuals involved in the incident, the patient's caregiver, as well as administrative representation, such as the risk manager or employee health nurse. Unfortunately, there is a tendency when delineating action plans to address only the immediate incident. It is the administrative representative's role to ensure that a broader perspective is taken and appropriate agency-wide actions are taken.

Safety

The JCAHO has dedicated an entire chapter in the 1995 standards manual to the function of managing the environment of care. The environment refers not only

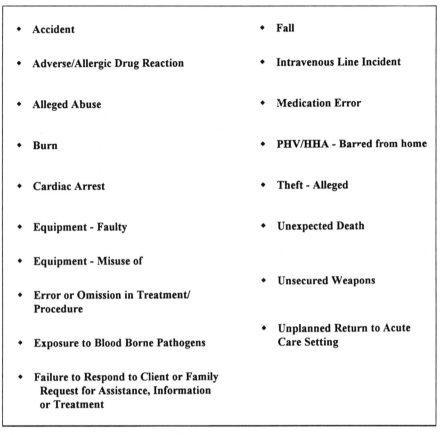

Figure 11.11 Sample incident types.

to the client's home but also to the office, warehouse, pharmacy, delivery van, or anywhere else patient care support activities take place.[23]

In the event of disasters, natural or otherwise, the JCAHO expects all home care agencies to have disaster preparedness plans in place. Furthermore, it expects these plans to be tested and the agency's performance assessed. In addition, the agency's clients must be informed of the agency's procedures during a disaster and the resources available to the client at such a time. It is best if this is discussed at the time of admission, backed up with written documentation such as emergency phone numbers, and then reviewed with the client on an as-needed basis.

In maintaining the integrity of medical devices and equipment, the organization must conduct functional testing as required by the manufacturer or as current practice dictates. In addition, the agency must maintain records of any preventive or other maintenance required on all pieces of equipment. Home care agencies are also bound by the Medical Devices Act to monitor and regularly report any malfunctions in equipment and devices that result in injury or death. Accrediting bodies will look closely for compliance with this legislation.

Education is an integral component of any safety program. Education for staff and clients should incorporate topics such as disaster preparedness, fire safety, equipment maintenance and malfunction procedures, and use, storage, and disposal of hazardous materials. Staff must be able to demonstrate competence in these fundamentals and must also assess and teach the client about them, as appropriate. Evidence of teaching and the client's response must be documented in the health record.

It is reasonable to expect that a surveyor will interview both staff and patients with regard to safety issues. With staff, the agency should expect that the surveyors will also ask about the agency's responsiveness to their environmental concerns. Thus, education of staff, maintenance of records, and complete documentation can provide the supporting evidence necessary for a successful review of the agency's ability to manage the environment of care.

Utilization Management

Given the focus on managed care in today's environment, significant time and space should be allotted to discuss utilization management (UM). However, this chapter will touch very briefly on this topic (also see the section on outcomes measurement).

UM "is a process by which appropriate utilization of services is validated in accordance with guidelines established by the payor source, including the efficient use of resources."[24] Although UM has traditionally been viewed as the review of claims and corresponding documentation before billing, in an era of managed care, the role of UM has grown significantly. UM can encompass, among other items, the review or examination of the following:

- Visit frequencies
- Visit frequencies for particular diagnoses
- Cost per visit
- Costs per member
- Appropriateness of discharge
- Appropriateness of admission to home care
- Integration of service

It is typically a significant component of any outcomes measurement project.

Infection Control

Infection control programs must strive to improve patient health outcomes through the identification of risks for infections among patients and staff. To accomplish this goal, the infection control program must consist of surveillance activities, be appropriate to the organization's patient population, and must address epidemiologically important issues.

Surveillance or monitoring must be conducted on an ongoing basis to ensure that staff first follow infection control policies and procedures and then establish baseline data by which to compare themselves. Monitoring employee infections is also necessary in meeting the intent of the JCAHO standard to reduce the risk of transmission of infections. Incident reporting is one mechanism by which to follow employee infections. Data collection methods will vary across agencies and will not be the focus of this section. Instead, the emphasis is to develop a monitoring system and then to use it consistently.

Organizations that supply equipment to patients must have well-defined cleaning and disinfection protocols. This even applies to organizations that provide only category 1 equipment. It is highly probable that the JCAHO surveyor will observe pickup, delivery, and storage methods of equipment to ensure adherence to fundamental infection control procedures.

Assessment and reporting of infection data should be conducted in a variety of ways, but should consistently follow epidemiological principles. One commonly used method is to calculate rates of infection (the number of infections per 1,000 patient days). Similar to the indicator measuring the frequency of complaints discussed earlier, it may also be beneficial to report infection rates by categories such as intravenous, wound, respiratory, urinary, and decubiti. Whatever categories are selected, they should reflect the patient and diagnosis mix. See Figures 11.12 and 11.13 for examples of rate-based statistical and graphical reports.

For purposes of educating staff, it is helpful to present rate-based information in a visual format. Graphical representation of increases and decreases in infection rates and then correlating these changes to particular occurrences, education, and other factors can be an extremely powerful teaching tool for staff. If rate-based information is too difficult to comprehend for all staff, the data should be presented in an understandable form. Instead of reporting that the rate of urinary infections during the first quarter was x infections per 1,000 patient days, consider saying, "Did you know that of x patients at risk for urinary tract infections, y patients actually developed infections?" Ensuring that staff understand the data is one of the key elements in preventing future infections.

	LIMITS	JAN	FEB	MAR	APR	MAY	JUN	JUL	AUG	SEP	OCT	NOV	DEC
IV													
Urinary													
Respiratory													
Wound													
Decubiti													
Other													
Average:													

Figure 11.12   Sample infection control report. (Reprinted with permission of Genesee Region Home Care, Inc., Rochester, New York.)

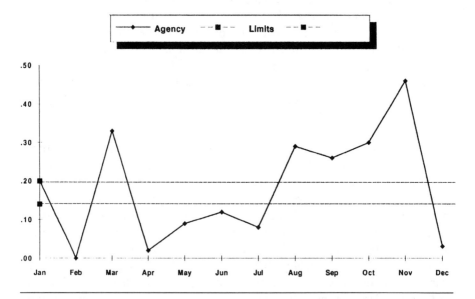

Figure 11.13   Sample graphical representation of infection control data for urinary infections (fictitious data). (Reprinted with permission of Genesee Region Home Care, Inc., Rochester, New York.)

Educating staff as to new practices and OSHA regulations is also required by the JCAHO. Other than being a regulatory requirement, it is obvious that this has some fundamental advantages, and therefore, techniques and principles of infection control should be reinforced on a periodic basis. Also, in keeping with JCAHO requirements, agencies should require that their home visiting staff be able to demonstrate competency in these procedures. Examples of competency testing can include handwashing, bag technique, and disposal of contaminated supplies.

The responsibility for education does not end with staff, however. Teaching clients and, most importantly, having them comprehend infection control procedures is also required. Agencies must be able to demonstrate through documentation in the patient record that teaching was conducted and the client was able to respond appropriately.

Once an organization has identified areas of risk or particularly problematic trends, it must develop action plans to reduce these risks. These actions can range from simple educational material to in-depth in-services on particular diseases or organisms to dramatic changes in agency practice.

Although infection control is a distinct function, the information gleaned impacts many other functions (e.g., care, treatment and service, and improvement of organizational performance). It also strengthens the need for efficiently operating functions, such as management of information, due to its dependence upon reliable and consistent data. It is obvious, then, that the identification and prevention of infections must be firmly integrated into a home care agency's systems for reasons of both positive patient outcomes and the protection of its staff.

Benchmarking

Defined as "an external focus on internal activities, functions or operations in order to achieve continuous quality improvement,"[25] benchmarking is emerging in leading-edge companies as a tool for obtaining competitive advantage. McNair and Leibfried[25] suggest that benchmarking embodies "the pursuit of excellence, the desire to be the best of the best."

The objective of benchmarking is to understand an existing process and then to identify an external standard by which the activity can be measured. Subsequently, management can make decisions about resource allocation and the strategic focus of the organization. Put another way, benchmarking facilitates the identification of best practice and adds value to the product or service by creating the same outputs with fewer inputs or more outputs with the same amount of inputs.[25]

Benchmarking is similar to the continuous improvement process in that it requires:

1. The identification of the problem or issue
2. The establishment of a baseline internal performance level
3. The gathering of external information
4. Analysis of data
5. Implementing changes in the process to reflect the results of benchmarking[25]

In fact, benchmarking is simply a systematic method that also closely follows the principles of the Shewhart cycle (Plan-Do-Check-Act). Therefore, benchmarking is in fact complementary to the continuous improvement process. However, "where continuous improvement is tweaking the existing process, benchmarking may result in throwing away existing practice and starting all over."[25]

When deciding who to benchmark against, it should be noted that there are essentially four levels. *Internal* benchmarking demands that the organization analyze existing practice within its departments and determine the best performance.[26] This methodology is useful when industry data are unavailable. One suggested use of internal benchmarking in home care is in the analysis of infection control. At this time, data on home care infection rates are limited, so an agency should consider calculating its own infection rates, establishing acceptable levels, and then comparing future rates to this acceptable level. In this way, continuous improvement can be promoted by decreasing the acceptable levels of infection rates over time.

Competitive benchmarking looks outward to identify how an organization's competitors are performing.[27] The key to this methodology is for the organization to first identify its own strengths and weaknesses. In situations where data from direct competitors are unavailable, a home care agency may decide to set up a consortium of agencies that have similar characteristics to the agency and its competitors (such as patient mix, population base, annual visits, number of employees) and use these data to make approximations or draw conclusions about its direct competitors.

Industry benchmarking suggests examining trends in the industry as a whole.[8] It should be noted that a uniform database for the home health care industry is currently being prepared by the National Association for Home Care.

Best-in-class benchmarking looks across industries in order to learn about innovative practices.[28] This type of benchmarking has been more evident in the area of customer service practice than in any other area. Manufacturing industries have learned about customer service from service industries and vice versa. Home care agencies should also look to other industries for this information. In addition, home care should not ignore the fact that much can be learned from within the health care industry itself, particularly from long-established fields such as acute and long-term care.

Reengineering

Hammer and Champy,[29] in their book *Reengineering the Corporation*, see reengineering as a way of reinventing an organization by making radical changes. Like benchmarking, reengineering and TQM are complementary as they both focus on customers and processes. Also, because they both emphasize process, they acknowledge that functions and processes cross departmental boundaries. Whereas TQM promotes incremental change, reengineering relies upon dramatic and perhaps rapid change. Whereas TQM keeps a process finely tuned, reengineering may require that the process be completely abolished and the organization start all over again.

Some characteristics of reengineered processes include:

1. Many jobs are combined into one. Imagine the effect on customer satisfaction if one individual were knowledgeable about all of a customer's needs.
2. Workers make decisions. It is important to recognize that workers are not merely empowered to make decisions, but rather it is a requirement of their job.
3. There are multiple versions of the same process. In this way, a simple request by a customer that can actually be handled quickly is not funneled through a series of unnecessary procedures that are appropriate for more complex requests.
4. Work is performed where it makes the most sense, even if that means breaking down traditional departmental barriers.
5. Checks and balances are reduced, specifically when they add no value to the product or service.
6. The number of external contact points in a process is reduced and, instead, a case manager serves as a single point of contact.
7. Departments are neither centralized nor decentralized. Instead, they are hybrid structures that connect all the various functions needed to complete a task. [29]

Because reengineering entails rethinking every aspect of a business, organizations must be serious about investing in this process. Also, the organization should not be arbitrary in its decisions to reengineer a process. It is crucial that an organization know the time and place when radical change is required for its continued survival. Coupled with continuous improvement, reengineering may be exactly what is needed to counter criticism that TQM is slow moving.

Conclusion

In an era of shrinking budgets and health care reform, home health care must carve out and secure a niche for itself. Traditional strategies to accomplish this goal involve the use of sound fiscal and operational practices. To truly be competitive in its market, and to guarantee its long-term viability, however, an organization's complementary strategy must be the management of the quality of its processes and functions.

The underlying requirements for effective quality management in any organization are a focus on the identification and satisfaction of customer needs, clearly evident commitment from leaders, employee participation in problem resolution, and integration of quality throughout the organization. In home health care, the basic structural elements of a quality management plan involve process and outcome indicator measurement, risk management, utilization review, staff development, infection control, and customer satisfaction. The quality management process itself should be built around a systematic, consistently utilized framework and the specific tools used for assessment must be scientifically based. Additionally, home care agencies must involve their customers and staff in problem solving and must then be willing to act on these recommendations. All the benefits of this effort can be lost if information is not disseminated to the organization's members and customers. Finally, it is most important to recognize that quality management is a never-ending, continuously driving process of investigation, action, and reinvestigation.

References

1. The Joint Commission on Accreditation of Healthcare Organizations, *1995 Accreditation Manual for Home Care,* Volume 1, JCAHO, Oakbrook Terrace, Illinois, 1995.
2. The Joint Commission on Accreditation of Healthcare Organizations, *Assessing and Improving Community Health Care Delivery*, JCAHO, Oakbrook Terrace, Illinois, 1994.
3. The Joint Commission on Accreditation of Healthcare Organizations, *Assessing and Improving Community Health Care Delivery*, JCAHO, Oakbrook Terrace, Illinois, 1994, p. 77.
4. Davis, E. R., *Total Quality Management for Home Care,* Aspen Publishers, Gaithersburg, Maryland, 1994.

5. Forsha, H. I., *Show Me: Storyboard Workbook and Template*, ASQC Quality Press, Milwaukee, Wisconsin, 1995.
6. Davis, E. R., *Total Quality Management for Home Care*, Aspen Publishers, Gaithersburg, Maryland, 1994, pp. 56–57.
7. Forsha, H. I., *Show Me: Storyboard Workbook and Template*, ASQC Quality Press, Milwaukee, Wisconsin, 1995, p. 3.
8. Kepner, C. H. and Tregoe, B. B., *The New Rational Manager*, Princeton Press, Princeton, New Jersey, 1981.
9. Forsha, H. I., *Show Me: Storyboard Workbook and Template*, ASQC Quality Press, Milwaukee, Wisconsin, 1995, p. 6.
10. Forsha, H. I., *Show Me: Storyboard Workbook and Template*, ASQC Quality Press, Milwaukee, Wisconsin, 1995, p. 14.
11. Forsha, H. I., *Show Me: Storyboard Workbook and Template*, ASQC Quality Press, Milwaukee, Wisconsin, 1995, p. 10.
12. Davis, E. R., *Total Quality Management for Home Care*, Aspen Publishers, Gaithersburg, Maryland, 1994, pp. 55–56.
13. Forsha, H. I., *Show Me: Storyboard Workbook and Template*, ASQC Quality Press, Milwaukee, Wisconsin, 1995, p. 5.
14. Davis, E. R., *Total Quality Management for Home Care*, Aspen Publishers, Gaithersburg, Maryland, 1994, p. 43.
15. Davis, E. R., *Total Quality Management for Home Care*, Aspen Publishers, Gaithersburg, Maryland, 1994, p. 46.
16. Forsha, H. I., *Show Me: Storyboard Workbook and Template*, ASQC Quality Press, Milwaukee, Wisconsin, 1995, p. ix.
17. Hampton, D. C., Implementing a managed care framework through care maps, *JONA,* 23(5):21–27, 1993.
18. Williams, J. K., Measuring outcomes in home care: current research and practice, *Home Health Care Services Quarterly,* 15(3):3–30, 1995.
19. Davidow, W. H. and Uttal, B., *Total Customer Service, The Ultimate Weapon*, Harper-Perennial, New York, 1989.
20. Davidow, W. H. and Uttal B., *Total Customer Service, The Ultimate Weapon*, Harper-Perennial, New York, 1989, p. 35.
21. Hayes, B. E., *Measuring Customer Satisfaction; Development and Use of Questionnaires*, ASQC Press, Milwaukee, Wisconsin, 1992.
22. Hayes, B. E., *Measuring Customer Satisfaction; Development and Use of Questionnaires*, ASQC Press, Milwaukee, Wisconsin, 1992, p. 8.
23. The Joint Commission on Accreditation of Healthcare Organizations, *1995 Accreditation Manual for Home Care,* Volume 1, JCAHO, Oakbrook Terrace, Illinois, 1995, p. 39.
24. Davis, E. R., *Total Quality Management for Home Care*, Aspen Publishers, Gaithersburg, Maryland, 1994, p. 247.
25. McNair, C. J. and Leibfried, K. H. J., *Benchmarking: A Tool for Continuous Improvement*, Oliver Wight Publications, Essex Junction, Vermont, 1992.
26. McNair, C. J. and Leibfried, K. H. J., *Benchmarking: A Tool for Continuous Improvement*, Oliver Wight Publications, Essex Junction, Vermont, 1992, p. 28.

27. McNair, C. J. and Leibfried, K. H. J., *Benchmarking: A Tool for Continuous Improvement*, Oliver Wight Publications, Essex Junction, Vermont, 1992, p. 29.
28. McNair, C. J. and Leibfried, K. H. J., *Benchmarking: A Tool for Continuous Improvement*, Oliver Wight Publications, Essex Junction, Vermont, 1992, p. 30.
29. Hammer, M. and Champy, J., *Reengineering the Corporation*, HarperBusiness, New York, 1994.

Other Readings

Albrect, K. and Zemke, R., *Service America!* Warner Books, New York, 1990.
Bellen, V., Employing a system approach to customer satisfaction, *J. Healthcare Quality*, 16(4):6–10, 1994.
Berwick. D., Continuous improvement as an ideal in health care, *New Engl. J. Med.*, 320(1):53–56, 1989.
Bone, D. and Griggs, R., *Quality at Work: A Personal Guide to Professional Standards*, Crisp Publications, Los Altos, California, 1989.
Joiner, B., *Fourth Generation Management—The New Business Consciousness*, McGraw-Hill, New York, 1994.
Quality Resources/The Kraus Organization, *Beyond the Basics of Reengineering: Survival Tactics for the '90's,* Industrial Engineering and Management Press, Norcross, Georgia, 1994.
Scholtes, R. R., *The Team Handbook: How to Use Teams to Improve Quality*, Joiner Associates, Madison, Wisconsin, 1988.
Shaughnessy, P. W. and Crisler, K. S., *Outcomes-Based Quality Improvement: A Manual for Home Care Agencies on How to Use Outcomes,* National Association for Home Care, Washington, D.C., 1995.
The Joint Commission on Accreditation of Healthcare Organizations, *1995 Accreditation Manual for Home Care,* Volume 2, Scoring Guidelines, JCAHO, Oakbrook Terrace, Illinois, 1995.

Pediatric Home Health Care

12

Sofia M. Franco, M.D.

In the past two decades, home health care has grown tremendously. In pediatrics, home health care has always been the predominant form of health care, with parents bearing the primary responsibility.[1] Caring for the ill child in the home setting is a tradition that predates scientific medicine. Families provided care to ill children in their home under the guidance of physicians. Hospitalization occurred only when the illness became life-threatening or surgery was necessary.

History

In the United States, the first multidisciplinary home health program began in 1946 when Montefiore Hospital in New York developed its "hospital without walls," an acute care program for patients after hospitalization. Further development of home care was enhanced when insurance companies began to include home nursing as a covered service.[2] Metropolitan Life was the first to provide such coverage in 1909, and by the 1920s many other insurance companies also reimbursed these services. However, the most significant impact on the development of home care in the United States was Title XVIII (Medicare) and Title XIX (Medicaid) of the Social Security Act of 1965, which became the primary sources of reimbursement for adult and pediatric home care services, respectively. Since then, pediatric home care has grown phenomenally. Today, it is more complex, involving advanced technology, coordination of multidisciplinary care, creative approaches to financing, and consideration of developmental needs of the child and family.[2]

Several factors have contributed to the growth of home care of children as we know it today. Great strides in medical knowledge and technology have led to improved prenatal and perinatal care as well as early diagnosis and treatment of children with serious problems. These advances brought about an increased population of chronically ill children with many complex medical problems. The system of prospective payment for hospital care based upon diagnosis-related groups (DRGs) resulted in a strong incentive for hospitals to discharge their patients quicker and sicker.[3] As a consequence, there arose a great demand for home health care as one solution to cost containment. Studies have documented that managed home care is more cost effective than keeping the child in the hospital. [4-9] For example, the average cost of caring for a ventilator-dependent child at home is 87% less than in a hospital, and home care costs are 70% less than hospital costs for other high-tech needs.[8,10] Health care cost has increased the awareness of both parents and professionals that a lifetime of hospitalization is not in the best interest of the child and family.[11] The development of pediatric home care practice has also been influenced by studies showing that family-centered coordinated home care reduced the psychosocial and behavioral sequelae of pediatric acute and chronic illness.[9,12-15] The chance for the child and the family to achieve optimal psychosocial growth and development is better when the child is at home rather than in a hospital.[4] The home environment provides more stable routines and normal social interactions, while hospitalization interrupts both and may result in developmental regression of the child. The sense that families may be able to regain some control over their personal lives and that of their ill children has added further impetus to using home care as an alternative.[16] The development of safer, more accurate technology used in home care[17,18] has led to an increased number of home-based high-technology care services.[19,20] All of these factors have shifted hospital care into the home setting.

Definition

Pediatric home care is defined as the provision of skilled care and support services to a child in his or her place of residence. It covers a wide array of professional and technical services and returns the care and responsibility to the family and the community within the dictates of safe medical practice.[4] It includes programs to avoid hospitalization for acute illness in otherwise healthy children and to monitor infants at risk for sudden infant death, as well as social support programs to promote maternal infant attachment or to prevent child abuse. Pediatric home health also provides visiting nurse services, physical therapy for stable patients, and organized hospice for chronically and terminally ill children.[21]

Although the formulation and framework of pediatric home care and adult home care are the same, there are differences between the two that require attention if the pediatric health agency is to succeed. The goal in pediatric home care is to teach the family caregiver to provide appropriate care to the child. In contrast, in adult home care, teaching is focused on the patient to increase his or her level of independent functioning. There is a rising need for medical social services in home care of the child, with approximately 90% of families being served through a pediatric home health agency requiring social service intervention.[22] This includes the support services of specially trained home health aides and volunteers to tend to the child's personal care needs and psychosocial development. Finally, there is greater medical liability in home care of children, as they get sick very quickly and there is less margin for error in their care compared with that of adults.

Types of Home Care Services

Professional and technical people describe two different types of home care for ill children. The differences and the boundaries of practice that exist between these two types of services are well defined.[23]

Professional home care is based upon scientific principles with professional standards of care. Professional home care providers receive formal instructions with licensure, certification, or documented qualification to provide quality home care. One of its basic characteristics is that it is a family-centered care with an interdependent relationship among the patient, family, and environment. There are three categories of professional home care:

1. Physician-directed, intermittent skilled care is delivered to homebound patients that is reasonable and necessary due to their diagnosis. The services are provided by a federally certified home health agency which may be composed of a highly skilled nurse; physician; occupational, physical, and speech therapist; social worker; and home health aide. Phototherapy for newborns with elevated bilirubin, apnea monitoring for high-risk infants, dressing changes, and parenteral nutrition are some examples of this category of professional home care.

2. Physician-directed hourly skilled care requires the use of high technology in the home. Commonly called "private duty" home care, the services provided are not necessarily through a federally certified home health agency. The services are delivered by highly skilled nurses, licensed practical nurses, or home health aides in the patient's home on an hourly (shift) basis. Examples of this type of care are infusion therapy, care of

the ventilator-dependent child, and multitherapy requiring hourly skilled intervention.
3. Hourly support services assist with respite care needs of families with chronically ill children. This may include short-term care of a mildly ill child who is unable to participate in a regular school or child care program. These services are provided either through a private duty agency or a registry. Care is delivered by a paraprofessional, usually a home health aide. Respite care for children with cystic fibrosis, muscular dystrophy, or cerebral palsy are examples of this type of care.

Technical home care, on the other hand, is product-driven care, with emphasis on monetary profits to providers. Care delivered is based primarily upon reimbursement guidelines, with no professional standards or regulations on how home care is delivered. Home equipment vendors of oxygen therapy, hospital beds, wheelchairs, and apnea monitors are a few examples of this type of provider. Professional standards and criteria that ensure sound patient management and quality patient care are lacking in technical home care. This is a significant difference from professional home care.

Parents and other family members are essential participants in home care and play a key role in the success of the home health care of their children. "While professionals can offer the expertise of their disciplines and knowledge gained from working with a number of children, parents are the only ones who can contribute information on their particular child in all settings."[24]

The Ad Hoc Task Force on Home Care of the American Academy of Pediatrics states the goal of a pediatric home care program is to offer comprehensive cost-effective health care within a nurturing home environment that maximizes the capabilities of the individual and minimizes the effects of the disabilities.[25]

Population Receiving Home Care

Early identification of the child as a candidate for home care and the use of appropriate medical and allied health resources in the hospital and the community settings are important steps to reduce fragmentation of services once the child is discharged to the home.[2] The children who benefit from home care programs are those with complex medical problems and those who are at risk in a hospital environment. At-risk children or those with diagnosed developmental disabilities can also benefit from home care programs.

Due to medical and technological advances, chronically ill children have survived who otherwise would have died. In the United States, about 10 million children are considered chronically ill.[8] These individuals may have a history of prematurity; low birth weight with chronic lung disease or neurologic sequelae; congenital defects that have been surgically corrected; and chronic conditions such as cancer, cystic fibrosis, muscular dystrophy, cerebral palsy, asthma, diabetes, and many others. Severity of these chronic illnesses ranges from mild, with minimal impairment of the child's functioning, to severe, requiring life-sustaining equipment and daily ongoing care by trained personnel. With pediatric home care programs, many of these children are able to receive much of their care in their homes. The Office of Technology and Assessment of the U.S. Congress[26] identified the clinical populations of children that are considered for home care (Table 12.1). The scope of pediatric home care continues to expand in services and clinical populations served. More recent pediatric home care services include those for infants and children with AIDS or born of mothers addicted to alcohol, cocaine, and other illicit drugs. A growing subspecialty in the home care industry is home care for normal newborns discharged from the hospital at 24 to 36 hours old. Early discharge may place a neonate at risk for undetected jaundice, undiagnosed sepsis, or heart defects that are not apparent in the first 36 hours of life. Mothers of such infants miss out on the health teaching of infant care skills traditionally taught by nurses when mothers and infants had a longer hospital stay after birth. Home health care for newborns will meet the needs of both the mother and infant. Home intervention programs have been developed to provide family support and medical surveillance for high-risk premature infants who likewise are discharged earlier from the hospital. The home health programs ensure postdischarge well-being and improve survival outcome during the first years of life.

Table 12.1 Clinical Populations Considered for Home Care

I.   Children dependent at least part of each day on mechanical ventilators.

II. Children requiring prolonged intravenous administration of nutritional substances or drugs (such as children with AIDS).

III. Children with daily dependence on other devices for nutritional or respiratory support including tracheostomy care, oxygen support, or tube feeding.

IV. Children with prolonged dependence on other medical devices that compensate for vital body functions and require daily or near daily nursing care. This group includes: infants that require cardiac and apnea monitoring; children requiring renal dialysis; or children requiring other medical devices such as urinary catheters or colostomy pouches as well as substantial nursing care in connection with their disabilities.

Source: Technical Memorandum, OT-TM-H-30, U.S. Government Printing Office, Washington, D.C., 1987, p. 17.

Table 12.2   American Hospital Association Home Care Constituents

Medical care and supervision	Speech therapy
Nursing care and supervision	Inhalation therapy
Social work services	Medical technician services
Physical therapy	Occupational therapy
Appliance, equipment, and sterile supply service	Pharmaceutical services
Nutritional guidance	Laboratory and radiology services
Transportation for patient and equipment	
Availability of hospital inpatient services	Homemaker and health aide services

From Friedman, J., *Home Health Care: A Complete Guide for Patients and Their Families*, W.W. Norton, New York, 1986, p. 16. With permission.

The American Hospital Association[27] provides a list of home health care services which are the basic components of home health care (Table 12.2). These services may be direct services such as dressing changes, drug administration, tracheostomy care, general nursing care, and evaluating therapy. Patient advocacy, education, and monitoring therapeutic programs are also important services[28] of home health.

Home Care Program Development

Comprehensive planning for all aspects of home health care and the coordination of all services in the home health care system are critical to achieving optimal physical, emotional, and developmental functioning of the child. It is also essential to minimize adverse effects on the family or unforeseen financial burdens.[25] Guidelines for home care of infants, children, and adolescents provided by the American Academy of Pediatrics' Task Force on Home Care[25] and other recommendations from the pediatric home care literature are shown schematically in Figure 12.1. Discussion of each guideline follows.

Discharge Planning

This process begins during the child's hospitalization and establishes the short- and long-term goals of home care in realistic measurable behavioral terms. The goals set will provide direction for the treatment plan. Such goals must be those of the child, the family, and the home care team. Once a child is identified as

DISCHARGE PLANNING

* Education of Client and Family
* Selection of Home Health Agency and Equipment Vendors
* Establishment of Community Support Network

* Identification of Family and Respite Support Groups
* Evaluation of Projected Costs for Home Care
* Organization of a Multidisciplinary Home Care Team

MULTIDISCIPLINARY HOME CARE TEAM

* Review patient's status and needs and family coping skills.
* Assess child and family readiness for home care.
* Prepare family and community to provide safe standards of home care.
* Evaluate program and assess outcome.
* Coordinate long term all home care services.
* Develop and implement an integrated home care plan.

INTEGRATED HOME CARE PLAN

* Identify a case coordinator and primary care physician.
* Define backup system for medical emergency.
* Arrange for educational services for school-age children.
* Monitor care plan through periodic review with parents and reevaluate as needed.
* Develop mechanism for making adjustments when needed.

INDIVIDUAL FAMILY SERVICE PLAN (IFSP)

* Statement of infant/child present level of physical, cognitive, language, speech and psychological development and self-help skills.
* Statement of family's strengths and needs related to enhancing child's growth and development.
* Statement of major outcomes expected to be achieved for child and family with criteria, procedures, and time lines to be used.
* Specific intervention services necessary to meet needs of children/family including frequency, intensity, method of delivery, projected dates of initiation, anticipated duration of services.

Figure 12.1 Pediatric home care program development.

a potential home health client, an initial assessment of the clinical status and needs in the hospital is done. If the assessment determines the child as a good candidate for home health, the discharge team begins to address several important steps during the discharge process.

The first step is to identify the education necessary for the child and family through an assessment of the family's understanding of the child's condition and treatment goals. The family's readiness and ability to provide home care improve when education is provided in the hospital setting prior to discharge. The family should be taught to recognize changes in the child's condition that would require consultation or modification of care. Teaching care for anticipated problems such as cardiopulmonary resuscitation is also essential. Finally, successful trial of care demonstrated by the home caregiver prior to discharge from the hospital, including the use of equipment and other supplies, is essential to the success of home care. A list of the facts and skills to be taught is kept and items are checked off when completed to coordinate teaching.[22]

Next, the discharge team chooses the home care agency and equipment vendor. The scope and quality of pediatric home care agencies vary; thus each agency should be investigated carefully as to its program development, supervision, quality assurance, and reimbursement issues. Equipment and supplies appropriate for home care must be selected and secured according to each patient's needs. The equipment vendor selected must guarantee continuous availability, emergency and routine maintenance, and replacement of equipment. The equipment and supplies to be used in the home should be used in the hospital first, so the family can be familiar with and proficient in their use. It is also important to determine whether or not the vendor has experience with the special needs of acutely and chronically ill children and their equipment requirements. The family must have immediate access to emergency backup and information. A prompt answering service and prompt delivery of equipment are imperative. Arrangements should be made for professional staff employed by the equipment vendor to conduct a home visit within 24 hours after a child's discharge to the home. Often this early home visit reduces the anxiety families may experience when procedures they learned in the hospital are finally put into operation in the home. The equipment vendor's professional staff can identify potential problems and facilitate communication between the family and the hospital.[29] They should also reinforce hospital discharge instructions, assist the family in adapting protocols to the home setting, and provide written instructions about the operation, care, and maintenance of the equipment. Because equipment for home care is not currently standardized, safety of equipment should be assessed when selecting the equipment vendor. The multidisciplinary home care team and the family should ask for service and maintenance records on equipment to ensure that it is in good working order.[29] Since there are no formal reviews of new technologies for their safety and effectiveness in the home setting, it is imperative that home care be delivered by professionals who are trained to handle this equipment and manage patient care in this independent environment.[10]

The third step is to establish a community support network. This is especially important for the child with complex medical needs or who is dependent upon technology. This support network includes the child's community physician who is responsible for primary care, the other members of the multidisciplinary home care team, the school or daycare center, equipment vendors, and specialized technical support such as a respiratory therapist. Community resources that are helpful in an emergency should be contacted, including the community's emergency rescue system, and notified that a child who is dependent upon technology will be moving into the area, so that emergency provisions for the child's care are established. Detailed directions to where the child lives may be necessary, especially if the child lives in a rural area. Area electrical and water companies should also be notified, so that interrupted services are returned on a priority basis.

The final step is to identify family and respite support groups. Parent support groups are valuable resources for families who need to talk with others who have been through the experience of providing home care for a child who is acutely or chronically ill. There are local, state, and national organizations and parent support networks related to the specific conditions for families of children with chronic problems. Examples include the Muscular Dystrophy Association, National Hemophilia Foundation, and Sick Kids (Need) Involved People (SKIP). The last group is an organization of families concerned with improving specialized pediatric home care especially for children dependent upon technology and with matching community resources to family needs. A number of other parent support groups are listed in Table 12.3. The discharge team can supply parents with the names and phone numbers of active local members of parent support groups or the team can directly contact the parent group with the family's permission. Participation in support groups is an effective form of therapeutic support because the parents' participation is a strong predictor of future adaptation.[30]

The immense work involved in providing care 24 hours a day may cause family caregivers to experience burnout unless respite care is provided. In this situation, respite care is defined as the provision of care for an ill child in the home by someone other than the parents or the usual caregivers. Although caregivers willing and able to care for ill children are scarce, parent organizations, church groups, and professional associations offer total family respite.

The projected cost for each child's home care plan must be evaluated in light of available resources.[17] Decisions regarding resource allocations should depend

Table 12.3   Selected Parent Support Groups

National AIDS Hotline
American Society Health Association
P.O. Box 13827
Research Triangle Park, NC 27709
(800) 342-2437
(800) 344-7432 (Spanish)

Association for the Care of Children's
Health
7910 Woodmont Avenue, Suite 300
Bethesda, MD 20814
(310) 654-6549

Cystic Fibrosis Foundation
6931 Arlington Road
Bethesda, MD 20814
(800) 344-4823 or (301) 951-4422
(301) 951-6378 (fax)

March of Dimes Birth Defects
1275 Mamaroneck Avenue
White Plains, NY 10605
(914) 428-7100

National Hemophilia Foundation
110 Greene Street, Room 303
New York, NY 10012
(212) 219-8180
(212) 966-9247 (fax)

Children's Hospice International
700 Princess Street, LL
Alexandria, VA 22314
(800) 242-4453 or (703) 684-0330
(703) 684-0226 (fax)

American Lung Association
1740 Broadway
New York, NY 10019
(800) 586-4872 or (212) 315-8700
(212) 265-5642 (fax)

Muscular Dystrophy Association
3300 E. Sunrise Drive
Tucson, AZ 85718-3208
(602) 529-2000
(602) 529-5300 (fax)

Neonatal Illness/Prematurity
Parent Care
9041 Colgate Street
Indianapolis, IN 46268-1210
(317) 872-9913 (voice/fax)

Parents of Chronically Ill Children
1527 Maryland Street
Springfield, IL 62702
(217) 522-6801

Threshold-Intractable Seizure Disorder
Support Group & Newsletter
26 Stavola Road
Middletown, NJ 07748-3728
(908) 957-0714

National Association for Sickle Cell
Disease
3345 Wilshire Boulevard, Suite 1106
Los Angeles, CA 90010
(800) 421-8453 or (213) 736-5455
(213) 736-5211 (fax)

SKIP (Sick Kids Need Involved People)
of New York
990 2nd Avenue
New York, NY 10022
(212) 421-9161

Spina Bifida Association of America
4590 MacArthur Boulevard NW, #250
Washington, DC 20007-4226
(800) 621-3141 or (202) 944-3285
(202) 944-3295 (fax)

National Association for Parents of the
Visually Impaired
P.O. Box 317
Watertown, MA 02272-0317
(800) 562-6265 or (617) 972-7441
(617) 972-7444

United Cerebral Palsy Association
7 Penn Plaza, Suite 804
New York, NY 10001

upon the patient's needs and be proportional to expected benefits. Financial eligibility of the family should be considered, taking into account family income and adjusting for medical expenses. To qualify for assistance, families must provide documentation that the cost of services delivered in the home does not exceed hospital or institutional costs. Title XIX (Medicaid) of the Social Security Act of 1965 and private insurance companies are the primary sources for pediatric home health services. A more recent funding mechanism, Title XIX Medical Model Waiver, now allows for services that in the past were covered by Medicaid in the hospital but not paid for in the home. The Health Care Financing Administration (HCFA) later developed an expanded Medicaid Home and Community Based Services Waiver Program (formerly known as the "Model Waivers") to include up to 50 technology-dependent children per state, removing the necessity of applying to HCFA for approval for each child.

Klug[16] published guidelines to assist the family and the discharge team in determining the home care services available through their private insurance carriers. A summary of these guidelines follows. (a) Benefits as described by the policy booklet should be verified during any hospitalization period by directly contacting the insurance company and obtaining accurate interpretation of the policy benefits. (b) The insurance company home care benefit may be interpreted differently for different cases; thus it is important to determine what language is most commonly used by the insurance company so that the same wording is used to support home care. (c) The financial limits of the insurance policy should be established and clarify whether the policy represents annual or lifetime expenditure. (d) Home care may not be listed as a separate benefit but may appear as private duty nursing or home care attendants. (e) The family should be aware that insurance companies will only verify coverage and not guarantee payment for services; payment of services will be based upon the submission of information with the first invoice and receipt of the letter of medical need. (f) A physician's letter of medical need should be submitted to the insurance company which shall then review the letter before approval of any home care. The letter of medical need should include the child's condition and current hospitalization, the nursing hours required, equipment needed, and the child's prognosis. A cost comparison of home care versus hospital care is also helpful. Prognosis plays an important role in determining how the insurance company will view the cost effectiveness of home care. If prognosis is poor but a cost reduction is shown by discharging the child home, the insurance company may still look upon home care favorably. Reimbursement for home care services by insurance companies is in part determined by the reviewer of medical need. Families must be prepared to pursue other avenues in case of rejection. Families can seek assistance from the State Department of Insurance, which works with policyholders and will advocate for individuals in particular cases. State and local legislators may be willing advocates for their constituents. The child's physician should be informed and kept abreast of any difficulties in securing insurance. The physician may be able to clarify any questions regarding the need for home care with a telephone call to the medical director of the insurance company.

One of the important steps in the development of a sound pediatric home care program is the organization of a *home care team*. Since many factors need to be considered, a team that is multidisciplinary will function best to address the many issues and services needed in a home care program. Composition of the team varies and may include a physician, nurse, social worker, and speech, physical, and occupational therapists. A developmentalist, psychologist, and teacher may be members of the team, as well as the equipment vendor and third-party insurers. The child and family are integral members of the home care team and form the nucleus around whom all activities revolve. Decision making is collaborative, with each profession bringing a core of knowledge and skills and respecting the unique contributions of the other disciplines.[30] In most multidisciplinary home care teams, the nurse functions as a generalist, child advocate, and case manager. In addition to coordination and liaison activities, the home health nurse provides direct patient care, teaches the family technical aspects of care and developmental needs of the child, and determines financial coverage of services. The nurse also ensures that the parents have identified a primary care physician and arranges for the child to receive routine screening and preventive health services on schedule.

The role of the team is to enable the family to take increasing responsibility for the care of their child and for the family to be able to institute services when required. The team begins its task when the child is first considered as a potential home care client. Each discipline in the home care team carefully reviews the patient's status and needs in the hospital, formulates goals and objectives for the patient, and develops a daily program to meet these goals in the home. Thereafter, all the disciplines meet to collaboratively formulate an integrated home care plan and make arrangements for its implementation. The home care team also needs to assess the child and family readiness for home care, prepare the family and community to provide safe standards of home care, provide ongoing support and assistance to the family, periodically evaluate the program, assess its outcome, and provide follow-up and long-term coordination of all home care services. Home visits by the team may initially be frequent, but as the parents gain confidence, the frequency may be reduced. Such visits build up trust between the family and the home care team. Families become more receptive to education and care in the home setting, while repeated visits permit teaching of the care of the child in the context of daily needs.[20]

Child and Family Readiness for Home Care

In determining the child and family readiness for home care, client, family, environment, and community factors need to be considered.[25]

Client Factors

The child's medical condition should be predictable and manageable without immediate physician involvement and additional diagnostic and treatment intervention.[30] Clinical stability is the cornerstone of successful home care. It is more difficult to formulate a home care plan if the child's condition is frequently changing. Clinical stability is based upon the child's physiologic status or on the assistance of technological equipment. Required levels of support and intervention within the home setting should be available. The risks for infection or deterioration of the medical condition within the home setting should be weighed against the potential benefits of home care.

Family Factors

The interest and willingness of the family to take the child home and provide care must be considered. Parents have a greater participatory role in this decision than in medical decisions for their hospitalized child.[1] If a family makes a reluctant decision to care for their child at home, they are at high risk of failure. The choice of home care should be made with the full range of options evident to the family to maximize the success of home care.[1]

The home care team also needs to assess the family's coping abilities, including the ability to learn and safely perform necessary procedures and make informed, clear decisions regarding courses of action. It is desirable to have at least two members of the extended family trained and fully able to care for the child in the home and able to work in collaboration with other members of the home care team. Other family members not residing in the home should also be considered for training so they can provide respite and backup when the primary caregiver is ill. McCarthy[31] recommends drawing a care contract when families are reluctant or unsure of participation in home care. The care contract outlines a goal, learning objectives, and responsibilities of the home care team and the family. This written contract obligates the team to provide appropriate instructions to parents and commits the parents to demonstrate an acceptable level of knowledge and skills. A decision regarding home discharge can be made following completion of the contract requirements by both parties. Care must be taken not to impose one's own values for health care on the family who will ultimately assume responsibility for it. It is essential that the family and the home care team have similar perceptions of readiness for discharge and home care for it to be successful. Early on and throughout the preparation for discharge, ongoing changes should be discussed with the family.[32]

Environmental Factors

Assessment of the environment includes the type (house, trailer, apartment) and location (urban or rural) of the residence; availability of electricity, running water, heating, and cooling; and adequacy of space for sleeping and for other activities of the child. Distance from emergency backup and presence of a telephone for emergency contacts should be evaluated. Physical modifications may need to be made to allow wheelchair access, additional electrical load, or other adaptive equipment. Transportation resources must be considered, and in rural areas, arrangements for provision of hospital, physician, pharmacy, or equipment vendor services must be made.

Community Factors

The medical, social, and educational resources play an important role in the success of home care. Their availability within the community is particularly important if the child has special equipment needs. The home care team can identify the necessary equipment needs and make arrangements for their delivery to the home. The telephone company and public utilities must be notified to provide continuous service in the event of an emergency. Community support may also include registered nurses, respiratory therapists, home health aides, and social workers who may be employed by state agencies, equipment vendors, or local organizations. Early involvement by community providers will maximize the potential for the family to become case managers and coordinate all their child's care.[32]

The Integrated Home Care Plan

After careful review of the patient's status and needs in the hospital, the home care team develops a comprehensive integrated home care plan. The essential components of the plan are shown in Figure 12.1. A primary case coordinator should be selected from among the members of the home care team to oversee and coordinate the program. The coordinator should be able to work closely with the family and the other team members. A primary care physician should also be identified to provide routine screening and preventive health services. These should include immunizations as well as acute illness care. The family should have access to a telephone at all times and a well-defined backup system for medical emergency should be in place.

The home care plan must include educational services for school-age children. No child should be disqualified from a home care program because of eligibility to attend an out-of home school, if home care is otherwise deemed necessary.[25] A safe medical plan must exist for the school as well as the home. Special arrangements may be needed by schools to accommodate the unique needs of these children.

The home care team should monitor the home care plan and periodically review it with the parents, evaluating the patient's status and needs as well as family coping mechanisms. This review should be done at intervals so that the plan is adjusted appropriately. The plan should also include an Individual Family Service Plan (IFSP) which is based on Public Law 99-457. This law provides for interdisciplinary assessment and evaluation of children from birth to 3 years old who are at risk for or have developmental delays. The IFSP has been widely accepted as an integral part of interdisciplinary health care team function for children of all ages. The basic components of an IFSP are shown in Figure 12.1.

Program Evaluation and Outcome Assessment

The goals or desired outcomes of the home care program form the basis for its evaluation. This evaluation process should be done on an ongoing basis from the time of discharge through to the end of the home care program. Both the family and the home care team as well any other professionals involved in the child's care evaluate the program. Data for review will be more helpful if obtained from several sources (parent, physician, school, community agencies). A better home care program can be developed when experiences are shared by those who are involved in the care of the child. The evaluation and assessment of outcome[17,30] should include the following: (a) the child's current status, need for subsequent hospitalization, developmental progress, and course of the underlying disease; (b) effects on the family members; (c) original goals, objectives, and the initial time lines; (d) effectiveness of planned interventions including adequacy of the home health community agencies; (e) actual versus expected utilization of resources; and (f) financial experience (cash flow and continued availability of benefits). Follow-up plans can be made based upon the results of this evaluation. Frequent reassessments and the flexibility to adjust to changing medical status or unanticipated social conditions will help to ensure a successful home care program.

Quality Assurance

The quality of patient care and the performance of the home care team must be monitored and evaluated through an ongoing process. Due to rapid changes in home care and increasing technology, this process should include the identification of important aspects of care[30] which should be monitored, evaluated, and incorporated into the quality assurance plan. This plan should clearly identify the method of collection, responsible persons, and reporting path for the outcomes. After data collection and analysis, follow-up action needs to be planned and implemented and the results of such action monitored to determine if the action plan was effective in changing the outcome.[30]

The aspects of care to be identified are either *high volume, high risk,* or *problem prone.* The ability of the parents to perform cardiopulmonary resuscitation or their compliance with protocol in the use of an apnea monitor are examples of aspects of care of high volume, that is, care occurring frequently or affecting large numbers of patients. A high-risk aspect of care is one that would deprive the patient of benefit or places the patient at risk of serious consequences if the care is not correctly provided, as in ventilator management or tracheostomy care. Medication management of a medically fragile patient is an example of an aspect of care that is problem prone or tended in the past to cause problems for the patient and the home care team.

Role of Physicians in Home Care

Physicians must become better informed about home care and the roles of the different members of the home care team.[33] The role of the physician in home care should be strengthened to collaborate with the home care team in implementing the care plan in the home.[34] Early involvement of the physician is essential from the time the child is considered for home care to the discharge planning and development of the home care plan. The physician should be closely involved in the coordination of medical care especially when the child has complex medical needs, such as those of a technology-dependent child. Before discharge to home care, the physician is responsible for determining the clinical stability of the child, which is essential to the success of home care. Before deciding whether or not to send a child home, the physician must also educate and negotiate with the family regarding home care and decide together on a mutually preferable course of action.[1] Personal values for health care should not be imposed on the family, who ultimately has to take responsibility for caring for the child in the home. The physician as well as the other professionals must be careful in deciding how vigorously to try to convince parents explicitly or by implication to assume obligations for home care of the child with complex life-support systems.[1] The physician involved in pediatric home care programs must determine that a competent home health care agency will be responsible for the care and advocacy of the child and family after discharge. The physician who will provide for the primary care of the child after discharge to home care should be encouraged to participate during the discharge planning. If this is not possible, documentation of the plans should be forwarded to the physician so he or she understands the reasons for all the decisions and actions as well as the roles and responsibilities of all the physicians involved.[35] The primary care physician will be encouraged to play an active role in home care if he or she has access to information from all the other members of the home care team. Early on in the child's hospital course, the primary care physician should communicate with the physician's hospital counterpart and begin to lay the groundwork for a collaborative relationship with the family. If the transfer of trust begins early, the family will be more likely to turn to the primary care physician when their child is home rather than continue to seek help from the hospital staff. Any difficulty in securing insurance coverage for home care should be shared with the primary care physician, who may be able to clarify any questions regarding the need for home care. A phone call or a letter to the medical director of the insurance company may resolve the problem of coverage. The letter of medical need, written and submitted to the insurance company prior to approval for home care, should be clear and precise to facilitate insurance coverage.

The physician should work together with the other members of the team in periodic reassessments of the home care plan and be responsive to the changing status and needs of the child and family. A careful review of quality assurance indicators will help the physician monitor the quality of patient care and the performance of the home care team and change practice patterns as indicated.

There are excellent resources to help the physician determine the appropriateness of home care services delivered.[36] There are also guidelines and recommendations available from several consensus activities.[25,37,38] Finally, the physician may need to be an advocate for community resources for patients with many needs.

New Horizon

Pediatric home health continues to evolve and there is great potential for further expansion in its scope. Health care reforms and the concept of managed care may bring about a new round of strategies for cost containment. New and more sophisticated technologies for home care continue to be developed. These factors will likely have a positive impact on home health.

In view of the continuing evolution of home care and the changes in health services for children that may occur with health care reforms, physicians caring for children should stay current in their knowledge of home health. They should be involved in the policy-making arena of health care and stay vigilant for the welfare of children.

References

1. Lantos, J. D. and Kohrman, A. F., Ethical aspects of pediatric home care, *Pediatrics*, 89(5):920–924, 1992.
2. Jackson, D. B. and Saunders, R. B., Eds., Home care of ill children, in *Child Health Nursing: A Comprehensive Approach to the Care of Children and Their Families*, J.B. Lippincott, Philadelphia, 1993, pp. 541–550.
3. Fox, D. M., Andersen, K. S., Benjamin, A. E., and Duratov, L. J., Intensive home health care in the United States, *Int. J. Technol. Assess. Health Care*, 3:561–573, 1987.
4. Kaufman, J. and Hardy-Ribakow, D., A model of a comprehensive approach for technology-assisted chronically ill children, *J. Pediatr. Nurs.*, 2(4):244–249, 1987.
5. Frates, R. C., Spaingard, M. L., and Harrison, G. M., Outcome of home mechanical ventilation for children, *J. Pediatr.*, 106:850-856, 1985.
6. Fields, A. I., Rosenblatt, A., Pollack, M. M., and Kaufman, J., Home care cost effectiveness for respiratory technology dependent children, *AJDC*, 145:729–733, 1991.
7. Donati, M. A., Guenette, G., and Auerbach, H., Prospective controlled study of home and hospital therapy of cystic fibrosis pulmonary disease, *J. Pediatr.*, 111:28–33, 1987.
8. Goldberg, A. I., Faure, E. A. M., Vaughn, C. J., Snarski, R. S., and Seleny, F. L., Home care for life supported persons: an approach to program development, *J. Pediatr.*, 104:785–795, 1984.
9. Strandvik, B., Hjelte, L., Malmborg, A. S., and Widen, B., Home intravenous antibiotic treatment of patients with cystic fibrosis, *Acta Paediatr.*, 81:340–344, 1992.
10. Humphrey, C. J. and Millone-Nuzzo, P., *Home Care Nursing, An Orientation to Practice*, C.T. Appleton and Lange, Norwold, Connecticut, 1991.
11. Feetham, S. L., Hospital and home care in the 80s, *Pediatr. Nurs.*, 12(5):383–386, 1986.
12. Korham, A., Pediatric Home Care: Ten Point Agenda for the Future: Home Care for the Children with Serious Handicapping Conditions, The Association for the Care of Children's Health, Washington, D.C., 1984.
13. Quint, R. D., Chesterman, E., Crain, L. S., Winkleby, M., and Boyce, T., Home care for ventilator dependent children. Psychosocial impact on the family, *AJDC*, 144:1238–1242, 1990.

14. Stein, R. E. K. and Jessop, J. D., Long term mental health effects of a pediatric home care program, *Pediatrics,* 88:490–496, 1991.
15. Stein, R. E. K. and Jessop, J. D., Does pediatric home care make a difference for children with chronic illness, *Pediatrics,* 73:845–853, 1984.
16. Klug, R. M., Understanding private insurance for funding pediatric home care, *Pediatr. Nurs.,* 17:197–198, 1991.
17. Morris, E. and Fonseca, J., Home care today, *Am. J. Nurs.,* 84:1342, 1984.
18. Haddad, A., *High Tech Home Care: A Practical Guide*, Aspen Publishers, Gaithersburg, Maryland, 1987.
19. Rawlin, A. and Shannon, K., PNPs case managers for technologically dependent children, *Pediatr. Nurs.,* 12(5):338–340, 1986.
20. Taylor, M., The effect of drugs on home health care, *Nurs. Outlook,* 33(6):288–289, 1989.
21. Stein, R., Home care: a challenging opportunity, Proceedings of Association for Care of Child Health Conference, Houston, 1984.
22. Maurano, L. W., Community and home care, in *Family Centered Nursing Care of Children*, 2nd edition, Betz, C. L., Hunsberger, M. M., and Wright, S., Eds., W.B. Saunders, Philadelphia, 1987.
23. Humphrey, C. J., The home as a setting for care—clarifying the boundaries of practice, *Nurs. Clin. North Am.,* 223:305–314, 1988.
24. Shelton, T. L., Jeppson, E., and Johnson, B., Eds., *Family Centered Care for Children with Special Health Care Needs*, 2nd edition, Association for Care of Children's Health, Washington, D.C., 1987.
25. Ad Hoc Task Force on Home Care of Chronically Ill Infants and Children, Guidelines for home care of infants, children and adolescents with chronic disease, *Pediatrics,* 74(3):434–436, 1984.
26. U.S. Congress Office of Technology Assessment, Technology Dependent Children: Hospital vs. Home Care—A Technical Memorandum, OT-TM-H-30, U.S. Government Printing Office, Washington, D.C., 1987.
27. Freidman, J., *Home Health Care: A Complete Guide for Patients and Their Families*, W.W. Norton, New York, 1986.
28. Lessing, D. and Latman, M. A., Pediatric home care in the 1990's, *Arch. Dis. Childhood*, 66:994–996, 1991.
29. Hartsell, M. and Ward, J., Selecting equipment vendors for children in home care, *Maternal Child Nurs.,* 10:26–28, 1985.
30. Urbano, M. T., Nursing care of children in the home, in *Child Health Care Process and Practice,* Castiglia, P. T. and Harbin, R. E., Eds., J.B. Lippincott, Philadelphia, 1992.
31. McCarthy, S., Discharge planning for the medically fragile children, *Caring,* 5(11):38–41, 1986.
32. Allen, N. L., Simone, J. A., and Wingebach, G. F., Families with a ventilator dependent child: transitional issues, *J. Perinatol.,* XXIV(1):48–55, 1994.
33. Health and Public Policy Committee, American College of Physicians: home health care position paper, *Ann. Intern. Med.,* 105:454–460, 1986.
34. Koren, M. J., Home care—who cares? *New Engl. J. Med.,* 314:917–920, 1986.

35. Goldberg, A. I. A., A new home care role for physicians. Mechanical ventilation outside the hospital, *Caring,* May:42–49, 1990.
36. Joint Commission on Accreditation of Healthcare Organizations, *Accreditation Manual for Home Care 1991*, Washington, D.C., 1991.
37. Donohue, W. J., Giovannoni, A. M., Goldberg, A. I., Keens, T. G., Make, B. J., Plummer, A. L., and Prentice, W. S., Long term mechanical ventilation: guidelines for management in the home and at alternative community sites, *Chest,* 90:15–37S, 1986.
38. Plummer, A. L., O'Donohue, W. J., and Petty, T. L., Consensus conference on problems in home mechanical ventilation, *Am. Rev. Respir. Dis.,* 140:555–560, 1989.

Home Care for Pediatric Respiratory Disorders

13

Nemr S. Eid, M.D.

Introduction

Home care is becoming a rapidly growing industry in the United States. Total home care expenditure was estimated to have been 3% of the total health care cost in 1994. This accounts for over 23 billion dollars.[1] Home care agencies refer to home health agencies, home care aide organizations, and hospices. The National Association for Home Care identified a total of 15,027 home care agencies in the United States in 1994. Children under 17 years of age account for 3.1% of home care recipients.[1] Percentage of current clients receiving home health and hospice care for diseases of the respiratory system include 6.5% for both adults and children.[2] According to the Health Care Financing Administration, home care in general accounts for the fastest growing component of personal health care spending and pediatric home care is its fastest growing segment.[3] This chapter reviews home care for the most common pediatric respiratory disorders. It also addresses the psychosocial and the ethical issues associated with home care.

In the past, pediatric home health care was mainly reserved for patients dependent upon advanced technological techniques for survival, such as patients needing home mechanical ventilation, oxygen therapy, and tracheostomy care. In the late 1980s and 1990s, the focus of home health care has shifted dramatically. Many children are discharged to home care services either for continued acute care or for rehabilitative care. Home care services are now provided for many respiratory disorders such as asthma, cystic fibrosis, pneumonia, sinusitis, apnea, and bronchopulmonary dysplasia. Many of these patients receive home care services which may include intermittent skilled nursing, infusion therapy, physical therapy, speech therapy, occupational therapy, medical social services, and dietary intervention. Many studies have shown the cost effectiveness of home care; therefore, in the cost-containment atmosphere of the 1990s, home care may become a forced necessity rather than an elective option.

General Guidelines for Pediatric Respiratory Home Care

Home care for respiratory diseases has been facilitated by the introduction of continuous monitoring devices and improved diagnostic and therapeutic modalities designed or adapted for home use.[4]

There are many steps to be taken prior to and after starting home care for respiratory diseases (Table 13.1). The first and most important step is patient selection. Selection criteria for each respiratory disease or condition must be identified, and long-term home care and goals must be defined. The child must be medically stable (e.g., a child with tracheostomy must have a mature tracheostomy and must have undergone tracheostomy changes after placement). Before discharge home, the patient and/or family must have adequate understanding of the patient diagnosis and prognosis. The parents must be willing and able to provide and meet the needs of the patient. They must have adequate training to successfully carry out specific care procedures and to react appropriately in a crisis situation. Prior to discharge, it is imperative that the appropriate home care team is selected and that the adaptive equipment is appropriate and functional. The role of each team member must be defined, and the family must

Table 13.1 Steps to Be Taken Prior to and After Starting Home Respiratory Care

- Patient selection: identify need for long-term respiratory care
- Define optimal goal
- Document physiologic stability
- Discharge planning
  - Assess family's capabilities to provide home care
  - Provide adequate family training
  - Explore financial and reimbursement issues
  - Select appropriate home care team
  - Define the role of each team member
  - Establish an ongoing line of communication
  - Establish a follow-up plan

have a clear understanding of the responsibility of the individuals and/or organizations that will be providing services at home. An ongoing line of communication and written instructions about home care must be given to the family, home care agency, and any other supplier involved in the home care of the patient. Usually, children with complex, chronic medical conditions, who are dependent upon medical technology to survive, are better served in a rehabilitation center for a finite period of time prior to discharge home. These centers have multidisciplinary teams that are suited to address the above concerns. Exploring financial and reimbursement issues must be addressed at the outset. This issue has far-reaching consequences in terms of the ability of the family to cope with chronic care, which sometimes can deplete all family resources. Finally, a medical follow-up must be established to monitor ongoing progress.

Home Mechanical Ventilation

General Guidelines

Home mechanical ventilation is becoming more common in pediatrics. Many patients with chronic respiratory failure can be potential candidates for home ventilation. Such conditions can be divided into three major categories: chronic lung disease, ventilatory muscle weakness, and decreased central respiratory drive (Table 13.2).

Table 13.2 Causes of Chronic Respiratory Failure in Children

- Ventilatory muscle weakness
  - Muscular dystrophy
  - Congenital or acquired myopathy
  - Diaphragmatic paralysis
  - Myasthenia gravis
- Chronic lung disease
  - Bronchopulmonary dysplasia
  - Cystic fibrosis
  - Fibrosing alveolitis
  - Asphyxiating thoracic dystrophy
- Decreased central respiratory drive
  - Congenital hypoventilation syndrome
  - Arnold-Chiari malformation
  - Spinal injury C1–C2
  - Transverse myelitis

Regardless of the condition which led to chronic respiratory insufficiency, medical stability is essential before the decision is made to consider home ventilation. Knowing that management of the ventilatory-dependent pediatric patient is rather complex, the initial task must begin with an assessment of each patient's survival potential and quality of life. Once the medical decision for home mechanical ventilation is reached, it is important to set the medical objectives for home ventilation. These objectives include, in addition to appropriate ventilatory setting and optimal oxygen delivery, appropriate growth and development and appropriate cardiorespiratory function. A multidisciplinary team of physicians, therapists, nurses, and other professionals is required to deliver optimal care. As a part of discharge planning, it is essential to define the role of each member of the team. The patient's family must be thoroughly educated in the child's care, and they must be involved in decision making from the outset. At this point, setting a goal would be crucial in understanding the full impact of what is being done at home. The family must understand and demonstrate skills in operating the equipment that is being considered. They must also demonstrate skills in feeding, tracheostomy care, and administering medications. While the equipment is being obtained, parents should undergo a training course at the bedside with a similar ventilator. It is also essential to discuss the potential for weaning from the ventilator if the clinical condition will permit in the future.

Mechanical home ventilation is a cost-effective service; however, it should be noted that the cost effectiveness is not the only rationale for home mechanical ventilation. In fact, it could be argued that home mechanical ventilation is a rather humane and compassionate way to deliver medical services in the patient's own environment, close to family and friends. Although there are many benefits of home ventilation, such as the reduction of risk of infection and the opportunity to be at home in a more relaxed, familiar environment, many difficult choices still need to be addressed. Most families report that they are glad to bring their child home, but many difficult adjustments are required in order to do so. The full nursing care that is needed to provide support to the patient may also intrude on the privacy of the family.[5] Furthermore, the financial burden of having a child on a ventilator at home can be a big stress on the family. Establishing parent–professional partnerships and providing for family support empowers parents to assume the responsibilities of caring for their children in a familiar, nonthreatening environment. In a recent study describing families' experiences in taking their ventilator-assisted children home, Allen et al.[6] found that despite the enormous social and economical impact, parents of these children would again make the same choice. This suggests that early collaboration between hospital staff, community-based providers, and families is essential to prepare the family for this option.

Mode of Ventilation

The most common mode of mechanical ventilation at home is positive-pressure ventilation. Many portable ventilators are available. Some models are small enough to be mounted on the back of a wheelchair. One of the major impediments to positive-pressure ventilation is the need for tracheostomy and the accompanying need for an external humidification source. The newer type of tracheostomy tubes have made complications less common. However, this procedure still generates many emotions and anxieties in the family (see next section). Indeed many families view the need for tracheostomy as an indicator of clinical deterioration and an impingement on the integrity of the body.

Other modalities of ventilation in children at home include negative-pressure ventilation. These devices are rather cumbersome and in many cases are considered uncomfortable. Negative-pressure ventilation is usually recommended for patients who have muscle weakness. Negative-pressure ventilators include tank respirators and the chest curases. These devices allow poor access to the patient, and, therefore, their use in pediatrics is becoming uncommon.

Still other modalities of providing mechanical ventilation at home include CPAP, or continuous positive airway pressure. Newer versions of this modality of ventilation include bilevel positive airway pressure (BiPAP®),* which in contrast to CPAP can be adjusted to deliver different pressures during inspiration and exhalation. This results in better tolerance for the patient while increasing tidal volume and minute ventilation.[7] Studies using BiPAP® have found it to be effective in pediatric patients with upper airway obstruction[8] and in children with respiratory failure.[9] Padman et al.[9] reported on the use of BiPAP® in 15 children (4 with cystic fibrosis and 11 with neuromuscular disease, who experienced acute ventilatory deterioration). All patients had chronic respiratory insufficiency. Significant improvement in dyspnea, increased activity tolerance, and improved quality of sleep were noted without major complications.

Outcome Measures

Field et al.[10] studied the outcome of home care for technology-dependent children and reported on community-based case management models. Their study included 28 patients from 8 hospitals, who utilized an independent community-based case management group to coordinate home care. After 26.3 months of follow-up, only 1 patient death was caused by complication of technology, and 56 children were weaned from technological support. Patients with chronic

---

* BiPAP® is a registered trademark of Respironics, Inc., Murrysville, Pennsylvania.

respiratory failure from central neurological dysfunction did poorly, as expected. Another study found similar clinical outcome between children on mechanical ventilation who were cared for by families and friends and those who were cared for by registered nurses.[11] The cost was much less when children were cared for by the family.

More recently, Canlas-Yamsuan et al.[12] evaluated the effectiveness of home care programs of Children's Hospital of Winnipeg for ventilatory-dependent children. Their study included 22 patients: 14 with primary neurologic disorder (Group A) and 8 with primary pulmonary disorder (Group B). The authors found the home care program to be effective, with few selective hospital readmissions. Factors such as diagnosis, type of family, home location, age at initiation of mechanical ventilation, and the initial duration of hospital stay did not influence morbidity and mortality in either group.

Although home ventilatory care has been shown to be safe and cost effective, and its outcome similar to the outcome of patients ventilated in the hospital, a few obstacles to discharge of ventilatory-assisted children from the hospital to home still exist. In a recent study, DeWitt et al.[13] showed that the greatest obstacle to hospital discharge was seeking approval for home care funding and for arranging out-of-home placement. Public funding agencies took significantly longer to approve home care funding than private insurance companies. Once ventilator-assisted children were medically stable, it took 184 days to obtain home care funding approval from public assistance agencies. Parent training took only 52 days and foster care placement took the longest, 369 days on average.

Home Tracheostomy Care

Tracheostomies are usually necessary in the management of upper airway obstruction in patients with prolonged intubation, in patients requiring long-term mechanical ventilation, and in patients needing frequent suctioning. Some of the most common indications for tracheostomy include severe laryngotracheomalasia, subglottic stenosis, vocal cord paralysis, laryngeal edema after burns, patients with bronchopulmonary dysplasia, and finally, patients with neuromuscular diseases. It should be noted that tracheostomy in children is not a benign procedure, and its related mortality has been reported to be as high as 10 to 27%. Reported mortality at home has ranged from 0.5 to 2 deaths per 100 months of home tracheostomy care.[14] The most common cause of severe respiratory distress and acute death in a child with tracheostomy is tube obstruction. As with other high-technology-related home care, parents of a child with potential tracheostomy should have a clear understanding of the indication and reason for their child's tracheostomy. They should be able to assess the signs of respiratory distress and be able to perform emergency tracheostomy changes. A child must never be left alone with a caregiver who is unable to perform such a procedure. In order to assess the impact of extensive parental education and home nursing care on tracheostomy-related mortality, Duncan et al.[15] reported their experience over a 9-year period with 44 children receiving tracheostomies. Their tracheostomy care regimen consisted of intensive parental training and tracheostomy management for a minimum of 10 days prior to discharge. Home nursing was arranged for at least 11 hours per day per patient in 77% of the patients; 83 of the patients had home apnea monitors. If parents failed to show adequate training and proficiency in tracheostomy management, discharge to home was delayed or canceled. With this regimen, there was no tracheostomy-related death in the hospital or after home discharge.

The most common type of tracheostomy tubes currently used in children are those constructed of polyvinyl chloride, which softens at body temperature, therefore conforming to the shape of the pediatric airway. The most commonly used types are Portex and Shiley. Pediatric sizes for these tubes range from 00 to 4. Tracheostomy tubes larger than size 4 must have an inner cannula. During periods of rapid growth, the size of the tracheostomy tube should be increased every 6 to 12 months. Tracheostomy tubes are usually labeled as disposable; however, with meticulous cleaning techniques, they can be reused as long as the tube's integrity persists. Two trained adults must be present for tracheostomy tube changes. Scissors and a clean tracheostomy tube should be kept by the patient's bedside at all times for emergency changes.

Since patients with tracheostomies no longer breathe through the nose, drying of the trachea can be a major problem if humidification is not provided. Units which provide humidification directly to the tracheostomy site are used in conjunction with tracheostomy collars. These units should be cleaned carefully to avoid bacterial contamination. Secretions must be suctioned from the tube as necessary. Parents should understand and assess the need for suctioning; however, they should be cautioned to avoid too frequent suctioning since this may lead to tracheal irritation and injury. Equipment for suctioning should be available at home at all times. The tracheostomy site should be cleaned at least twice daily to minimize irritation and granulation tissue formation. All standing water presents a hazard to the child with tracheostomy; however a child with a tracheostomy can be bathed in a tub with 1 to 2 inches depth of water.[16] A child with tracheostomy must never be left alone near water, and this includes swimming pools, bathtubs, toilets, and even buckets. The most common reason for obstructive tracheostomy tubes is mucus plugging. Parents should be instructed to recognize the signs of mucus plugging. These include retractions, agitation, severe respiratory distress, cyanosis, and nasal flaring. Another cause of tracheostomy tube obstruction may be unsupervised siblings who may insert foreign objects into the tube.

Children with tracheostomies are at risk for delayed speech; therefore, speech and early verbal stimulation should be instituted at an early age. A fenestrated tracheostomy tube, which has an opening in the superior aspect of the outer cannula, or a Passey-Muir one-way valve increases air through the upper airway, therefore permitting vocalization. Finally, a frequently asked question by parents of infants or children with tracheostomy is when to take the tube out. In order for tracheostomy decannulation to be successful, the underlying condition for which the tracheostomy was placed should be resolved.

Home Oxygen Therapy

Home oxygen programs have evolved to facilitate the discharge of children with chronic lung disease from intensive care nurseries. In this group of patients, there is the possibility for improvement, and even recovery. A second growing group of patients on home oxygen therapy includes patients with irreversible lung diseases, such as cystic fibrosis or fibrosing alveolitis. In these patients, the goals of oxygen therapy are to provide some improvement in exercise tolerance, improve quality of life, and decrease breathlessness. Oxygen delivery at home is provided most commonly by nasal cannulae, which seems to be well tolerated by small infants and children. There are, however, some problems associated with nasal cannulae. These include nasal crusting, obstruction, irritation, epistaxis, discomfort, and finally, inadvertent displacement during sleep.

Many other innovative oxygen delivery systems have been described for use in the home environment. Zinman et al.[17] used an "inverted tent" that lines the walls and floor of the crib into which oxygen is flowed via an entrainment device. With this method, up to an FiO_2 of 0.40 was able to be delivered with a low-flow oxygen source from a concentrator. Coates et al.[18] used a simple tubing connected to the tracheostomy tubes of infants with tracheostomies and bronchopulmonary dysplasia (BPD) through a specially created hole. This system allows the safe administration of oxygen while minimizing the risk of accidental decannulation. More recently, Panitch and Isaacson[19] described the first pediatric use of oxygen via a transtracheal catheter inserted directly into the tracheal lumen in a 3-year-old girl with BPD. This mode of oxygen delivery has been used successfully in adults since the early 1980s. Because the catheter is inserted directly in the trachea, and therefore bypasses the upper airways, the oxygen flow rate is reduced, irritation of the nostrils is avoided, and breathlessness is reduced.[20,21]

Home oxygen sources include compressed gas cylinders, oxygen concentrators, and liquid oxygen reservoirs. Liquid oxygen is preferred over the large compressed tank because of its safety and because patients can be provided with small portable units that are easily refilled from a large reservoir. The choice of the system, however, is dictated by the flow needed to provide adequate oxygen saturation. Oxygen concentrators are typically used for a 1- to 3-liter-per-minute flow and liquid oxygen can be provided at up to 5 liters per minute. With all systems used in children, humidification should be provided. Weaning from oxygen should be attempted in small increments under the supervision of a pediatric pulmonologist. This is usually accomplished at home while keeping oxygen saturation above 94%. Usually oxygen is first weaned during waking hours and only kept at night and during periods of increased activity, such as feeding. Nighttime oxygen is gradually weaned in the same manner.

Home oxygen therapy has been shown to promote weight gain and growth in infants with BPD.[22] It has also been found to permit safe early discharge, even of extremely low birth-weight infants.[23] Oxygen therapy has been shown to improve right ventricular function and prevent pulmonary hypertension and core pulmonale in patients with chronic lung disease.[24,25]

Since BPD is a common disorder affecting 2 per 1000 live births, the cost saving from early discharge cannot be overemphasized. McAleese et al.[26] showed that the median cost for home oxygen therapy was only $5195 compared with a projected cost in the hospital of $46,920 for the same period in infants with BPD. It should be noted, however, that home oxygen therapy alone for small premature infants with BPD is not enough for optimal outcome. Very low birth-weight infants require significant nursing care at home. The efficacy of home nursing care on medical utilization indicates that there are fewer hospitalizations and fewer emergency room visits, and this appears to improve the health of high-risk premature infants and may also be less stressful for parents.[27] Other investigators have found similar results. Casiro et al.[28] found that a community-based program designed to provide individualized support and education for families of low birth-weight infants was cost effective and had a positive influence on the care environment.

Home Apnea Monitors

Apnea is usually defined by cessation of airflow and respiratory pause. This respiratory pause can be either central, obstructive, or mixed. The most common apnea encountered in pediatrics relates to apnea of prematurity, which is defined as periodic breathing with pathological apnea in the premature infant younger than 37 weeks gestation. Apnea of infancy is similar, but occurs in infants who are older than 37 weeks gestation at the time of onset.[29] Other conditions requiring apnea monitors include apparent life-threatening events (ALTE) previously referred to as near-miss sudden infant death syndrome (SIDS). These episodes are usually a combination of apnea, change of color, hypotonia, and choking or gagging. Finally, obstructive sleep apnea is seen in infants and mainly in children with upper airway obstruction. Apnea monitors are not indicated for patients with obstructive apnea since cessation of airflow occurs with continued respiratory efforts; thus, the monitor will interpret the child's effort against an obstructive airway as respirations. Another form of apnea occurring in infants and children is central apnea, which is seen in patients with central hypoventilation syndrome (Ondine's curse) and in patients with Arnold-Chiari malformation. In this form of apnea, cessation of both airflow and respiratory effort occurs.

The most common candidates for home apnea monitors include survivors of a severe ALTE, infants with low birth weight, infants with BPD, infants with tracheostomy tubes, and infants with central hypoventilation syndrome. As with any high-technology equipment, strict guidelines should be followed, as detailed in Table 13.1. Furthermore, limitations of the alarms should be fully explained to the parents prior to discharge. It should be stated clearly that the alarms will help identify rather severe episodes that need parental intervention. Parents should not believe that monitoring an infant will make their lives easier. Instead, they should recognize that it is a full-time job that requires constant dedication by the caregiver. In addition, parents should recognize that monitoring can cause accidental risk, mainly entangled wire and electric shock. Rosen et al.[30] have shown that preterm infants with persistent episodes of apnea, bradycardia, and cyanosis beyond 36 weeks gestation remain at risk for future serious episodes for several months, even when they are monitored at home. In their observation of 83 preterm infants, they found that 16% had serious episodes that required parental intervention, including mouth-to-mouth ventilation in one infant. Ironically, home apnea monitors have not been shown to decrease the incidence of SIDS. Although many factors contribute to these results, they mainly were due to parental noncompliance with monitoring technique and limitations of the monitors themselves.[31,32] An elegant study on parental compliance was recently performed by Cordero et al.,[33] who used monitors with electronic memory to allow for more objective evaluation. Their study included 30 premature infants. Of 26 parents who recalled never leaving their infant unmonitored, 70% missed at least one night and 30% missed at least three or more nights. The authors also found that the decline in use of home monitors progressed as time went by. Some of the babies were unmonitored more than 30% of the day and 15% were unmonitored at night.

Home Pharmaceutical Services

Home pharmaceutical services are now more widely used in respiratory disorders. These services include home intravenous antibiotic infusion and aerosolized antibiotic for the treatment of pulmonary infections of cystic fibrosis. They may also involve aerosolized bronchodilator and anti-inflammatory drugs for the treatment of childhood asthma and home intravenous antibiotics for the treatment of acute respiratory infections.

Home Intravenous Antibiotic Therapy for Cystic Fibrosis

Patients with cystic fibrosis experience frequent exacerbations of their pulmonary infection. This usually leads to long periods of hospitalization, requiring intravenous antibiotic therapy in addition to frequent postural drainage and nutritional intervention and support. Several studies have demonstrated the feasibility of home intravenous antibiotic treatment in patients with cystic fibrosis.[34-37] Clinical improvement was clearly demonstrated and patients seemed to prefer home treatment over hospital admission.[34] In addition to the psychosocial advantage, the cost effectiveness was substantial in most of these studies. For example, in one study, the average saving per course of home intravenous antibiotic therapy was $5017, or $618 per day.[35] The frequent use of peripherally inserted central venous catheters (PICC) has made home intravenous antibiotic therapy more acceptable to many patients and their families. These silastic long lines are superior to conventional cannulas in terms of patient tolerance and reduction in number of hospital admissions, number of repeated venepunctures, and local complications.[36] Most patients on this therapy are usually able to attend school or work. Although home intravenous antibiotic therapy has been found to be effective, few control comparisons of clinical outcome between home and hospital therapy have been conducted. A recent study by Pond et al.[37] found no significant difference in improvement in forced vital capacity, forced expiratory volume in one second, C-reactive protein, plasma viscosity, total white cell count, absolute neutrophil count, total immunoglobulin G concentration, chest x-ray score (Northern), Shwachman-Kulczyki score, and weight gain. Further, in this study, most patients were found to prefer home treatment and a minority of patients refused any hospital admission.

In addition to cystic fibrosis, home intravenous antibiotic therapy is now being given for a wide array of pulmonary and respiratory infections such as acute sinusitis and acute pneumonia. Usually patients are admitted to the hospital for a few days and then sent home to continue therapy. Before such practices become widely accepted, however, additional studies to determine outcome criteria, such as rehospitalization rates, average length of home care service per diagnosis, and compliance issues, should be conducted.

Home Aerosolized Antimicrobial Therapy for Cystic Fibrosis

The use of home inhaled antibiotics in patients with cystic fibrosis is now becoming the standard of care in many North American and European cystic fibrosis centers. Aerosolized antibiotics are usually used for mild to moderate pulmonary exacerbation or for prophylaxis, in order to avert pulmonary deterioration. The most commonly used aerosolized antibiotics are tobramycin and colistin. Wall et al.[38] reported on the efficacy of inhaled tobramycin and ticarcillin in nine patients with worsening cystic fibrosis lung disease. All patients were treated for 5 to 15 months with 80 mg of tobramycin and 1 g of ticarcillin, administered twice daily with a hand-held nebulizer. Hospital admissions rates decreased after active treatment, and weight gain improved. No emergent resistance to tobramycin was noted during or immediately after the study period. The authors concluded that prophylactic inhalation of antibiotics may lead to a significant improvement in the lifestyle of certain patients with cystic fibrosis. MacLusky et al.[39] demonstrated that inhaled tobramycin arrested or delayed pulmonary deterioration in some patients with cystic fibrosis colonized with *Pseudomonas aeruginosa*; however, in the 32-month study period, 33% of patients treated with nebulized tobramycin (80 mg, three times daily) acquired resistant organism after treatment. More recently, a high dose (600 mg) of preservative-free tobramycin given via ultrasonic nebulizer three times a day for 28 days was shown to be efficacious and safe treatment for endobronchial infections in stable cystic fibrosis patients.[40] In these studies,[38-40] tobramycin was found to be safe, with no renal or ototoxicity. However, in some susceptible individuals, inhaled gentamicin has been shown to cause bronchospasm.[41] Therefore, patients receiving inhaled antibiotics should be monitored closely. The other inhaled antibiotic widely used is colistin. Littlewood et al.[42] showed that children with cystic fibrosis had a reduced frequency of positive *Pseudomonas aeruginosa* cultures after inhalation of colistin. Jensen et al.[43] found that colistin-treated patients had better clinical score and pulmonary function and less inflammatory mediators than patients treated with placebo.

Home Care for Childhood Asthma

Asthma is one of the most prevalent chronic illnesses in childhood. It affects 9 to 12 million persons in the United States.[44] Minority groups and the poor population appear to be involved disproportionately in the number of hospitalizations and mortalities related to asthma. In addition to the enormous personal and social costs, asthma places a significant burden on health care resources. The total care for asthma was estimated to be 1% of the total U.S. health care expenditure.[45] No other pediatric problem has such far-reaching consequences. Asthma is generally treated in an outpatient setting. Given the high cost of hospital inpatient care, it seems that a less intensive alternative to hospital treatment for asthma is needed, in order to reduce the cost for asthma care.

Effective treatment of asthma revolves around proper outpatient management and the use of anti-inflammatory agents as the primary drug therapy. Unfortunately, until recently, guidelines for the treatment of asthma and outcome measures have been lacking. Furthermore, cost–benefit studies for asthma management have also been lacking. In 1989, the National Asthma Education Program (NAEP) was established by the National Heart, Lung and Blood Institute, and in 1991 a booklet which contained the guidelines for measurement of asthma was released.[46] It was the desire of the NAEP that effective control of asthma should be promoted through modern science-based treatment and education programs and by encouraging partnership among patient, general practitioner, specialist, and other health care providers.

Home care for asthma is a rather new entity. It revolves mainly around families treating their children. Home care agencies are now involved in the home treatment of childhood asthma. They provide durable medical equipment, such as nebulizers needed to deliver aerosolized bronchodilators and anti-inflammatory drugs. They also provide nursing services to instruct on medication usage, to assess compliance, and to check the home environment for the presence of triggers.

The efficacy and safety of home nebulizer therapy for children with asthma were studied by Zimo and colleagues[47] in 1989. The safety of nebulized beta agonists used in the homes of 22 children was assessed. Significant reduction in the number of emergency department visits and hospital admissions and shorter courses of prednisone therapy occurred when home nebulizer therapy was provided. The younger the patient, the more frequently improvement occurred.

Carswell et al.[48] assessed the efficacy of using a home visiting asthma nurse in the treatment of childhood asthma. Their study, done in Bristol, England, looked at the clinical asthma outcome measures when a community nurse who had specific training in asthma visited the homes of patients. During the 6-month study, these children developed and sustained higher peak flow expiratory rates than 43 control asthmatics.

More recently, Butz et al.[49] studied the use of community health workers to obtain health, social, and environmental information from African-American inner-city children with asthma; 140 school-age children with asthma were recruited and enrolled in a program to receive home visits by community health workers. The study found that appropriately recruited and trained community health workers are effective in obtaining useful medical information from inner-city families with children with asthma and in providing basic asthma education in the home.

A more comprehensive study in the care of asthma was conducted by Hughes et al.[50] Their 2-year randomized, controlled trial involved 95 children. Intervention for the study group during the first year included 3 months of clinic visits, education, and home visits by a specially trained research nurse. The control subjects continued to receive their regular care from their family doctors or their pediatricians. Study subjects had less school absenteeism than control subjects and showed significantly better small airway function after 1 year. The severity of asthma also improved in 13 study subjects. Study subjects exhibited better technique in using their metered dose inhalers and had fewer hospital admissions than control subjects. The authors concluded that comprehensive ambulatory programs for childhood asthma management can improve objective measures of illness severity.

The potential saving as a result of the shift from more expensive inpatient hospital care to less expensive ambulatory care seems to be the way of the future. A close partnership between patient, general practitioner, and specialist; proper allocation of health care resources according to the severity of the illness; and proper use of outpatient setting, home care services, and program education would ultimately lead to reduced cost and better outcome measures in childhood asthma.

Psychosocial Impact of Home Respiratory Care

Caring for a chronically ill child at home is not easy. Despite the potential advantages of home care cited earlier, families of technology-dependent children experience a high level of stress which may impair their coping mechanisms. When home health care involves the use of advanced medical technology, it strains the traditional conceptions of parental responsibility to care for the health of children at home.[51] Quint et al.[52] studied the impact of providing home care for ventilator-dependent children in 18 northern California families. Primary caretakers in this sample showed significantly reduced coping subscale scores with a longer duration of home ventilatory care. Another study examined 29 parents' perceptions of coping for their chronically ill child at home and found that increased caregiving burden (when parents were primarily responsible for their children's care regimen) was associated with greater stressfulness and the use of fewer helpful coping strategies.[53] Other investigators found similar results in parents of medically fragile children cared for at home.[54] Of 57 families studied, 59% of the mothers and 67% of the fathers reported a significant level of distress symptoms, which seem to increase with increased family responsibilities for home care.

Many families experience social isolation because of their care commitments at home.[16] They may experience family disruption, which can lead to poor health. Ahmann et al.[55] examined 12 aspects of family life among 93 families with infants considered at high risk for SIDS and on home apnea monitors. Mothers of such infants were found to have increased risk of poor health when compared to controls. Other predictors of family stress have been identified in parents of ventilator-assisted children. These include families with financial problems, families with large numbers of extended family members in the household, and families without designate nurse care managers.[56]

Physicians should have a complete understanding of the impact of home health care on the family, especially when it involves technology-dependent devices. Clinicians and health policymakers should address the long-term effects on family life and then target extra support services for families identified to be at risk in these areas.[57] Successful home care depends upon the ability of the family to cope with this option, the ability of the community to provide the necessary services to the family, and a comprehensive care plan that provides education for both the family and the caregivers.

Conclusion

In conclusion, home care for respiratory disorders is a compassionate way to deliver care to patients in their own environment. It can be a rewarding experience for both the patient and the physician. It is feasible, cost effective, and even medically effective in many instances. However, respiratory home care is not without problems. The physician who refers his or her patient to home care services must understand that he or she alone is ultimately responsible for that patient. Therefore, choosing a home health care agency is extremely important. The physician must rely upon written reports, phone conversations, and team conferences to assess the response of the patient to therapy. Managing a patient in such a way can sometimes be frustrating.

Another problem is quality assurance. The physician must rely upon proper equipment delivered by the home care agency and the proper functioning of the equipment. Paradoxically, and despite the important role of physicians in initiating and implementing home care, inadequate and limited reimbursement remains an issue. Goldberg et al.[58] believe that home care will be the "next frontier" in pediatric practice and that future changes in health care delivery should encourage the participation of physicians in program development in order to implement cost-efficient home care.

Finally, home respiratory care involves teamwork among many players; the patient and the family are at the center, then the physician, and multiple health care providers are included on the team. All team players must work together closely in order to deliver optimal, safe, and cost-effective treatment.

References

1. Halamandaris, V. J., *Basic Statistics About Home Care 1994*, National Association for Home Care, Washington, D.C., 1994.
2. Strahan, G., Overview of Home Health and Hospice Care Patients: Preliminary Data from the 1992 National Home and Hospice Care Survey, Advance Data from Vital and Health Statistics, Number 235, National Health Statistics, Hyattsville, Maryland, 1993.
3. Vladeck, B. D., From Health Care Financing Administration: Medicare home health initiative, *JAMA*, 271:1566, 1994.
4. Goldberg, A. I., Pediatric high technology home care, in *Intensive Home Care*, Rothkopf, M. M. and Askenazi, J., Eds., Williams and Wilkins, Baltimore, 1992, pp. 199–213.
5. Aday, L. A. and Wegener, D. H., Home care for ventilator-assisted children: implications for the children, their families and health policy, *Children's Health Care*, 17:112–120, 1988.
6. Allen, N. L., Simone, J. A., and Wingenbach, G. F., Families with a ventilator-assisted child: transitional issues, *J. Perinatol.*, 14:48–55, 1994.
7. Waldhorn, R. E., Nocturnal nasal intermittent positive airway pressure (BiPAP®) in respiratory failure, *Chest*, 101:516–521, 1992.
8. Teague, W. G., Kervin, L. J., DiWadkar, V. V., and Scott, P. H., Nasal bi-level positive airway pressure BiPAP acutely improves ventilation and oxygen saturation in children with upper airway obstruction (Abstract), *Am. Rev. Respir. Dis.*, 143:A505, 1991.
9. Padman, R., Lawless, S., and Von Nessen, S., Use of BiPAP® by nasal mask in the treatment of respiratory insufficiency in pediatric patients, *Pediatr. Pulmonol.*, 17:119–123, 1994.
10. Field, A. I., Cobble, D. H., Pollack, M. M., and Kaufman, J., Outcome of home care for technology-dependent children: success of an independent, community-based case management model, *Pediatr. Pulmonol.*, 11:310–317, 1991.
11. Frates, R. C., Jr., Splaingard, M. L., Smith, E. O., and Harrison, G. M., Outcome of home mechanical ventilation in children, *J. Pediatr.*, 106:850–856, 1985.
12. Canlas-Yamsuan, M., Sanchez, I., Kesselman, M., and Chernick, V., Morbidity and mortality patterns of ventilator-dependent children in a home care program, *Clin. Pediatr.*, 32:706–713, 1993.
13. DeWitt, P. K., Jansen, M. T., Davidson-Ward, S. L., and Keens, T. J., Obstacles to discharge of ventilator-assisted children, from hospital to home, *Chest*, 103:1560–1565, 1993.
14. Okamoto, E., Fee, W. F., Boles, R., et al., Safety of hospital vs home care of infant tracheostomies, *Trans. Am. Acad. Ophthal. Otol.*, 84:92–99, 1977.
15. Duncan, E. W., Howell, L. J., DeLorimer, A. A., Adzick, N. S., and Harrison, M. R., Tracheostomy in children with emphasis on home care, *J. Pediatr. Surg.*, 27:432–435, 1992.

16. Zander, J. H., Comprehensive home care, in *Respiratory Disease in Children: Diagnosis and Management*, Loughlin, A. M. and Eigen, H., Eds., Williams and Wilkins, Baltimore, 1994, pp. 783–794.

17. Zinman, R., Franco, I., and Pizzuti-Daechsel, R., Home oxygen delivery system for infants, *Pediatr. Pulmonol.*, 1:325–327, 1985.

18. Coates, A. L., Blanchard, P. W., and Schloss, M. D., Simplified oxygen administration in tracheotomized patients with bronchopulmonary dysplasia, *Int. J. Pediatr. Otorhinolaryngol.*, 10:87–90, 1985.

19. Panitch, H. B. and Isaacson, G., Transtracheal oxygen use in a young girl with bronchopulmonary dysplasia, *Pediatr. Pulmonol.*, 18:255–257, 1994.

20. Heimlich, H. J. and Carr, G. C., The micro-trach. A seven-year experience with transtracheal oxygen therapy, *Chest*, 95:1008–1012, 1989.

21. Banner, N. R. and Govan, J. R., Long term transtracheal oxygen delivery through microcatheter in patients with hypoxemia due to chronic obstructive airways disease, *Br. Med. J.*, 293:111–114, 1986.

22. Groothuis, J. R. and Rosenberg, A. A., Home oxygen promotes weight gain in infants with bronchopulmonary dysplasia, *AJDC*, 141:992–995, 1987.

23. Hudak, B. B., Allen, M. C., Hudak, M. L., and Loughlin, G. M., Home oxygen therapy for chronic lung disease in extremely low birth weight infants, *AJDC*, 143:357–360, 1989.

24. Abman, S. H., Wolfe, R. R., Accurso, F. J., Koops, B. L., Bowman, C. M., and Wiggins, J. J., Pulmonary vascular response to oxygen in infants with severe bronchopulmonary dysplasia, *Pediatrics*, 75:80–84, 1985.

25. Halliday, H. L., Dumpit, F. M., and Brady, J. P., Effects of inspired oxygen on echocardiographic assessment of pulmonary vascular resistance and myocardia contractibility in bronchopulmonary dysplasia, *Pediatrics*, 65:536–540, 1980.

26. McAleese, K. A., Knapp, M. A., and Rhodes, T. T., Financial and emotional costs of bronchopulmonary dysplasia, *Clin. Pediatr.*, 32:393–400, 1993.

27. Zahr, L. K. and Montejo, J., The benefit of home care for sick premature infants, *Neonat. Network*, 12:33–37, 1993.

28. Casiro, G. O., McKenzie, M. E., McFadye, N. L., Shapiro, C., Seshia, M. M., McDonald, N., Moffatt, M., and Cheanj, M. S., Earlier discharge with community-based intervention for low birth weight infants, a randomized trial, *Pediatrics*, 92:128–134, 1993.

29. Beckerman, R. C. and Goyco, P., Sudden infant death syndrome, in *Pediatric Respiratory Disease: Diagnosis and Treatment*, Hilman, B., Ed., W.B. Saunders, Philadelphia, 1993, pp. 579–584.

30. Rosen, C. L., Glaze, D. G., and Frost, J. D., Home monitor follow-up of persistent apnea and bradycardia in pre-term infants, *AJDC*, 140:537–550, 1986.

31. Meny, R. G., Blackmon, L., Fleischmann, D., Gutberlet, R., and Naumburg, E., Sudden infant death and home monitors, *AJDC*, 142:1037–1040, 1988.

32. Cain, L. P., Kelly, D. H., and Shannon, D. C., Parents perception of the psychological and social impact of home monitoring, *Pediatrics*, 66:37–41, 1980.

33. Cordero, L., Morehead, S., and Miller, R., Parental compliance with home apnea monitoring, *J. Perinatol.*, 13:448–452, 1993.

34. Gilbert, J., Robinson, T., and Littlewood, J. M., Home intravenous antibiotics treatment in cystic fibrosis, *Arch. Dis. Child.*, 63:512–517, 1988.

35. Kane, R. E., Jennison, K., Wood, C., Black, P. G., and Herbst, J. J., Cost savings and economic considerations using home intravenous antibiotic therapy for cystic fibrosis patients, *Pediatr. Pulmonol.*, 4:84–89, 1988.

36. Pradeepkumar, V. K., Waseem, E., Shortt, C., Barry, D., and Watson, J. B., Home intravenous therapy using a silastic long line catheter in cystic fibrosis, *Ir. Med. J.*, 85:110–111, 1992.

37. Pond, M. N., Newport, M., Joanes, D., and Conway, S. P., Home versus hospital intravenous antibiotic therapy in the treatment of young adults with cystic fibrosis, *Eur. Respir. J.*, 7:1640–1644, 1994.

38. Wall, M. A., Terry, A. B., Eisenberg, J., McNamara, M., and Cohen, R., Inhaled antibiotics in cystic fibrosis, *Lancet*, 1:1325, 1983.

39. MacLusky, I. B., Gold, R., Corey, M., and Levison, H., Long-term effects of inhaled tobramycin in patients with cystic fibrosis colonized with *Pseudomonas aeruginosa, Pediatr. Pulmonol.*, 7:42–48, 1989.

40. Ramsey, B. W., Dorkin, H. L., Eisenberg, J. D., et al., Efficacy of aerosolized tobramycin in patients with cystic fibrosis, *New Engl. J. Med.*, 328:1740–1746, 1993.

41. Dally, M. B., Kurvis, S., and Breslin, A. B., Ventilatory effects of aerosol gentamicin, *Thorax*, 33:54–56, 1978.

42. Littlewood, J. M., Miller, M. G., Chonheim, A. T., and Ranmsden, C. H., Nebulized colomycin for early pseudomonas colonization in cystic fibrosis, *Lancet*, 1:865, 1985.

43. Jensen, T., Petersen, S. S., Barrie, S., et al., Colistin inhalation therapy in cystic fibrosis patients with chronic *Pseudomonas aeruginosa* lung infections, *J. Antimicrob. Chemother.*, 19:831–831, 1987.

44. Evans, R., III, Mullally, D. I., Wilson, R. W., et al., National trends in the morbidity and mortality of asthma in the U.S., *Chest*, 91(Suppl.) 6:655–745, 1987.

45. Weiss, K. B., Gergen, P. J., and Hogdson, T. A., An economic evaluation of asthma in the United States, *New Engl. J. Med.*, 326:862–866, 1992.

46. National Asthma Education Program Expert Panel Report, Publication Number 91-3042A, National Institutes of Health, Bethesda, Maryland, 1991.

47. Zimo, D. A., Gaspar, R. M., and Akhter, J., The efficacy and safety of home nebulizer therapy for children with asthma, *AJDC*, 143:208–211, 1989.

48. Carswell, F., Robinson, E. J., Hek, J., and Shenton, T., A Bristol experience: benefits and cost of an asthma nurse visiting the homes of asthmatic children, *Bristol Medico Chirugical J.*, 104:11–12, 1989.

49. Butz, A. M., Malveaux, F. J., Eggleston, P., et al., Use of community health care workers with inner-city children who have asthma, *Clin. Pediatr.*, 33:135–141, 1994.

50. Hughes, D. M., McLeod, M., Garner, B., and Goldbloom, R. B., Controlled trial of a home and ambulatory program for asthmatic children, *Pediatrics*, 87:54–61, 1991.

51. Lantos, J. D. and Kohrman, A. F., Ethical aspects of pediatric home care, *Pediatrics*, 89:920–924, 1992.

52. Quint, R. D., Chesterman, E., Crain, L. S., Winkleby, M., and Boyce, W. T., Home care for ventilator-dependent children. Psychosocial impact on the family, *AJDC*, 144:1238–1241, 1990.

53. Ray, L. D. and Ritchie, J. A., Caring for chronically-ill children at home: factors that influence parents' coping, *J. Pediatr. Nurs.*, 8:217–225, 1993.

54. Leonard, B. J., Brast, J. D., and Nelson, R. P., Parental distress: caring for medically fragile children at home, *J. Pediatr. Nurs.*, 8:22–30, 1993.

55. Ahmann, E., Wulff, L., and Meny, R. G., Home apnea monitoring and disruption in family life: a multidimensional controlled study, *Am. J. Public Health*, 82:719–722, 1992.

56. Wegener, D. H. and Aday, L. V., Home care for ventilator-assisted children: predicting family stress, *Pediatr. Nurs.*, 5:371–376, 1989.

57. Ahmann, E., Meny, R. G., Wulff, L., and Fink, R., Home apnea monitoring and risk factors for poor family functioning, *J. Perinatol.*, 13:310–318, 1993.

58. Goldberg, A. I., Gardner, H. G., and Gibson, L. E., Home care: the next frontier of pediatric practice, *J. Pediatr.*, 125:686–690, 1994.

Home Health Care of Chronically/Terminally Ill Child

14

Salvatore J. Bertolone, M.D.

Introduction

Although parents have traditionally provided care at home for routine childhood illnesses (vomiting, diarrhea, and colds), they are increasingly called upon to deliver more health care at home as "routine health care" takes on new meaning. Hospitalization of children occurs rarely and usually only after extreme circumstances. When hospitalization does occur, it alters the customary division of authority between parents and professionals. Home care for the technology-dependent child represents neither traditional hospital care nor traditional home care.[1] It is this aspect of home health care that continues to widen and thereby change the traditional paradigm.

Private and public care health funding policies of the 1930s and 1940s encouraged hospital- and office-based care while creating payment and clinical management disincentives for care in the home. However, medical progress has resulted in the survival of children with previously fatal illnesses who can frequently be cared for by the family in the home. Unfortunately, while home-based care has been described by the Health Care Financing Administration as the fastest growing component of health care, physician participation has been discouraged by an inadequate knowledge base.[2] Involvement requires education that is not usually available in medical schools and postgraduate programs. Issues of quality and risk management require physician attention to appropriate candidate selection, preparation in training of patients and families, and commu-

273

nication among physicians, home care service providers, payors, and family members.

Specific physician competencies have been identified by Goldberg et al.[2] and include understanding and utilizing the required community resources. The physician must specifically determine which resources are medically appropriate for individual patient and family needs and reevaluate the medical necessity periodically. Physicians should be familiar with current costs and reimbursement issues in home health care. They also should remain current about public and private funding policies and supplemental funding sources. Primary care physicians should understand the principles of life support treatments and monitoring that can be accomplished at home. Medical devices have been designed and adapted for home use which make possible intravenous antibiotics, chemotherapy, blood product administration, metabolic endocrine support, cardiopulmonary monitoring, and maintenance of vital organ functions. The physician should be aware of research-validated state-of-the-art technology and understand the relationship among primary versus specialty care providers, physician versus other home health care members, and hospital- versus community-based services. Also, physicians should be aware of all elements of home care and their specific criteria to meet the needs of individual cases: medical, psychosocial, environmental, technical, organizational, and financial. Physicians should be actively involved in hospital discharge planning and management of the patient as a team effort. A physician should understand the collaborative team model and be aware of the skills and abilities of all team members. He or she must approve the educational plan for the family and caregivers and participate in the preparation of the child and family for care. Written records should include integrated information about the family, the ambulatory setting, and the hospital care for the patient. Family-centered care is the key to success for home care. Many families are capable of major management roles in partnership with professionals. Physician and team members should be able to determine the availability and reliability of the family unit, including friends, neighbors, and other neighborhood primary caregivers. Physicians must understand the risk of caregiver burnout and identify the need for and capability of supplemental support for families (i.e., respite care and self-help groups).

Home Health Care/Hospice and the Oncologic Patient

In the United States, approximately 100,000 children die each year. Major causes of death vary according to age. In the first year of life, the leading causes of death are birth defects, sudden infant death syndrome, and problems related to pregnancy, childbirth, and the period immediately after birth. Accidental injury is the leading cause of death in all children over the age of one and accidents actually account for more than 25,000 deaths each year in children and young adolescents.[3] Approximately 10% of all deaths during childhood are related to cancer. It is not surprising, then, that hospice has played an important role in home health for the oncologic patient.

Dr. Ida Martinson's pioneer work reported on alternatives to hospitalization for children dying with cancer.[4–6] More recent studies have included care for children with other terminal conditions.[7,8] Caring for the dying child at home is both cost effective and desirable. The actual time required to care for a dying child with incurable cancer, inoperative heart disease, or birth defects is often of such short duration that there is little rationale for not providing families with the opportunity to do so. With improved methods of pain control and other effective system management techniques (i.e., the use of beepers and/or portable telephones and the support of the hospice team), families should be able to be co-managers of the care of their dying child.

When Americans turned most of the care of dying patients over to hospitals in the middle third of this century, observers became concerned about the consequences of that action. Evidence mounted showing that health care workers were uncomfortable with taking care of dying patients.[9,10] Nurses and other hospital staff members were observed to avoid contact and discussions of death with the terminally ill. In an attempt to solve these problems, the hospice concept was introduced in this country in the early 1970s. Saunders[11] describes the hospice movement as a *concept* of care rather than as a *site* of care. Dedicated to total family care, hospice attempts to alleviate pain and responds to the dying patient in a holistic manner. There is special attention to physical, social, emotional, and spiritual needs of the dying patient. A number of organizational models have been developed and tested. Dr. Martinson's original work calls for a change in both the goal for terminal care and a means for accomplishing that goal. The changed goal was to provide comfort and care for children with terminal illness and to provide that care in the child's home rather than in the hospital. This called for two important changes in prevailing practices. First, there was a change to a nurse-directed rather than a physician-directed care program. Second, parents assumed the role of primary caregivers, with health care professionals serving as consultants and giving assistance upon request of the parents.[7,12–14] Many adjustments in the care of dying children in acute care hospitals have taken place, but this care is still at odds with most of the dying child's needs. Hospital technology, protocols, and professionals have cure or restoration as their goal. Patients with diseases that fail to respond do not seem to fit into the acute care hospital setting. Dying children in particular want to be at home and not subjected to unneeded intrusive procedures.

A mid-1980s study[15] showed that home care services were offered by approximately 85% of pediatric institutions that cared for seriously ill children. Half of these institutions administered their own programs; the other half relied upon community-based services. Institutions that provided their own services offered home care to a greater proportion of eligible patients, had a larger proportion of families accept this option, and had a smaller proportion of children return to the hospital to die than institutions that used community agencies.

Dr. Martinson's studies have demonstrated the changing roles of the family, physician, and nurse. The expanded role of the nurse includes teaching health assessment, procurement of medical equipment, facilitating physician care, performing technical treatment, and providing emotional counseling. Telephone support is also frequently provided. Initial studies demonstrated the desirability and feasibility of home care for children dying of cancer, and subsequent studies have dealt with the issues of continuing experimental therapy in the home health care and hospice settings. Martinson presents readers with arguments that families deserve the option to continue therapy even if the chances of cure are small.[16,17]

Family Decision Making: Home or Hospital?

The parents' decision on how terminal care should be given will be affected by a number of variables, primarily the child's and their own desires and abilities to provide care. A retrospective survey of parents who had cared for their dying child at home revealed that the parents perceived their ability to provide care as second in importance only to the child's desire to be at home. Other areas that ranked high were the desires of siblings and parents to have the sick child at home.[18] The factors that had a low influence on a parent's decision were cost and suggestions from friends and other parents of hospitalized children. Factors reported to influence the decision for terminal home care include the availability of 24-hour nursing, the open-door policy of allowing a child to return to the hospital at any time, and the child's perceived concern that he or she could not receive adequate care at home.[19] Common concerns among parents in this setting were the negative factors of fear, of not being able to control their child's pain, and extreme anxiety over what would occur at the moment of death and the effects of a child dying at home on their healthy siblings. Lauer et al.[20] reported their findings concerning children's perceptions of their sibling's death at home versus in a hospital. Children who participated in home care described a significantly different experience than those whose siblings died in the hospital. All children involved in home care reported full awareness that their sibling was dying. In contrast, only 30% of children whose siblings were hospitalized reported an awareness that their sibling was dying. Children in the home care group were more than twice as likely to have spoken to their sibling about his or her impending death. Recently, Martinson et al. examined the self-concept of bereaved siblings.[21] Their findings indicate that the self-concept ratings of these siblings were significantly higher than would be expected from normal children. These data are preliminary and the number of patient subjects is small, but the results would indicate that healthy siblings may benefit in their grief process and self-image when they participate in the home care of a sibling dying at home. When various aspects of a palliative home or hospital care program have been evaluated, components of the program deemed most satisfactory were being able to care for the child at home, having access to a palliative care nurse, and having access to a pediatric clinical pharmacist.[22] The National Hospice Organization and Children's Hospital International described their support and philosophy of palliative care as one that affirms life. Corr and Corr[23] explore this concept of pediatric hospice care in which hospice care is a philosophy and attitude or an approach to care, rather than a place. Because hospice affirms life, those interested in the hospice philosophy care not only for the dying child but also for the parents, siblings, and friends of the child who is dying. Although do not resuscitate (DNR) orders are available (which means not initiating cardiopulmonary resuscitation), many parents still want aggressive supportive care to include blood products, antibiotics, daily blood work, continued diagnostic procedures, and palliative chemotherapy and/or radiotherapy. Hospice of Louisville trains its nurses in this state-of-the-art technology. However, when a child is terminal, arrangements are made with the parents and primary care hospice nurse to alert the medical examiner of an impending death. When the child dies, his or her body can be taken directly to the funeral home once the medical examiner has been notified because these arrangements have been made in advance. The police and medical examiner are avoided, which helps the family maintain its level of intimacy and privacy. The death certificate is forwarded from the funeral home to the primary physician's office, where it is signed.

Currently the use of indwelling central line catheters has changed the management of pain and related issues for patients in the homebound setting. Many terminal pediatric patients have thrombocytopenia and recurrent anemia. With the use of central venous catheters, it is possible to administer antibiotics, intravenous fluids, and blood products to include red blood cells and platelets, as well as continuous drip opiates if necessary. The relatively recent addition of Fentanyl® patches also allows for transdermal continuous pain medication, which can be supplemented with home infusion pumps of opiate boluses.

Home Health Care and Bone Marrow Transplantation

One reads with amazement and dismay the following catching headline: "bone marrow transplantation as an outpatient treatment." Certainly anyone in the medical field or a related field realizes that bone marrow transplantation is not an outpatient procedure. However, in this day and age of cost containment, the medical profession is constantly striving to look for new ways to perform old procedures more cost efficiently.

There are three types of bone marrow transplants (BMTs). Autologous BMT involves a collection of the patient's own bone marrow during a known remission of the patient's disease. The patient usually has a solid tumor with no bone marrow involvement or metastasis. Bone marrow stem cells and/or peripheral stem cells can be harvested either from the bone marrow in the traditional operating room setting or harvested from the various pheresis machines that are available (Cobe, Fenwal, Hemanetics). Using neutrophil growth factor to stimulate marrow white counts, the patient's neutrophil counts will rise to 30,000 to 60,000 per cubic millimeter. This allows for the collection of numerous CD34+ stem cells. BMT will have engraftment and/or earlier neutrophil production using a combination of bone marrow and peripheral stem cells.

Allogeneic BMT involves the procurement of bone marrow from an HLA-identical individual (usually a sibling) and/or finding an HLA match through the Matched Unrelated Donor Program of the National Bone Marrow Registry Program, which currently has over 1.5 million individuals registered who have identified themselves as willing bone marrow donors. These individuals are taken to the operating room and bone marrow is harvested from them as donors who are HLA matched with a recipient who needs the bone marrow. The bone marrow cells are then reinfused into the patient after high-dose myeloablative chemotherapy and/or radiation therapy. This type of transplantation usually has more complications due to potential problems related to graft vs. host disease.

Another type of marrow transplant involves syngeneic BMT in which the marrow donor is an identical twin of the recipient. Once a patient is admitted for BMT, he or she undergoes the preparative regimen, which usually consists of high-dose chemotherapy and/or radiotherapy. This totally ablates the patient's bone marrow and all its blood-forming cells. Depending upon the regimen and the side effects, the patient is seen as an outpatient the morning of the bone marrow harvest and taken to the operating room as an outpatient. The marrow is then harvested through multiple bone marrow aspirations—as many as 50 to 100. The patient then receives the myeloablative therapy as an inpatient or an outpatient with close monitoring.

Whether the transplant is autologous or allogeneic, there may be a "honeymoon" period in which it takes approximately 4 to 7 days for the white count and platelet count to drop to absolute zero levels. It is during this time that the patient may be monitored in a nearby outpatient facility close to the hospital with appropriate personnel trained in evaluation of the patient. With a noncomplicated autologous solid tumor transplant, it is entirely possible for the absolute neutrophil counts to be >500 per square millimeter in 14 to 21 days. This is the theory behind following some of these patients in an outpatient setting. The more toxic regimens, allogeneic regimens, mismatched transplants, and matched unrelated donor transplants will require much closer monitoring and longer inpatient hospitalization.

As identified by Randolph,[24] there are three keys to the successful and safe discharge of a BMT patient: communication, collaboration, and continuity of patient care. Continuous updates from the BMT team are necessary for the outpatient care providers so that accurate and timely patient problems can be identified and/or adverted. In most instances, when the BMT team discharges a patient, it is discharging the patient to an extension of its own team (i.e., not a routine home health care team, but rather outpatient members of the unified team who have been specially trained in the seriousness of complications associated with BMT). Key participants in the program include primary nurses, clinical pharmacists, dietitians, and social workers. One such program is Critical Care America, which launched a nationwide home health care program for BMT patients in early 1991. All nurses take part in competency-based programs specific to BMT, as well as oncology, chemotherapy, and pediatrics. Primary nursing ensures consistency in assessments, compliance with scheduled medicines, and prompt recognition of changes in the patient's status. Any alterations in the patient's health are promptly communicated to members of the transplant team. Because pharmacists are specifically and specially educated in BMT, they recognize correct pharmaceutical management of these patients and complications of their infusion therapies.[24] The complexity of the BMT patient is driven by the high level of susceptibility to infection and multiple organ damage associated with BMT. This backup team of outpatient caregivers must be available 24 hours a day and have 24-hour-a-day, 7-day-a-week access to BMT physicians specifically and specially trained in caring for these patients. BMT is not a stand-alone outpatient procedure but rather is a very complicated high-tech procedure that requires intensive inpatient and outpatient supervision.

Hemophilia and Home Therapy

Hemophilia, the absence of blood clotting Factor VIII or Factor IX, in male patients has been the prototype for home infusion therapy. Dr. Richard Haulden as medical director of the Blood Center in Texas wrote a letter recalling his efforts to stimulate home transfusions in the Texas area in 1960.[25] These early attempts were usually for geographical reasons. It is reported that patients in Scandinavia living many miles from the nearest hospital were encouraged to store fresh frozen plasma at home. With the introduction of cryoprecipitate and subsequently large-scale fractionation of Factors VIII and IX, home therapy became universally available in developed countries.[26,27] While it might have been argued initially that parents were incapable of treating their children, physicians not caring for hemophiliacs, the medical community in general, and the lay public did not understand the restrictions imposed on hemophiliacs dependent upon hospital therapy and did not appreciate the scope of home therapy. A home hemotherapy program is a generic term that covers injection by patients themselves or by suitably trained parents or guardians. More importantly, it means therapy on their terms and in their time frame.[28] It means convenient therapy to allow for school and/or work attendance. It provides coverage for holidays and business travel whether on demand or crisis. For the hemophilia community, this came to be known as comprehensive care. Federal funding of hemophilia centers in the United States has shown the average days lost from school or work in the year after the introduction of comprehensive care to fall between 58 and 86% of previous lost days.[29,30] The three rules of hemophilia therapy that have stood the test of time remain (1) the earlier the treatment is given, the better; (2) when in doubt, treat; and (3) a shot in time saves Factors VIII or IX. Along with Factors VIII or IX infusion for classic hemophiliacs, any of the purified factor concentrates for factor-deficient patients are available for home use.[31]

In 1985, the American Association of Blood Banks (AABB) began investigating home transfusion as an extension of outpatient therapy. The scientific commission of the AABB has now set forth and published a pamphlet of suggestive protocols and documentation forms for the initiation of a home transfusion program.[32,33] Pluth[33] reports a zero incidence of either transfusion or posttransfusion reaction during the administration of 350 units of red blood cells and 65 units of platelets to 40 clients over a 2-year period. General patients selected for home hemotherapy include those with a history of previous transfusion and no adverse reactions and patients in stable medical condition without any major cardiovascular compromise also with adequate venous access. In tandem with this, the home environment requires a working telephone, a capable primary caregiver to be present during the transfusion, ready access to emergency medical services, as well as ready access to a primary physician during transfusion and ready access to the transfusion team. Average nursing time in some studies has been approximately 9 hours, with 4.5 hours representing actual home visit time and 4.5 hours in travel time to and from the patient's home and the blood bank.[34]

Technology

None of the above would have been possible without the development and implementation of the new infusion pumps as well as numerous central venous catheters. Permanent central venous catheters have become standard in the management of children with malignancies. They are commonly placed in patients with cystic fibrosis, short gut syndrome, hemophilia, sickle cell disease, and HIV patients, to name a few. The insertion of PIC (peripheral inserted catheter) lines can be used to facilitate short courses of home antibiotics for patients with cystic fibrosis, appendicitis, osteomyelitis, and in general any disease entity where 7 to 14 days of antibiotic therapy through peripheral parental access is necessary.[35] Most pediatric hospitals as well as major tertiary medical centers have access and extensive experience with external catheters of the Broviac or Hickman type. Also, the use of completely implanted venous ports in adults as well as pediatrics has shown a decreased incidence of infection and greater patient satisfaction compared with the use of external catheters.

Oncology Patient

One of the first programs to give chemotherapy in the patient's home was the program at the Children's Hospital of Philadelphia in which intravenous infusions of methotrexate were performed.[36] The use of infusion pumps and possible subcutaneous infiltration were a major concern. With the newer venous access port systems and external Broviacs and Hickmans, greater volumes of fluid as well as various chemotherapy agents can now be administered. Jayabose et al.[37] have shown that other chemotherapy agents can be safely administered at home. When parents of patients are routinely trained to administer heparin flushes through central venous catheters, selected chemotherapeutic agents such as cytosine arabinoside, vincristine, actinomycin D, and methotrexate have been given at home. In their study, all patients were required to have a central venous catheter in place and well-trained parents to administer the intravenous heparin flushes. Only one patient had an implantable intravenous port. As a rule, only those drugs that do not have any immediate side effects (i.e., allergic reactions, hypothermia, or anaphylaxis) should be used in such a program. In any home chemotherapy infusion program, the rule of safety requires that the first few doses be given in the hospital so that any side effects can be observed. The severity of vomiting is accessed, and appropriate antiemetics and duration of intravenous fluids when needed can be determined. Patients who tolerate these infusions without serious vomiting can usually receive subsequent doses at home. When dealing with any chemotherapeutic agents in the home, it is important that parents be taught how to deal with any spillage by using gloves, masks, protective eye wear, and disposable gowns.[37] The hallmark of any successful home infusion chemotherapy program involves a communication network established among the attending pediatric oncologist, the oncology clinical nurse specialist, and an experienced team of home care pharmacists and nurses. Within our own clinic setting, we have established a policy that requires our staff to personally educate and train any home health care provider in the administration of any product to our patients in the home. This would include neutrophil growth factor, intravenous fluids, and safe handling of catheters as well as chemotherapeutic agents, aerosolized pentamidine, and red cell and platelet transfusions. It is one thing to say that these services can be done at home but it is another to specifically have a home health care provider with nurses specifically trained to deal with pediatric patients who have high-tech hardware.

Catheter devices have expanded our ability to deliver care at home but they frequently become infected. The incidence of catheter infections in cancer patients ranges from 10 to 60%.[38,39] Extensive data are lacking regarding types of catheters, degree of aggressive chemotherapy, and support services. Ulz et al.[40] reported a 44% incidence of infection in a series of immunosuppressed patients at high risk due to allogeneic BMT. The variability of infection may depend upon degree of immunosuppression, type of hematologic malignancy, type of catheter,[38,41–44] and to some extent types of fluids that are to be administered. The specific criteria used to establish a central line infection are not standard. Rizzari et al.[45] report a higher incidence of central venous catheter infections in patients who were on home management as opposed to hospital management. Although the difference was not statistically significant, they conclude that the care given to the catheters by the parents was good on the whole but that home management was less safe and reliable than hospital management. In general, most institutions and major centers that deal with tertiary care pediatrics would agree that the selection of a central venous catheter must take into account the patient's age, difficulty of peripheral venous access, intensity of the chemotherapy, and the severity of the disease stage. Their study also confirmed, as did other studies, that systematic and intensive training of the parents and nurses and better measures of aseptic handling of central venous catheters can further reduce all catheter-related infections, both inpatient and outpatient alike.

In this age of managed care and low-cost bidding, it behooves the primary care provider to assure him or herself that the patient can be safely managed at home by the health care team that has been designated by the managed care provider to perform the services. While a plethora of adults are receiving home health care from numerous agencies, the child who needs home health care services is best served by a home health care agency that has a specific pediatric team that has been specifically trained and has enough experience with pediatric patients on a regular basis. More often than not, this is usually not the case unless these home health care organizations have some relationship with a pediatric tertiary care hospital. Wolfe[46] has enumerated a model system for the integration of services for cancer care in children. While specifically reported as being developed for children with cancer, this system really embraces a philosophy for all home health care for children. It describes a seamless relationship that places the patient at the center of care and addresses the major boundaries that patients face. The inpatient–outpatient boundary has been effectively breached by an inpatient care manager and a rotation of the inpatient nurse to the outpatient area for specialty training. Discharge planning is improved by sharing a nurse with the clinic's major home health care company, providing a direct clinic/home health liaison for the patient. Boundaries to continuity of care exist with each episodic illness or therapy in an inpatient or outpatient setting. Integration of inpatient/outpatient information and scheduling are essential. As is the case at our clinic, a nurse clinician in the outpatient setting is responsible to make rounds with physicians and house staff to provide continuity between inpatient and outpatient services. The nurse clinician visits the patients, reviews changes in the conditions of the patients, and discusses ways of dealing with ongoing problems or new problems in an outpatient setting. As patients often leave the hospital with many ancillary medicines and coordination necessary, the discharge planning process has become more complex and the key to any continuity of care program. In our clinic setting, the central high-tech device necessary for outpatient care is the oncology clinical nurse specialist, who rotates her time between clinic and rounds.

Along with infusion pumps and central lines, another essential piece of equipment necessary in a home health program is a fax machine. Through the use of the fax machine, orders can instantly be transmitted from hospital or clinic to any home health care organization which allows for same day turnaround and delivery of any medical support services. Currently there is a fax machine in our oncology ward, in the outpatient clinic, and in the hospital pharmacy, as well as in the home health care organization. This allows for instantaneous transmission of all orders in an accurate fashion. Any mistakes, misinterpretations, or misrepresentations can be immediately addressed.

Home Health Care at What Price?

The cost savings of pediatric home care are well documented. The increase in savings is usually proportional to the complexity of the medical condition. A ventilator-dependent child may save 40 to 60% in costs when home care services are matched against inpatient hospital care.[47,48] Certainly the most common form of insurance is through traditional insurance policies in which the family has health insurance from either the mother or father's employer. Not all health insurance plans currently cover home health costs. This is one area where health care reform can provide mandated language that requires all insurance companies to provide the same standard of home care benefits. Medicaid coverage in pediatrics is also available to state patients, although the coverage guidelines are different in each state. It is important to call the state Medicaid office to establish the exact terms of any home care policy. As it does in private insurance companies, the language can vary. Usually the main criterion for entitlement under a Medicaid program is financial eligibility, as opposed to private insurance where the main criterion is payment of health premiums either by the employer and/or the employee. If someone is not eligible through the spend-down process (poverty level), coverage may be available if the state has a Medicaid waiver. Each state may apply to the federal Health Care Financing Administration. Waivers are currently designed to fill the gap in coverage for pediatric patients.[49] Eligibility is based upon the child's income rather than the parents'. Eligibility for Medicaid reimbursement is often limited to those cases in which the cost of the home care is equal to or less than the cost of hospital care. Therefore, it is necessary to present the mathematics to the state Medicaid office very clearly.

Medicaid waivers enable the child's income to be considered for financial eligibility, thus expanding the Medicaid eligibility criteria to include middle and upper income families whose private insurance benefits have either capped out or do not reimburse for home care.[50]

The cost of home care borne by parents includes home remodeling, increased utility charges, lost income from work, transportation, child care, and training of family members. Out-of-pocket expenses and loss of family leisure time can be major causes of stress.

Enrollment in health maintenance organizations (HMOs) has grown steadily over the past decade; they now serve more than 30 million members.[51] The HMO primary care physician should be able to arrange for the most appropriate array of health care services to meet a child's needs. Children with special needs typically require more specialized, long-term medical and nonmedical interventions which may not be available through the HMO system. Fox et al.[52] report that while HMOs have several advantages over traditional fee-for-service plans, for families whose children have special health needs, HMOs did not always operate effectively to service these children. Most HMO policies are structured to limit the enrollee's use of home health care benefits. Less than half of the HMOs in this study permitted the provision of home health care services on a physician's referral alone. Given the gatekeeping philosophy of HMOs, it is not surprising that 85% of the plans reviewed in this study required their primary care physicians to make all referrals to in-plan specialists. This is extremely alarming since many children who require home health care are usually tertiary care pediatric subspecialist patients (i.e., cystic fibrosis, hemophilia, pediatric oncology, and pediatric AIDS patients).

Certainly HMOs streamline the process. For the HMO patient, the final home care plan would be similar to that of the traditional insurance model. However, the advantage of the HMO would be the steps saved and the quicker entry into the HMO medical department.[49] Various studies have shown that home health care may save up to $300,000 per year, with a mean cost of only 50% of institutional costs on respiratory technology-dependent children.[53–55] The third-party payors frequently will not reimburse fully for the coverage of services for home health care. This shifts the financial burden to the family.

Who Benefits the Most from a Pediatric Home Care Program?

Families with lower coping resources benefited comparatively more from home care intervention when defined in terms of social rather than medical factors. Data recently published show that maximum benefit was evidenced when the illness burden was small but coping resources were low. This finding suggests that the conventional priority of allocating existing intervention resources to the maximally most burdensome cases may not always be maximally beneficial.[56] The methodology of medical cost measurement, while widely studied, results in a wide range of disparate costs when one looks at the cost of home health care. While legislators and policymakers make decisions about policy based upon program data and program contributions to public expenditures, the costs to the family are usually hidden and overlooked. Although hidden, they are nonetheless real. In this context, cost cutting may be cost shifting. Policies relating to programs and institutions affect the family costs for chronically ill and handicapped children.[57] Family caregiver costs can be separated into (1) direct out-of-pocket home costs for recurring items, (2) direct travel costs related to the patient's condition, (3) cost for durable equipment and home renovation, and (4) indirect costs for transportation, caregiving, and increased utility costs. Family members give up time from work and other activities in order to provide care for the child. Usual cost methodology studies focus on the time lost from work and place a value equal to how much family members would have earned had they worked. Leisure time given up is seldom included. Four studies looked at the expense of caring for a child with cancer at home. The figures are disparate by approximately $5000 at the low end.[58–60] This burden was not strictly a function of families in the United States. A single U.K. study showed family costs to be approximately 20% of income.[61]

A renewed interest in pediatric home care because of public and private health care funding policies has encouraged hospital and primary gatekeeper pediatricians to thoroughly review all aspects of health care. The introduction of home health care agencies, newer technologies, different delivery systems, and venous access, as well as the transdermal administration of pain medicine, has allowed and pushed the delivery of many high-technologically-dependent children out of the hospital and into the home care setting. Children with chronic conditions dependent upon high-tech medical technology have found care at home possible because of the advances in continuous monitoring and new diagnostic and therapeutic modalities designed or adapted for home use. The growth of the self-help movement of the 1980s has resulted in more individuals and families taking responsibility for their own health care. Cost-containment efforts have encouraged faster discharge of sicker patients. Medicare diagnostic-related groups (DRGs) have resulted in a 40% increase in earlier discharges of sicker patients.[62]

Who is responsible? Pediatricians are ultimately responsible for initiating, supervising, and terminating home care. Each pediatric patient who requires home care needs someone to assume responsibility for his or her primary care and collaborative management as well. Currently very little is taught about home health care principles in academic centers which provide residency training.[2] A collegial association of community-based pediatricians and academic centers is needed to provide continuing education of the future physicians who will practice primary care in this country. Residents should have broad-based exposure to community-based organizations, including public and managed care foundations as well as nursing agencies and home medical equipment suppliers. Residents should also be taught about family-centered care and parent–professional collaboration. Pediatric home care is the next frontier in pediatric practice. It is with us today and plays an ever-changing role.

References

1. Lantos, J. D. and Kohrman, A. F., Ethical aspects of pediatric home care, *Pediatrics*, 89(5):920–924, 1992.
2. Goldberg, A. I., Gardner, H. G., and Gibson, L. E., Home care: the next frontier of pediatric practice, *J. Pediatr.*, 125(5, Part 1):686–690, 1994.
3. National Center for Health Statistics: Advanced Report of Final Mortality Statistics, 1989, Monthly Vital Statistics Report, Hyattsville, Maryland, Public Health Service, 39(Suppl.):7–13, 1990.
4. Martinson, I. M., Moldow, D. G., Armstrong, G. D., et al., Home care for children dying of cancer, *Res. Nurs. Health*, 9:11–16, 1986.
5. Martinson, I. M. and Henry, W. F., Home care for dying children: costs and consequences for the family, *Hastings Cent. Rep.*, 10:5–7, 1980.

6. Martinson, I. M., Why don't we let them die at home? *Regist. Nurse*, 39:57–65, 1976.
7. Lauer, M. E. and Camitta, B. M., Home care for dying children: a nursing model, *J. Pediatr.*, 97:1032–1035, 1980.
8. Martin, B. B., Pediatric hospice care: an update, *Caring*, 5:5–6, 1986.
9. Glaser, B. G. and Strauss, A. L., *Awareness of Dying*, Aldine Publishing, Chicago, 1966.
10. Sudnow, D., *Passing On*, Prentice-Hall, Englewood Cliffs, New Jersey, 1967.
11. Saunders, C., *The Management of Terminal Illness*, Hospital Medicine Publication, London, 1967.
12. Mulhern, R. K., Lauer, M. E., and Hoffmann, R. G., Death of a child at home or in the hospital: subsequent psychological adjustment of the family, *Pediatrics*, 71:743–747, 1983.
13. Dufour, D. F., Home or hospital care for the child with end-stage cancer: effects on the family, *Issues Compr. Pediatr. Nurs.*, 12:371–383, 1989.
14. Edwardson, S. R., Physician acceptance of home care for terminally ill children, *Health Serv. Res.*, 20(1):85–101, 1985.
15. Lauer, M. E., Mulhern, R. K., Hoffmann, R. G., and Camitta, B. M., Utilization of hospice/home care in pediatric oncology: a national survey, *Cancer Nurs.*, 9(3):102–107, 1986.
16. Martinson, I., Hospice care for children: past, present, and future, *J. Pediatr. Oncol. Nurs.*, 10(3):93–98, 1993.
17. Martinson, I. M., Moldow, D. G., Armstrong, G. D., Henry, W. F., Nesbit, M. E., and Kersey, J. H., Home care for children dying of cancer, *Res. Nurs. Health*, 9:11–16, 1986.
18. Edwardson, S., The choice between hospital and home care for terminally ill children, *Nurs. Res.*, 32(1):29–34, 1983.
19. Carlson, P., Simacek, M., Henry, W., and Martinson, I., A model home care program for the dying child, *Issues Compr. Pediatr. Nurs.*, 8(1–6):113–127, 1985.
20. Lauer, M., Mulhern, R., Bohne, J., and Camitta, B., Children's perceptions of their siblings death at home or hospital: the precursors of differential adjustment, *Cancer Nurs.*, 8(1):21–27, 1985.
21. Martinson, I., Davies, E., and McClowery, S., The long-term effects of sibling death on self-concept, *J. Pediatr. Nurs.*, 2(4):277–335, 1987.
22. Duffy, C. M., Pollock, P., Levy, M., Budd, E., Caulfield, L., and Koren, G., Home-based palliative care for children. Part 2. The benefits of an established program, *J. Palliative Care*, 6(2):8–14, 1990.
23. Corr, C. A. and Corr, D. M., Children's hospice care, *Death Studies*, 16:431–449, 1992.
24. Randolph, S. R., Bone marrow transplant therapy in the home, *Caring*, 11(9):68–70, 1992.
25. Jones, P., *Haemophilia Home Therapy*, Pitman, London, 1980.
26. Pool, J. G. and Shannon, A. E., Production of high-potency concentrates of anti-haemophilic globulin in a closed bag system, *New Engl. J. Med.*, 273:1443, 1965.

27. Rabiner, S. F. and Telfer, M. C., Home transfusion for patients with hemophilia-A, *New Engl. J. Med.,* 283:1011–1015, 1970.
28. Strawczynski, H., Stachewitsch, A., Morgen, G., and Shaw, M. E., Delivery of care to hemophilia children: home care versus hospitalization, *Pediatrics,* 51:986–991, 1973.
29. Levine, P., Efficacy of self-therapy in haemophilia: a study of 72 patients with haemophilia A and B, *New Engl. J. Med.,* 291:1381–1384, 1974.
30. Britten, A. F. H., A concept of home treatment for haemophilia, in Proc. Workshop on Haemophilia, Paterswolde, Smit Sibinga, C. Th., Ed., Drukkerij Schut, Groningen, 1980.
31. Jones, P., Haemophilia home therapy, *Haemostasis,* 22:247–250, 1992.
32. Snyder, E. and Menitove, J., Eds., *Home Transfusion Therapy,* American Association of Blood Banks, Arlington, Virginia, 1986, pp. 61–69.
33. Pluth, N. M., A home care transfusion program, *Oncol. Nurs. Forum,* 14:43–46, 1987.
34. Crocker, K. S. and Coker, M. H., Initiation of a home hemotherapy program using a primary nursing model, *J. Intravenous Nurs.,* 13(1):13–19, 1990.
35. Stovroff, M. C., Totten, M., and Glick, P. L., PIC lines save money and hasten discharge in the care of children with ruptured appendicitis, *J. Pediatr. Surg.,* 29(2):245–247, 1994.
36. Lange, B. J., Burroughs, B., Meadows, A. T., and Burkey, E., Clinical and laboratory observations, *J. Pediatr.,* 112(3):492–495, 1988.
37. Jayabose, S., Escobedo, V., Tugal, O., Nahaczewski, A., Donohue, P., Fuentes, V., Devereau, G., and Sunkara, S., Home chemotherapy for children with cancer, *Cancer,* 69:574–579, 1992.
38. Becton, D. L., Morris, K., Golladay, E. S., Hathaway, G., and Berry, D. H., An experience with an implanted port system in 66 children with cancer, *Cancer,* 61:376–378, 1988.
39. Cairo, M., Spooner, S., Sowden, L., et al., Long-term use of indwelling multipurpose silastic catheters in pediatric cancer patients treated with aggressive chemotherapy, *J. Clin. Oncol.,* 4:784–788, 1986.
40. Ulz, L., Petersen, F., Ford, R., Blakeley, W., Bennett, L., Grimm, M., and Hickman, R.O., A prospective study of complications in Hickman right-atrial catheters in marrow transplant patients, *J. Parent. Enter. Nutr.,* 1:27–30, 1990.
41. Gyves, J., Ensminges, W., Niederhuber, J., et al., A totally implanted injection port system for blood sampling and chemotherapy administration, *JAMA,* 251:2538–2541, 1984.
42. Strum, S., McDermed, J., Korn, A., and Joseph, C., Improved methods for venous access: the Port-A-Cath, a totally implanted catheter system, *J. Clin. Oncol.,* 4:596–603, 1986.
43. Brincker, H. and Saeter, G., Fifty-five patient years' experience with a totally implanted system for intravenous chemotherapy, *Cancer,* 57:1124–1129, 1986.
44. Pegelow, C., Narvaez, M., Toledano, S., et al., Experience with a totally implantable venous device in children, *AJDC,* 140:69–71, 1986.

45. Rizzari, C., Palamone, G., Corbetta, A., Uderzo, C., Vigano, E. F., and Codecasa, G., Central venous catheter-related infections in pediatric hematology-oncology patients: role of home and hospital management, *Pediatr. Hematol. Oncol.*, 9:115–123, 1992.
46. Wolfe, L. C., A model system: integration of services for cancer treatment, *Cancer*, 72:3525–3530, 1993.
47. Briggs, N. and Cummings, B. S., Insurance reimbursement of pediatric home care, *Pediatr. Nurs.*, 12(6):449–457, 1986.
48. Wheeler, T. W. and Lewis, C. C., Home care for medically fragile children: urban versus rural settings, *Issues Compr. Pediatr. Nurs.*, 16:13–30, 1993.
49. Fields, A. I., Rosenblatt, A., Pollack, M. M., and Kaufman, J., Home care cost-effectiveness for respiratory technology-dependent children, *AJDC*, 145:729–733, 1991.
50. Murray, J. E., Payment mechanisms for pediatric home care, *Caring*, 8(10):33–35, 1989.
51. Stiver, H. G., Telford, G. O., Mossey, J., et al., Intravenous antibiotic therapy at home, *Ann. Intern. Med.*, 89:690–693, 1978.
52. Fox, H. B., Wicks, L. B., and Newacheck, P. W., Health maintenance organizations and children with special health needs: a suitable match? *AJDC*, 147:546–552, 1993.
53. Burr, B. H., Guyer, B., Todress, I. D., Abrahams, B., and Chiodo, T., Home care for children on respirators, *New Engl. J. Med.*, 309:1319–1323, 1983.
54. Frates, R. C., Splaingard, M. L., and Harrison, G. M., Outcome of home mechanical ventilation for children, *J. Pediatr.*, 106:850–856, 1985.
55. Goldberg, A. I., Faure, E. A. M., Vaughn, C. J., Snarski, R., and Seleny, F. L., Home care for life-supported persons: an approach to program development, *J. Pediatr.*, 104:785–795, 1984.
56. Jessop, D. J. and Stein, R. E. K., Who benefits from a pediatric home care program? *Pediatrics*, 88(3):497–505, 1991.
57. Jacobs, P. and McDermott, S., Family caregiver costs of chronically ill and handicapped children: method and literature review, *Public Health Rep.*, 104(2):158–163, 1989.
58. Lansky, S. B. et al., Childhood cancer: nonmedical costs of the illness, *Cancer*, 43:403–408, 1979.
59. Bloom, B. S., Knorr, R. S., and Evans, A. E., The epidemiology of disease expenses, *JAMA*, 253:2393–2397, 1985.
60. McCollum, A. T., Cystic fibrosis: economic impact upon the family, *Am. J. Public Health*, 61:1335–1341, 1971.
61. Bodkin, C. M., Pigott, T. J., and Mann, J. R., Financial burden of childhood cancer, *Br. Med. J.,* 283:1542–1544, 1982.
62. Christianson, J. B., The evaluation of the national long-term care demonstration, *Health Serv. Res.*, 23:1, 1988.

Care of the Patient Receiving Radiation

15

William J. Spanos, Jr., M.D.

General Considerations

The effect of radiation on patients varies with the site treated, volume radiated, and patient condition. Some effects of radiation are seen early, such as nausea or vomiting with upper abdominal radiation. Most side effects have a gradual onset, such as skin inflammation, diarrhea, hair loss, etc. These effects result from the cumulative tissue reaction to radiation and their time of onset will vary depending upon the nature of radiation (e.g., electron, photon, beam energy), the amount of radiation per treatment, and the number of treatments per week.

Although there is some variability in the time of onset of side effects between individual patients, the appearance of a side effect significantly earlier than expected should be investigated promptly for the possibility of additional factors superseding or compounding the radiation effect. One example is the early onset of brisk skin erythema in a postoperative patient. An inflammatory process such as cellulitis may be a superseding factor. Recognition of that possibility may lead to antibiotic therapy appropriate for the infection, whereas supportive anti-inflammatory care for radiation effect would allow the infection to progress.

The course of radiation with curative intent usually consists of five treatments each week and a radiation dose of 170 to 200 centigrays (cGy) per dose for a duration of 5 to 7 weeks. For the purpose of discussion of timing of symptoms, this dose schedule will be assumed. For palliative care, the dose per treatment is usually higher (250 to 350 cGy) for a duration of 2 to 4 weeks. These accelerated treatment schedules frequently result in radiation symptoms not appearing until the patient has completed the course of radiation. The same spectrum of symptoms described in the following sections will still apply, but the patient and family will need to be alerted to the likely appearance of these symptoms after the patient has been discharged from radiation. Additionally, the appearance of radiation symptoms after radiation is completed may lead the patient or caregiver to attribute the symptoms to causes other than radiation, thus affecting management of the symptoms.

Nutritional Considerations

Good nutritional maintenance is important to the overall well-being of the patient and to the ability to tolerate and recover from the effects of radiation on normal tissue. For some sites (e.g., breast, skin, extremities), the side effects of radiation do not interfere with normal appetite or ability to eat. For other sites, such as head and neck, lung, and abdomen, radiation often produces a direct physiologic response that affects the ability to eat or secondary depression of appetite, which may significantly interfere with nutrition if allowed to progress without intervention. The specific nutritional needs related to the site radiated will be discussed in the following sections. The details of nutritional recommendations are outside the scope of this chapter. Specific nutritional guidelines and recipes can be found in several sources.[1-4]

Nutritional status needs to be monitored closely in the patient receiving radiation. Assessment of weight change provides a valuable and accurate measure of nutritional stability during radiation. For patients receiving radiation to sites not affecting appetite or ability to eat, weekly weights are sufficient. However, patients receiving radiation to sites listed above that are likely to produce significant effect on intake, daily weights should be monitored. Nutrition should also be assessed by serum albumin. An initial serum albumin should be obtained at the start of radiation and subsequent values obtained as indicated by patient progress or suspicion of poor intake.

Patient motivation for food can decline for a multitude of reasons other than radiation, including depression and secondary effects from the cancer. It is important to proceed with nutritional counseling and encouragement along with changes in food types to accommodate the specific physiologic changes in any patient exhibiting weight loss or loss of appetite, regardless of the etiology.

Site-Specific Radiation Changes

Skin Changes from Radiation

The skin is affected in all external beam radiation. The magnitude of effect depends upon the modality (orthovoltage, electron beam, high-energy photon beam) and the dose. For patients treated with high-energy photon beams (≥ 6 MV) for deep-seated targets, skin reactions are usually mild or not clinically apparent. One exception is skin tangential to the beam (e.g., vulvar or perineal skin included in pelvic treatment, breast treated with oblique fields), where the skin receives a higher dose because of internal scatter. Lower energy photon beams and electron beams frequently are associated with clinically significant skin reactions.

Radiation-induced skin reactions will range from erythema to moist desquamation depending upon dose and beam arrangement. In addition to the visible changes, there is an accompanying decrease in natural skin oils with associated dryness. If the dose to the dermis is high enough, there will be loss of epithelium, resulting in serous production (moist desquamation). For standard fractionation, the erythema usually starts after 10 to 15 treatments. If the radiation dose to the skin is sufficient to produce moist desquamation, the moist desquamation first appears in scattered patches and is usually not seen before 20 to 25 treatments. This will progress to confluent regions if radiation continues. For short-course intense schedules, the skin changes may not reach their peak until after the radiation course is completed.

Skin Care

General

Radiated skin should be kept dry as much as possible. Skinfold areas such as the groin, perineum ductal folds, and inframammary sulcus tend to stay moist and will develop more intense reactions. Loose clothing that wicks moisture (cotton) is the preferred covering for skin that cannot remain exposed to the air. It is acceptable to allow water to run over the radiated skin. Soaking in a bathtub for prolonged periods is not advised. The use of soap is not advisable as it increases skin dryness. Following shower or bath, the radiated skin should be gently patted dry (not rubbed). In some very sensitive areas such as the perineum, air drying with a hair dryer set on cool will achieve more complete drying with less irritation and discomfort.

Erythema and Dry Desquamation

Replacement of oils with a moisturizer will significantly improve patient comfort and aid in healing. The use of a moisturizer during radiation should be accompanied by careful instructions or supervision. A thin layer of oil over the treatment area may compromise the skin-sparing effect of some radiation energies. Therefore, application of lotions should be avoided within 3 to 4 hours prior to each radiation treatment. In addition, externally applied oils may dissolve the skin marks that define treatment borders. Therefore, care must be taken to apply any lotion carefully so as to avoid marked borders. Once the radiation course is completed, the application of moisturizers should be done at least three to four times per day until the reaction has healed.

Erythema and dry desquamation changes should heal by 2 to 3 weeks following radiation. If prominent erythema persists, the possibility of a secondary source such as infection needs to be considered.

Radiation will permanently decrease the number of sebaceous glands, depending upon the dose of radiation to the skin. Therefore, some degree of long-term application of a skin moisturizer is advisable to maintain the health and appearance of the skin. There are also structural changes to the epithelium and dermis that make the skin more susceptible to sunburn. Previously radiated skin that is in a region of the body frequently exposed to sun should be protected with shade, cover, or high SPF sunblock lotion.

Moist Desquamation Care

The skin changes associated with moist desquamation are similar to those seen with partial thickness thermal burns. However, in almost all patients developing moist desquamation, radiation leaves clonogenic cells that subsequently form skin islands and eventually coalesce to recover the area. During the moist desquamation phase, the patient is susceptible to infection. Therefore, the application of an antibiotic barrier cream, such as silver sulfadiazine, or porus physical barrier, such as Vigilon™, is important. Elective use of antibiotics is not indicated. However, in the event the areas show signs of infection with production of purulent discharge, systemic antibiotics should be used along with regular cleaning of the area with dilute (1:2 peroxide:water) hydrogen peroxide solution. Once the area is reepithelialized, regular application of moisturizing agent will help keep the skin healthy and pliable.

Head and Neck: Radiation Effects on Oral Cavity and Oropharynx

Radiation to the oral cavity, oropharynx, and larynx frequently produces inflammatory changes that range from mild inflammation to exudative denuding of the mucosa (mucositis). A varying amount of salivary gland tissue is included in most radiation of the head and neck region. The quality of saliva is important in the health of the oral mucosa because of its lubricating and antibacterial properties, in addition to assistance with digestion. Therefore, changes in the saliva from radiation produce a cascade of secondary problems, including more difficulty swallowing because of thicker, more tenacious saliva and increased risk of infection with loss of antibacterial qualities.

Taste is affected relatively early (approximately 2 to 3 weeks), and specific types of taste are lost at varying times, leaving the patient with aversions to many foods he or she previously enjoyed.

The combination of oral pain from erythema, salivary changes, and loss of taste or taste abnormalities creates a significant barrier to eating and maintaining nutrition. If swallowing becomes significantly impaired, the patient will become dehydrated. Dehydration will result in thicker, more tenacious saliva, further compromising swallowing. This pattern can easily become a vicious cycle, producing malnutrition and increasing dehydration.

Management of Oral Reactions

Nutritional Considerations—As swallowing difficulty and loss of taste progress, the patient will need to modify diet to maximize nutrition and maintain ease of swallowing. Initially, soft bland foods are indicated. As symptoms progress, transition to a high-calorie liquid supplement is often necessary.

If dehydration is suspected, 1 or 2 liters of lactated Ringer intravenously will often produce a dramatic improvement in symptoms. Serum electrolyte levels including assays for trace metals should be obtained in the presence of dehydration or suspected electrolyte imbalances. Close monitoring of the patient's hydration and electrolyte balance is particularly important in the presence of reduced intake, vomiting, or diarrhea. Recording urinary output is particularly useful and easily monitored in the home environment. Urinary output should equal 50 cc or more per hour and should not appear dark or concentrated. If in doubt about concentration, a hygrometer may be used to check the specific gravity of the urine. The specific gravity normally ranges from 1.015 to 1.025. Cloudy urine and urine with unusual odors should be submitted to the laboratory for urinalysis. In the presence of bacteria and excessive leukocytes on microscopic examination, a urine sample collected under sterile conditions should be submitted fresh to the laboratory for culture and the determination of antimicrobial drug sensitivities.

Mucositis—The gradual buildup of debride, tenacious secretions, and thickened saliva in the lining of the oral cavity can provide a medium for fungal or bacterial growth. This bacterial proliferation will increase the oral cavity reaction.

It is important to keep this debride clear with frequent use of a dilute saline solution (1 teaspoon salt plus 1 teaspoon baking soda in a quart of water) for rinsing and gargle. Using a stream with force can help dislodge buildup that will not respond to simple rinse. A forceful stream can be obtained by using a commercial power spray device or by placing the solution in a bag with a hose and hanging it high enough to allow gravity to provide the force. The rinsing process should be done a minimum of three to four times a day.

Additionally, a medicated mouth rinse which contains an antifungal agent, anti-inflammatory agent, and topical anesthetic is helpful for providing relief. Varying formulas are available. One effective formula is as follows:

Nystatin slurry (100,000 units/ml)	120 cc
Benadryl liquid (12.5 mg/5 ml)	120 cc
Hydrocortisone (60 mg)	————
Makes	240 cc

Dose: 1 to 2 teaspoons, swish and swallow

This solution can be used three to four times per day as long as symptoms persist.

A number of common food and drink products are responsible for increasing the oral reactions. The following partial list is to be avoided or minimized: alcohol, smoking, coffee, carbonated beverages, and mouthwashes with alcohol base.

Patients may develop odynophagia (pain on swallowing) which does not respond to the above measures. It is critical that they keep their caloric intake high enough to maintain weight within 10 lb or 10% of body weight (whichever comes first). Initial steps to help with swallowing can be accomplished with a topical anesthetic such as lidocaine hydrochloride viscous 2% 10 to 15 minutes a.c. If this does not provide sufficient relief, the addition of a liquid narcotic (without alcohol base) 20 to 30 minutes a.c. will frequently allow the patient to continue to maintain oral feedings. Because of the intensity of reaction or lack of motivation, some patients will not be able to maintain a sufficient caloric intake. These patients should be considered for a gastrostomy or percutaneous gastronomy tube if their weight falls below the 10% or 10-lb margin.

Mediastinal Radiation

The mediastinum is usually included in radiation for any cancer with gross mediastinal involvement or risk of subclinical spread to the mediastinum. Common examples include lung cancer, Hodgkin's and non-Hodgkin lymphomas, and esophageal cancers.

The most significant symptom from mediastinal radiation is esophagitis. As with the previous sites, the symptoms are due to progressive inflammation and are gradual in onset. Indeed, with some of the more common palliative schemes (high dose per fraction and short treatment course), the esophagitis will not become clinically significant until the treatment course is completed.

Early esophagitis is usually described by the patient as feeling a "knot" or "lump" in the throat or upper chest on swallowing. As the severity progresses, the intensity of this discomfort increases. Paradoxically, patients frequently have more difficulty with water than with soft solids or thicker liquids.

Eventually, if the esophagitis progresses, the patient will be unable to complete the swallow because of tertiary contractions and will regurgitate. Nutrition becomes a major consideration in patients with moderate or severe esophagitis, and appropriate steps need to be taken early to ensure the patient's ability to maintain adequate nutrition. Fortunately, esophagitis produced by most radiation schedules is readily managed by symptomatic treatment with low-intensity outpatient medications.

Any esophagitis that is unusually severe, has early onset, or does not resolve soon after radiation is completed should be suspect for compounding factors. One of the most common of these factors is esophageal candidiasis. Esophageal candidiasis is more commonly seen in the immune compromised patient, but can happen in any patient.

Management of Esophagitis

The rapidity of onset of esophagitis as well as the severity can be modified by modification of diet. Patients should be cautioned to avoid drinks at temperature extremes or drinks that may be irritating, such as coffee, carbonated beverages, or alcohol. As esophagitis appears, a switch to soft foods will decrease irritation.

Symptomatic medication can significantly improve the patient's willingness to maintain adequate nutrition. In the early phases of esophagitis, Aspergum™ provides both topical and systemic anti-inflammatory effect. Additional anti-inflammatory help can be obtained from liquid antacids. As the esophagitis progresses, temporary topical anesthesia can be obtained by swallowing 1 to 2 teaspoons of lidocaine hydrochloride viscous 2% 10 minutes prior to meals.

When esophagitis becomes moderate or severe, topical agents are inadequate, and systemic liquid narcotics taken before meals may be the only way to allow adequate nutrition. Since narcotics often suppress appetite, therapy should be reserved for patients who do not respond to topical agents.

If the onset, severity, or persistence of the esophagitis suggests the possibility of candida esophagitis, a trial of a systemic antifungal agent such as Diflucan™ or Nizoral™ is the most efficient way to verify the assumption. If this does not produce prompt improvement, esophagoscopic examination may be indicated, particularly for esophagitis persistent long after completion of radiation.

Upper Abdominal Radiation

Varying volumes of the upper abdomen will be included in radiation of the para-aortic nodes, pancreas, or stomach. The largest abdominal volume treated is seen with whole abdominal radiation used in treatment of ovarian cancer and some cases of endometrial cancer. Often unanticipated is the abdominal effect of the exit dose from palliative radiation for the lower thoracic or upper lumbar spine metastases from other primary sites.

Unlike the gradual onset of symptoms described in previous sections, abdominal radiation may produce early onset of nausea and/or vomiting. The intensity of this symptom is usually, but not necessarily, associated with the volume of the stomach affected. The effect is also dose per fraction dependent, which explains the less common nausea and vomiting with whole abdominal radiation than with para-aortic radiation because of the lower dose per fraction.

Radiation produces varying changes in small bowel epithelia, with shortening or loss of villi and changes in absorption of bile salts, flat carbohydrates, proteins, water, and electrolytes.[5-9] The cumulative effects of abdominal radiation may produce gastritis or enteritis. Symptom of gastritis will include early satiety, nausea, and upper abdominal pain. Symptoms of enteritis include abdominal soreness, mild abdominal pain, and intermittent diarrhea. Enteritis may progress to ileus. Additionally, patients with prior abdominal surgery are at risk for intestinal obstruction. If the abdominal pain becomes moderate or severe and is associated with abdominal distension or vomiting, ileus or obstruction should be suspected. The patient should be evaluated promptly for hospitalization, as this can be a life-threatening situation.

Management of Abdominal Symptoms

Nutritional Considerations—Because of the inflammatory, atrophic, and absorptive changes from radiation of the stomach and intestinal tract, the content of feeding significantly affects the health of the gastrointestinal tract and influences the severity and onset of radiation symptoms. Animal and human studies with elemental feedings and blind bowel segments have suggested that minimizing residue and bile transit significantly reduce radiation effects.[10-12]

Since it is not practical to place most patients on elemental feedings, a low-residue diet is an important step in minimizing intestinal reaction to radiation. Gastritis can be minimized by eliminating gastric irritants such as alcohol, coffee, and spices.

Nausea and Vomiting—If the only symptom is nausea without vomiting, a time-release antiemetic such as prochlorperazine spansules (15 or 30 mg) may be sufficient to alleviate the symptoms. However, if the patient is vomiting, the level of antiemetic available from time-release medication is frequently lower than necessary. Usually radiation produces a pattern of vomiting closely associated with the time of radiation. Therefore, the antiemetic should be timed to produce peak levels close to the timing of radiation. One effective scheme is to prescribe an antiemetic such as prochlorperazine (10 mg, not time release) approximately 1 hour before radiation and again within $1/2$ hour or 1 hour after radiation. Although this medication spacing is closer than used in nonradiation settings, it is quite effective and usually results in the patient not requiring additional doses during the day. Preradiation antiemetic schedule also gives the patient a better chance of keeping medication down.

If the intensity of vomiting is such that oral antiemetic cannot be kept down, the patient should be provided suppositories and monitored closely as he or she may need to be hospitalized for intravenous fluid replacement and intravenous antiemetic.

Susceptibility to gastritis or enteritis may be modified by diet to reduce or eliminate irritants such as coffee, alcohol, and spices and to convert to low-residue diet. Gastritis usually responds to antacids and H2 blocking agents similar to nonradiation gastritis.

Symptoms of enteritis should be monitored closely for signs of abdominal pain, tenderness, or distension, which might suggest ileus or intestinal obstruction. The radiated patient may not produce the same intensity of peritoneal signs as a nonradiated patient. Therefore, the index of suspicion must be higher. If ileus or intestinal obstruction is suspected, radiation should be discontinued and the patient hospitalized until the clinical picture is evaluated and managed.

Pelvic Radiation

The pelvis contents are radiated in the treatment of cervical, vaginal, prostatic, endometrial, rectal, and bladder cancers. Pelvic radiation is also a part of palliative treatment of pelvic bones. The pelvis includes the bladder, rectum, sigmoid colon cecum, and small bowel. Pelvic radiation may produce symptoms of proctosigmoiditis, cystitis, and enteritis. These symptoms are gradual in onset, and severity will depend upon volume, dose, and patient factors.

Proctosigmoiditis is usually manifested by diarrhea. Diarrhea is usually progressive in frequency of stools and development of loose or watery stools. Early in the course of radiation, diarrhea is usually intermittent. The symptoms will usually not become persistent before 10 to 15 treatments of standard fractionation. The appearance of persistent moderate or severe diarrhea early in the course of radiation should be investigated for other contributing or causative factors. The term diarrhea is often misunderstood by patients. They may deny having diarrhea because of the lack of watery stools but may be having six to eight stools per day. Thus, it is important to verify stool frequency as well as consistency with the patient.

Cystitis is manifested by increased frequency and/or dysuria. Radiation-induced cystitis symptoms are usually not seen before 10 to 15 treatments of standard fractionation. Radiation cystitis symptoms are identical to urinary tract infection. Since urinary tract infections are relatively common, any patient with symptoms of cystitis should have a urinalysis.

Management of Pelvic Symptoms

Nutritional Considerations—Through the same mechanism as abdominal radiation, radiation causes inflammation atrophy and partial loss of intestinal mucosa. The health of intestinal mucosa and susceptibility to irritability and infection are partially dependent upon the content of the gut. Since the pelvis contains both small and large bowel, minimizing bile transit and residue in the gut significantly reduces the radiation effects. Therefore, a low-residue diet is important in minimizing intestinal reaction to radiation. Additionally, patients should eliminate colonic irritants and colonic stimulants such as spicy foods and coffee.

Proctosigmoiditis—Early symptoms of proctosigmoiditis will be intermittent loose stools and increased frequency of stools. As long as the symptoms are intermittent, as-needed use of antidiarrheal medication such as diphenoxylate hydrochloride (2.5 mg) or Loperamide (2 mg, 1 to 2 tablets every 4 hours) is appropriate. However, when diarrhea becomes a daily occurrence, a regular schedule of antidiarrheal medications will improve control of diarrhea. Scheduled antidiarrheal medication should be timed to meals. The recommended schedule is one to two tablets of diphenorxylate hydrochloride or Loperamide, 30 minutes a.c. and h.s. titrated to the patient's needs. For mild diarrhea, only one tablet before breakfast and/or dinner may be sufficient. For the majority of patients, one dose before each meal is usually sufficient. The additional use of a fiber supplement with psyllium will improve the control of diarrhea by absorbing liquid in the colon and providing bulk to decrease the colon transit time. Anti-inflammatory agents that inhibit prostaglandin activity have been shown to significantly decrease diarrhea intensity and frequency in radiated patients. The most common drug in this category is acetylsalicylic acid.[13]

If diarrhea severity is not controlled with eight tablets per day of diphenorxylate hydrochloride or Loperamide, additional factors contributing to the diarrhea should be considered. If the diarrhea onset is early in the course of treatment, watery, and the patient has been on antibiotics, the possibility of *Clostridium difficele* infection should be considered. This can be determined by stool culture and toxin assay. If suspected, radiation is to be stopped and the patient hospitalized until the condition has been verified and treated, as this can be a life-threatening condition.

Proctosigmoiditis may persist for several weeks after radiation, with symptoms of rectal urgency rather than diarrhea. If the patient has symptoms of urgency, a course of steroid enemas for 1 to 2 weeks frequently provides symptomatic relief. In addition, maintaining the patient on a fiber supplement will keep the stools bulky and soft and decrease the rectal irritation.

Cystitis—Cystitis symptoms can be improved with a urinary tract analgesic agent such as Phenazopysidine (200 mg t.i.d.). Cystitis intensity may be reduced or delayed by eliminating bladder irritants such as smoking or caffeine. High-volume fluid intake (2 quarts) is recommended to keep the urine dilute and the bladder well irrigated. Increased urinary frequency and burning are also symptoms of urinary tract infection, and urinalysis is indicated. If urinary tract infection is demonstrated, appropriate antibiotic therapy should be started.

References

1. Thiel, H. J., Fietkau, R., and Sauer, R., Malnutrition and the role of nutritional support for radiation therapy patients, *Cancer Res.*, 108:205–226, 1988.
2. Aker, S. and Lenssen, P., *A Guide to Good Nutrition During and After Chemotherapy and Radiation,* 2nd edition, Fred Hutchinson Cancer Research Center, Seattle, 1979.
3. Pennington, J. A. T., *Food Values of Portions Commonly Used,* 15th edition, Harper & Row, New York, 1989.
4. Block, A. S., Ed., *Nutritional Management of the Cancer Patient,* Aspen Publishers, Gaithersburg, Maryland, 1990.
5. Reeves, R. J., Cavanaugh, P. J., Sharpe, K. W., Thorne, W. A., Winkler, C., and Sanders, A. O., Fat absorption studies and small bowel X-ray studies in patients undergoing ^{60}Co teletherapy and/or radium application, *AJR*, 94:848–851, 1965.
6. Reeves, R. J., Sanders, A. P., Isley, J. K., Sharpe, K. W., and Baylin, G. J., Fat absorption from the human gastrointestinal tract in patients undergoing radiation therapy, *Radiology*, 73:398–401, 1959.
7. Stryker, J. A., Hepner, G. W., and Mortel, R., The effect of pelvic irradiation on ileal function, *Radiology*, 124:213–216, 1977.
8. Stryker, J. A., Mortel, R., and Hepner, G. W., The effect of pelvic irradiation on lactose absorption, *Int. J. Radiat. Oncol. Biol. Phys.*, 4:859–863, 1978.
9. Tarpila, S., Morphological and functional response of human small intestine to ionizing radiation, *Scand. J. Gastroenterol.,* 6(Suppl. 12):9–52, 1971.
10. Yeoh, E. K., Lui, D., and Lee, N. Y., The mechanism of diarrheoa resulting from pelvic and abdominal radiotherapy; a prospective study using selenium-75 labelled conjugated bile acid and cobalt-58 labelled cyanocobalamin, *Br. J. Radiol.*, 57:1131–1136, 1984.
11. Heusinkveld, R. S., Manning, M. R., and Aristizabel, S. A., Control of radiation induced diarrheoa with cholestyramine, *Int. J. Radiat. Oncol. Biol. Phys.*, 4:687–690, 1978.
12. Mulholland, M. W., Levitt, S. H., Song, C. W., Potish, R. A., and Delaney, J. P., The role of luminal contents in radiation enteritis, *Cancer*, 54:2396–2402, 1984.
13. Mennie, A. T., Dalley, V. M., Dinneen, L. C., and Collier, H. O. J., Treatment of radiation-induced gastrointestinal distress with acetylsalicylate, *The Lancet*, Nov.:942–943, 1975.

Home Health Care for the Head and Neck Cancer Patient

16

David S. Robinson, M.D.

Introduction

Head and neck cancer care involves an extended collaboration between the patient, his or her doctors, hospital-based therapists, outpatient health care workers, and the patient's family. If such a program is to be successful, it must involve home health care that begins early with a plan initiated by the primary caregiver, usually a head and neck surgeon, and continues through a course of recognized treatment extending in time well beyond the norm of most patients, often lasting years. Continuity and communication are the vital links with not only surgeons and radiation oncologists, but with dentists, nurses, speech therapists, psychosocial specialists, maxillofacial prosthodontists, and medical oncologists. In its broadest sense, it embraces more than planned visits by home health care professionals and becomes woven into the fabric of the patient's life. Consequently, the distinction between inpatient and outpatient care fades; the approach of this chapter reflects that model directed toward a seamless amalgam.

Taken in its broadest sense, home health care must take a long-term look at all phases of rehabilitation. This often complex challenge requires a real *commitment from the patient* and his or her family. At the risk of repeating areas of care covered elsewhere in this text, those issues of special interest to care of the head and neck patient will be surveyed in this chapter. They include: (1) pulmonary care and tobacco cessation; (2) routine dental care, maxillofacial prosthetics, and prosthodontics; (3) nutritional care; (4) speech and swallowing therapy; and (5) psychosocial rehabilitation.

Pulmonary Care and Tobacco Cessation

Lung disease is often a comorbid factor for the head and neck cancer patient. Because tobacco is a known carcinogen of both aerodigestive and pulmonary cancer, it is not surprising that many patients are smokers of some significance. Joyce and McQuarrie[1] noted that 90% of their patients smoked more than one pack of cigarettes per day. Cessation in this population is poor. With regard to its influence on reconstruction, surprisingly, unlike flaps outside the head and neck area for which smoking shows a clear-cut difference in flap survival, the consequences of smoking in head and neck reconstruction are mixed.[2,3] Nevertheless, it is clear that smoking after radiation therapy bears a greater risk of recurrence.[4] Moreover, pulmonary function analyses may reveal a level of chronic obstructive pulmonary disease that can determine success or failure of an operative procedure; studies demonstrate that patients with FEV_1/FVC ratios of less than 50% show a marked increase in complications due to chronic obstructive pulmonary disease. When it is successful, preoperative counseling in an attempt to diminish, if not stop, cigarette smoking and outpatient respiratory therapy over a 2-week preoperative period has an impact on early postoperative outcome. Psychosocial services focusing on tobacco addiction with the invocation of family assistance in the home setting are important.

Dental Care

The dentition of many patients with head and neck cancer is poor. Lockhart and Clark[5] note that 97% of dentulous patients at the time of presentation needed dental care before radiotherapy. As part of the initial plan, the patient should be seen by a dentist who becomes part of the team for assessment and restoration of any dental and periodontal disease. Usually, the patient's local dentist is that important partner. Because operative intervention may involve resection of teeth, bone, and alveolar mucosa, the patient's dentist should be made aware of the surgical plan so that impressions, should they be needed, can be taken preoperatively. In addition, stents made preoperatively for skin graft bolsters are essential to the early success of such procedures as maxillectomy.

　　The home health care dental component, both in the preoperative and postoperative periods, is important because the risk of infection from devitalized and chronically infected tissues may have a significant impact on postoperative wound healing. In addition to compliance with proposed dental restoration, the patient needs to begin management at home of the intraoral environment. While many inpatient services use a positive-pressure aerosol spray, this is not practical in the home setting. Preoperative education of postoperative oromucosal wound care and the purchase of a water jet appliance is important. A jet irrigation system (e.g., Water Pik®) at a *low* pressure level, initiated at the time of discharge, will maintain a clean intraoral operative site. The use of half- or third-strength hydrogen peroxide in warm water followed by a warm tap water cleansing is important in posthospitalization continued home care.

Finally, long-term surveillance and proper dental hygienic maintenance are crucial for the dentulous patient who will receive postoperative radiation therapy. Xerostomia in one study occurred 81% of the time in those patients receiving two ports of radiation therapy to a level of 40 to 75 Gy.[6] The decreased bathing of the oral cavity by saliva, absent in the postradiation setting, gives rise to higher rates of dental and periodontal infectious disease. Therefore, patients undergoing radiation therapy should be fitted for and taught the use of fluoride carriers to protect the remaining teeth.[7] Many of these patients will also require the relatively constant administration of artificial saliva made of carboxymethylcellulose solutions that many find unsatisfactory.[8] Because there is almost no recovery of significant salivary function after 2 years of xerostomia, the administration of artificial saliva may be a chronic, ongoing element of self-care and, consequently, of home care. Certainly, both careful dental restoration and continued ongoing observation by the patient's dentist are important to maintain the best results and decrease the possibility of osteoradionecrosis secondary to a radiation therapy.

In the past, the devastating impact of facial disfigurement from curative head and neck surgery drove many patients to hermetic existences. Today, facial restoration through alloplastic maxillofacial prosthetics has changed that circumstance for many who now maintain socially integrated, active lives. The maxillofacial prosthodontist combines compassion with artistic talent and technical skill to hollow cast prostheses that are consequently both light and speech resonant. The advancement in soft silastic materials and pigments can now produce a more natural translucent skin appearance, texture, and color than ever before. The result is the rehabilitation of a patient who feels that he or she can return to society without becoming an object of public curiosity. In addition to the building of lifelike noses, eyes, periorbital prostheses, and ears, there has been a significant advance through the use of osseointegrated implants.[9] This advance has fostered not only the development of complex, soft moulage prostheses, but also the creation of intraoral dental prosthetics that otherwise would not have been possible. Such patients have undergone masticatory restoration that simply could not be accomplished with standard dentures because of often resected or shallow, resorbed alveolar bone.

Communication is very important between the patient, the surgeon, and the maxillofacial prosthodontist before, during, and after the operation, if there is to be successful prosthodontic rehabilitation.[10] The patient should view this as an ongoing and continued collaboration that may last a lifetime in evaluation and remodeling of both the prosthesis and the patient's response to it as soft tissues and bone change with time. In addition, the patient should undergo periodic surveillance of the osseointegrated implants for possible complications.

The role and wisdom of the osseointegrated implantation prior to or following radiation therapy remains in question. Granstrom et al.[11] report several complications of patients who had titanium implants placed for skin-penetrating prostheses prior to radiation therapy. If postirradiation placement is entertained, Visch et al.[9] recommend a 6- to 12-month recovery period before implantation following radiation. This evolving technology, its timing, and the employment of such adjunctive treatment programs as hyperbaric oxygen remain to be resolved.

Nutritional Care

It is estimated that more than 80% of head and neck cancer patients develop a significant weight loss during multimodal therapy,[12] and one-third of patients with advanced head and neck cancer are severely malnourished when first seen.[13]

The nutritional assessment of the head and neck patient is an important part of the presenting evaluation that may well direct and guide the management and outcome for many patients. Brookes,[14] in assessing both laboratory and anthropomorphic measurements, reports that weight change and other anthropometric indices were the most reliable measurements of nutritional status. Goodwin and Torres[15] suggest that a prognostic nutritional index calculated from the serum albumin, triceps skinfold thickness, serum transferrin, and delayed hypersensitivity reactions provides an objective measure of nutritional status that will identify patients at high risk for complications. In their analysis, Linn and Robinson[16] compared the admission clinical assessment of the preoperative head and neck patient (history and physical examination) with both anthropomorphic measurements and laboratory parameters. They discerned that the initial clinical evaluation was the most reliable index when all the data sets were compared to one another; that is, a patient's history of significant weight loss and the physical signs of inanition (e.g., temporal wasting) are as reliable determinants of malnutrition as more expensive and sophisticated laboratory measurements and anthropomorphic data.

By attempting to quantify and analyze malnutrition, all of these authors tried to discern which patients would benefit from preoperative nutritional support. This came with a growing awareness in the past 25 years that nutritional intervention in both the preoperative and postoperative periods could decrease the morbidity from multimodal treatment. Many studies generated during that time report the benefit of preoperative total parenteral nutrition;[17–19] Jensen[20] extended this concept to suggest that the beneficial effects may not be limited to malnourished patients undergoing complex multimodal treatment in that a number of patients who are not malnourished become so during the course of therapy. However, there is a problem with all of this: total parenteral nutrition (TPN) as an adjuvant to treatment requires patients to be hospitalized for 1 to 2 weeks prior to surgery for the receipt of this support delivered through a central intravenous line. In another paper, Linn and Robinson[21] addressed one practical aspect of this question in evaluating the outcome of such patients who are candidates for preoperative treatment before and after the advent of diagnosis-related groups (DRGs), which limit the number of in-hospital days; they reported that nutritionally deficit patients fared more poorly following the advent of DRGs because they did not receive in-hospital TPN prior to treatment. Another approach needs to be considered.

During the rise of TPN, a number of reports presented the concept of home-administered enteric hyperalimentation given before, during, and after radiation therapy. Some authors have cited a significant benefit from this mode of nutritional intervention for more advanced patients,[22] while others could find no significant difference for those patients taking oral liquid supplementation.[23] The weight of evidence in reports presented over the last decade would suggest that in a controlled setting, patients do benefit from preoperative and preradiation therapeutic nutritional support. We would advocate the administration of home enteric tube administered nutritional support for more malnourished preoperative patients, for all patients about to undergo radiation therapy for head and neck cancer, and for postoperative patients not yet able to receive adequate nutrition by mouth.

To produce the best plan for the patient, a nutritional assessment outlining a balanced approach should be undertaken by a nutritionist who is part of the management team. Because most patients will not tolerate a long pretreatment period after diagnosis, this plan should be developed as soon after the initial assessment as possible. Consequently, outpatient nutritional supplementation should be initiated by the nutritionist–dietitian within 1 to 2 weeks prior to the operation. Most authors advocate a combination of glucose at 30 to 40 kcal/kg and 1 g of protein per kilogram per day. These can be administered orally in the preoperative setting as commercially available enteric supplements if the patient is able to receive them. If the patient has more advanced disease, then enteric nutritional support should be administered by a soft silastic nasogastroduodenal tube or by percutaneous gastrostomy tube (PEG). TPN in the home setting is not recommended because of the high expense, the possibility of infection in the home health setting, the difficulty in control of serum glucose, and because a central line, usually through a subclavian site, may fall within the proposed operative and/or radiation therapy field.

Enteric nutritional support can be administered in bolus fashion through a hanging bag if the patient is not able to accept it orally. In both the preoperative and postoperative home health setting, the visiting home nurse becomes very important in instructing the patient and his or her family as well as in determining any problems that occur during the course of the prolonged treatment program. For patients who may not be able to quickly accept oral feedings, we advocate use of the silastic weighted feeding tube passed through the nasopharynx to the stomach and duodenum. The tip of this tube must be confirmed in its placement through a chest x-ray. One complication that might be encountered is possible migration. Coracoid chondritis, found with firmer red rubber and other stiffer tubes placed at the end of an operation, is usually not seen with the soft silastic feeding tube, but reflux and aspiration do occur just as they may following the placement of a PEG. Because the soft silastic tube is well tolerated, it may be left in place for a long period; that may be useful for the patient undergoing a prolonged postoperative recovery or for the slow repair of an orocutaneous fistula. Clearly, there are some patients with advanced disease who are unable to accept the passage of any tube to the upper aerodigestive pathway.

In addition to hypercaloric feedings, nitrogen balance may be best maintained by exercise. Often when a head and neck cancer patient with more advanced disease presents, his or her state of inanition may have evolved to the point where malaise and lethargy have decreased the level of exercise significantly. If this patient is to have a good outcome, it is suggested that some form of exercise is fundamental to maintaining muscle mass.

Finally, there are reports advocating the use of PEGs in patients with advanced disease after all other treatment has been completed or cannot be given. Campos et al.[24] suggest that home enteral feeding via tube gastrostomy enables patients with advanced malignant disease who might be otherwise unable to maintain themselves at home nutritionally to be independent in the home setting. They note that of 39 patients with advanced head and neck cancer, 28% were never readmitted and 24% needed one readmission because of home-administered enteric nutrition. They also note that patients with significantly advanced disease are not candidates for this process, especially those considered too sick to go home again.

In all, nutritional advances have had a significant impact in decreasing morbidity and mortality in head and neck cancer care. In our current environment of shrinking health dollars, home management of nutritional enteric care in the perioperative period, during the course of radiation therapy, and in the phase of advanced disease for palliation provides enhancement to the patient's life.

Speech and Swallowing Care

We retain our uniqueness in part because of our ability to communicate; voice communication is a fundamental, rudimentary quotient of that capacity. Without it, we feel estranged and isolated from friends, family, and our community. In fact, for many of us, the ability to vocally communicate is vital not only to our jobs but to our lives. Consequently, voice preservation (when possible) is the optimal approach to treatment of early laryngeal carcinoma. Benninger et al.[25] found that voice preservation was achieved in 83% of patients. The authors also noted that continued smoking after radiation therapy carried a significantly greater risk of recurrence. For other patients, the voice may be salvaged through preservation of a portion of the larynx by supraglottic or hemiglottic laryngectomy without radiation therapy. Here, the quality of voice is rougher and deeper, but the speech preserved is spontaneous. Still, for a number of patients who either fail voice preservation or have more advanced disease, laryngectomy is the optimal course. It is this group of patients who will need ongoing speech therapy and assistance of family members at home.

While carcinoma of the larynx can often be cured by laryngectomy, the issue of which approach to take in regaining speech is of interest. It is estimated that approximately 40 to 50% of patients use a vibrating electrolarynx, while 20 to 30% of laryngectomees employ esophageal speech.[26] Most of the remaining laryngectomy patients employ a tracheoesophageal fistula with a variety of prostheses.[27–29] A small cohort of patients remain unable to vocally communicate and will either write or sign. A preoperative evaluation by a speech therapist knowledgeable in all of these techniques is an important part of long-term care and planning well beyond the hospital setting and into the home. The therapist will assist the patient in the postoperative period to select the best approach in establishing vocal communication. Usually, patients will begin with an electrolarynx; some will then learn esophageal speech. Many women prefer to continue using the electrolarynx because it sounds more pleasing than the guttural sound of esophageal speech. For the patient who is unable to learn esophageal speech and does not wish to carry an electrolarynx, a tracheoesophageal fistula and one of the phonation devices is recommended.

Most patients will receive initial instruction and will usually not return to the speech therapist after the first month. Consequently, little is often gained at home for most patients after the third postoperative month.[30] With specific reference to the issue of family support in the home setting, Gibb and Achterberg-Lawlis[31] observed that those patients who learned esophageal speech more quickly and who had a better quality of voice had spouses who were more likely to disagree verbally with them, addressed them in a way that encouraged long verbal answers, and showed compassion and affection.

For the patient who will retain his or her larynx but will undergo resection of part of the tongue, floor of the mouth, pharynx, nose, or sinuses, speech presents a different problem. Here, the vocal sound is present, but the quality is thick, inarticulate, or nasal. These patients may require an ongoing relationship with a speech therapist on an outpatient basis as well as with a maxillofacial prosthodontist to work toward improving the quality of voice.

Swallowing problems may be difficult for some patients and a few may require a feeding tube at home for a considerable period, until they can take enough by mouth without aspiration to sustain themselves. Initially, in the hospital, it is easier for patients relearning to swallow to lift a semisolid bolus of food back to the pharynx with the tongue than it is to drink liquids which may run around the epiglottis to be aspirated. Consequently, it is often recommended that patients at home purée virtually all solid foods (each separately) with a food processor to the point of a paté-like consistency before attempting to swallow. This preserves the flavor and the communal feature of sharing food with other members of the household. As such, this approach may be important to the patient who feels a sense of estrangement brought on by the disease and its treatment. Swallowing problems may last for a very long time, and most patients find a level of adaptation after several months of care at home.

Psychosocial Rehabilitation

For any cancer patient, dealing with the illness, its treatment, and its consequences is often overwhelming. Add to that facial disfigurement, the profound loss of communication skills, and a decreased capacity to socially interact, then it is little wonder that patients who have had head and neck cancer often withdraw. Furthermore, as Hermann and Carter[32] state, "Patients are discharged from the hospital with elaborate home care regimens to follow and little support to follow through with them." Consequently, it is important that someone with the skill and time pursue these aspects in the home with the patient and family. Often in today's setting, that person is a home health care nurse who not only tends to the somatic needs of wound care, nutritional issues, and the administration of medications, but who can deal with the social and emotional needs as well. It can be argued that home social workers should have an opportunity to look at the home setting and determine if the appropriate components are available to provide for the patient's global needs; unfortunately, in this managed-care world, it is unlikely that there will be adequate financial support for this evaluation in most circumstances.

All too often, support is not sustained over a long period of time. The expected mourning of the loss of (if nothing else) a prior way of life, the need to find assistance for the more difficult as well as the simpler day-to-day problems, the possible issue of coping with addiction to tobacco and alcohol, the estrangement because of disfigurement and mastication changes, and the decreased ability to communicate all make the life of a postoperative head and neck patient difficult. In an attempt to reestablish a life of quality, "...most people will manage the cancer experience without formal counseling because of their inherent strengths and family support."[33] Still, others may benefit from some form of intervention. At our institution, we have established such a psychosocial head and neck support group managed in the same fashion as a colostomy club or a laryngectomee organization. At least one enthusiastic very long-term surviving patient volunteer, a social worker, and a member of the psychooncology staff meet with recently treated patients on a weekly basis just outside the hospital setting to share mutual issues of support and to offer help to those who are recovering from major craniofacial therapeutics.

How should our goals be directed to assist in the recovery of such patients? Argerakis[33] states, "A sense of being needed and wanted, that is what life is about. All of our rehabilitation efforts should be directed towards that goal...." As Hermann and Carter[32] note, "Survivorship, regardless of duration, is immeasurably enhanced by the power of a positive, human connection between doctors, patients, and families, as they struggle to manage the challenge of living with cancer."

References

1. Joyce, L. D. and McQuarrie, D. G., Application of contemporary reconstructive techniques in head and neck surgery for anterior oral-facial cancers, *Surgery,* 80(3):373–378, 1976.
2. Macnamara, M., Pope, S., Sadler, A., Grant, H., and Brough, M., Microvascular free flaps in head and neck surgery, *J. Laryngol. Otol.,* 108(11):962–968, 1994.
3. Lovich, S. F. and Arnold, P. G., The effect of smoking on muscle transposition, *Plastic Reconstr. Surg.,* 93(4):825–829, 1994.
4. Benninger, M. S., Gillen, J., Thieme, P., Jacobson, B., and Dragovich, J., Factors associated with recurrence and voice quality following radiation therapy for T_1 and T_2 glottic carcinomas, *Laryngoscope,* 104(3P1):294–298, 1994.
5. Lockhart, P. B. and Clark, J., Pretherapy dental status of patients with malignant

conditions of the head and neck, *Oral Surg. Oral Med. Oral Pathol.,* 77(3):236–241, 1994.

6. Liu, R. P., Fleming, T. J., Toth, B. B., and Keene, J. H., Salivary flow rates in patients with head and neck cancer 0.5 to 25 years after radiotherapy, *Oral Surg. Oral Med. Oral Pathol.,* 70(6):725–729, 1990.

7. Beumer, J., III, Curtis, T., and Harrison, R. E., Radiation therapy of the oral cavity: sequelae and management. Part 2, *Head Neck Surg.,* 1(5):392–408, 1979.

8. Nelson, R. and Fox, P., Salivation, in Rehabilitation of Head and Neck Cancer Patients: Consensus of Recommendations from the International Conference on Rehabilitation of the Head and Neck Cancer Patients, Mathog, R. H., Ed., *Head and Neck,* 13(1):1–13, 1991.

9. Visch, L. L., Scholtemeijer, M., Denissen, H. W., Kala, W., and Levendag, P. C., The use of implants for prosthetic rehabilitation after cancer treatment: the clinical experiences, *J. Invest. Surg.,* 7:291–303, 1994.

10. Martin, J. W., Lemon, J. C., and King, G. E., Maxillofacial restoration after tumor ablation, *Clin. Plastic Surg.,* 21(1):87–96, 1994.

11. Granstrom, G., Tjellstron, A., and Albrektsson, T., Postimplantation and radiation for head and neck cancer treatment, *Int. J. Oral Maxillofacial Implants,* 8(5):495–501, 1993.

12. Chencharick, J. D. and Mossman, K. L., Nutritional consequences of the radiotherapy of head and neck cancer, *J. Cancer,* 51:811–815, 1983.

13. Goodwin, W. J., Jr. and Byers, P. M., Nutritional management of head and neck cancer patient, *Med. Clin. North Am.,* 77(3):597–610, 1993.

14. Brookes, G. B., Nutritional status—a prognostic indicator in head and neck cancer, *Otolaryngol. Head Neck Surg.,* 93(1):69–74, 1985.

15. Goodwin, W. J., Jr. and Torres, J., The value of prognostic nutritional index in the management of patients with advanced cancer of the head and neck, *Head Neck Surg.,* 6(5):932–937, 1984.

16. Linn, B. S. and Robinson, D. S., Predictors of Complications after Head and Neck Surgery in the Old, Annual Scientific Meeting Program of the Society of Gerontology, Miami Beach, Florida, 1985.

17. Burt, N. E., Stein, T. P., Schwade, J. G., and Brennan, M. F., Whole-body protein metabolism in cancer-bearing patients. Effect of total parenteral nutrition and associative serum insulin response, *Cancer,* 53(6):1246–1252, 1984.

18. Nayel, H., el-Ghoneimy, E., and el-Haddad, S., Impact of nutritional supplementation on treatment delay and morbidity in patients with head and neck tumors treated with radiation, *Nutrition,* 8(1):13–18, 1992.

19. Daly, J. M., Massar, E., Giaco, G., Frazier, C. H., Mountain, C. F., Dudrich, S. J., and Copeland, E. M., 3rd, Parenteral nutrition and esophageal cancer patients, *Ann. Surg.,* 196(2):203–208, 1982.

20. Jensen, S., Clinical effects of enteral and parenteral nutrition preceding cancer surgery, *Med. Oncol. Tumor Pharmacol.,* 2(3):225–229, 1985.

21. Linn, B. S. and Robinson, D. S., The possible impact of DRG's on nutritional status of patients having surgery for cancer of the head and neck, *JAMA,* 260(4):514–518, 1988.

22. Arnold, C. and Richter, N. P., The effect of oral nutritional supplements on head and neck cancer, *Int. J. Radiat. Oncol. Biol. Phys.,* 16(6):1595–1599, 1989.
23. Enig, B., Winther, E., and Hessov, I., Changes in food intake and nutritional status in patients treated with radiation for cancer of the larynx and pharynx, *Nutr. Cancer,* 7(4):229–237, 1985.
24. Campos, A. C., Butters, M., and Meguid, M. M., Home enteral nutrition via gastrostomy in advanced head and neck cancer patients, *Head Neck,* 12(2):137–142, 1990.
25. Benninger, M. S., Gillen, J., Thieme, P., Jacobson, B., and Dragovich, J., Factors associated with recurrence and voice quality following radiation therapy for T1 and T2 claudic carcinomas, *Laryngoscope,* 104(3):294–298, 1994.
26. Mathog, R. H., Rehabilitation of head and neck cancer patients: consensus on recommendations from the International Conference on Rehabilitation of the Head and Neck Cancer Patient, *Head Neck,* January–February, 1991.
27. O'Leary, I. K., Heaton, J. M., Clegg, R. T., and Parker, A. J., Acceptability and intelligibility of tracheoesophageal speech using the Gronigen valve, *Folia Phoniatr. Logoped.,* 46(4):180–187, 1994.
28. Amatsu, M., Kinishi, M., and Jamir, J. C., Evaluation of speech of laryngectomees after the Amatsu tracheoesophageal shunt operation, *Laryngoscope,* 94(5, Part 1):969–701, 1984.
29. Li, F. L., Functional tracheoesophageal shunt for vocal rehabilitation after laryngectomy, *Laryngoscope,* 95(10):1267–1271, 1985.
30. Pauloski, B. R. et al., Speech and swallowing function after oral and oropharyngeal resections: one year follow-up, *Head Neck,* 16(4):313–322, 1994.
31. Gibb, H. W. and Achterberg-Lawlis, J., The spouse as facilitator for esophageal speech: a research perspective, *J. Surg. Oncol.,* 11(2):89–94, 1979.
32. Hermann, J. F. and Carter, J., The dimensions of oncology, social work, intrapsychic, interpersonal, and environmental interventions, *Semin. Oncol.,* 21(6):712–717, 1994.
33. Argerakis, G. P., Psychosocial considerations of the postoperative treatment of head and neck cancer patients, *Dental Clin. North Am.,* 34(2):285–305, 1990.

Mental Health Needs of the Homebound and Their Caretakers

17

Danielle Turns, M.D.

In his "Historical Perspectives on Home Care," Benjamin[1] reviews the sociocultural, demographic, economic, medical, and legislative factors that have shaped home care as we know it today, i.e., a vital part of health services. In 1980, approximately 10.8 million persons with severe or moderate disabilities required long-term care, a number expected to reach over 14 million by the year 2000.[2] It is now estimated that, due to increased longevity and prevalence of chronic disease, 6 million people will need home care services. According to Axelrod,[3] of those presently receiving such care, 70% suffer from medical illnesses, 30% from psychiatric disorders, and 90% are elderly. The vast majority of these patients are homebound.

This chapter offers an overview of the homebound population. The mental health needs of patients, their caretakers, and caregivers (the latter defined as health professionals) are addressed. Assessment and interventions, program evaluation, and, in the last sections, special issues arising during the care of such patients are discussed.

Definitions and Overview

Definitions

For the purpose of this chapter, the following definition of homebound is offered: persons who, because of physical, psychiatric, or mixed disabilities, need help or supervision with activities of daily living (ADL) and cannot leave their living quarters without assistance. Medicare and Medicaid eligibility criteria further specify that going out of the home must be physically taxing and create a potential risk for the patient. While these descriptions evince the image of an elderly demented patient, the population it covers is much more varied. The characteristics explored below are useful when assessing the needs of patients and caretakers and devising appropriate plans for care.

Characteristics

Age

Although most homebound are older adults or elderly, a significant number include children and young adults: those with severe developmental disabilities including mental retardation,[4] posttraumatic or postinfection syndromes, autism, and, more rarely, immunity deficiency syndromes and cancer. Their care is emotionally, physically, and financially draining. The parents who care for them, as is usually the case, face a lifelong ordeal and eventually the dilemma of the child's future after their demise.

Type of Illness

Adults and the elderly constitute a large population that may suffer from any of the following diseases:

1. **Physical conditions**—Rheumatoid arthritis, advanced cardiovascular or pulmonary disease, degenerative neurological and poststroke syndromes, terminal cancer, and AIDS cover most of the cases. Patients with the HIV spectrum diseases present special mental health needs associated with the course of the disease, its stigma, and other social consequences of their diagnosis.[5]
2. **Dementias**—Dementias, when nonposttraumatic or infectious, strike mostly people over 50; Alzheimer's disease and arteriosclerotic dementia are prime examples.
3. **Psychiatric conditions**—These are simply listed here as they will be considered in more detail later. Chronic schizophrenia and, to a lesser extent, severe agoraphobia and obsessive compulsive disorder are the most frequently encountered.
4. **Mixed conditions**—Patients with incapacitating medical conditions are at high risk for depression, debilitating anxiety, organic brain syndromes secondary to the primary illness or its treatment, and substance abuse.

Such conditions tax the resiliency of caretakers and, most of the time, require specialized intervention.

Course of Illness

The course of illness is to be considered as well. Is the patient terminal or is his or her condition compatible with prolonged life? Terminal illness in the elderly may be easier to bear for patients and caretakers alike, as an end is in sight. Facing such an end is more difficult when the patient is a child or young adult. In either case, grief work is essential here. Chronic, lifelong conditions (quadriplegia, stable vegetative states, profound mental retardation, or severe cerebral palsy) call for another set of interventions.

Patient's Living Conditions

The patient's living conditions must be taken into account. Is the patient living alone or with caretakers? In the former instance, patients are totally dependent upon outside help and "the good will of strangers." Social and emotional isolation are of concern here, as is safety. If the patient lives with caretakers, the strengths and weaknesses of the latter must be realistically evaluated. The support network has needs of its own that must be addressed for an acceptable outcome. Many caretakers will need assistance in making the decision to institutionalize the patient when their resources are overwhelmed.[6]

Mental Health Issues and the Homebound Patient

Psychiatric Disorders as a Cause of Homebound Status

Severe schizophrenia usually results in institutionalization, particularly when associated with agitation or violent behavior. However, many schizophrenics who may be totally dysfunctional, yet of mild disposition, are cared for at home. Their care entails specialized psychiatric treatment modalities. Medications such as long-acting haloperidol or fluphenazine decanoate with monthly or biweekly injections usually control the more dramatic symptoms (hallucinations, delusions). Schizophrenia "negative symptoms" (withdrawal, apathy, self-neglect, uncommunicativeness) respond less well. Clozapine has shown effectiveness, but the mandated weekly blood count monitoring needed to identify early signs of agranulocytosis makes its use unwieldy. Other medications such as respiridone have shown promise, yet their effectiveness in chronically disabled patients remains moot. Visiting psychiatric nurses play a vital role in the care of such patients. They administer medications, identify bothersome side effects such as tardive dyskinesia, monitor changes in the patient's condition, and provide support and education for the family.

Reclusiveness is not a psychiatric disorder per se. However, a certain number of persons characterized by eccentricity or avoidant or schizoid personality traits may de facto become homebound. Such patients are usually very resistive to attempted intervention.

Severe agoraphobia is an anxiety disorder that results in seemingly self-inflicted homebound status. Such patients are paralyzed by overwhelming anxiety when confronted with crowds or open spaces. Leaving the home or sometimes a room within the home is unfeasible, even in the face of actual danger.

Severe obsessive compulsive disorder may render patients with lengthy and multiple rituals (unceasing handwashing, repetitive checking) unable to perform ADL or leave their home for days on end. Specialized interventions are needed in such cases. Medications such as antidepressants (MAO inhibitors, chlormipramine, fluoxetine) and the benzodiazepine alprazolam have shown dramatic results. Behavioral interventions have been found useful[7] and the counseling of spouses essential.[8]

When not posttraumatic or infectious, dementias most often strike people over 50. The most frequent, Alzheimer's disease, is a prime example of a steadily deteriorating condition, as is the much rarer Huntington's chorea. Arteriosclerotic or multi-infarct dementia is another frequent condition, but with a more fluctuating course. Disorientation, memory loss, incontinence, inability to perform ADL, loss of communicative skills, and erratic and violent behavior characterize the end stage. Incontinence, wandering, and violent behavior are the frequent heralds of institutionalization.[9] Medications aimed at restoring cerebral function (hydergine, tacrine) have not proven to be reliably effective. Small doses of major tranquilizers such as haloperidol are useful in the control of agitation, sundowning (when, due to sensory deprivation, the patient experiences hallucinations and disorientation in the evening), and insomnia. They are preferable to short-acting benzodiazepines (e.g., lorazepam), which are effective but may induce dependence. Perhaps the most difficult times for caretakers are in the early and middle stages of the disease, when flashes of the former self fan hope and require a tightrope adjustment of the caretaker's response.

Mental Health Problems Associated with or Resulting from Homebound Status

Becoming or being homebound entails a number of psychological and emotional stages that must be addressed for a successful adaptation. Patients who do not reach that goal are candidates for bonafide psychiatric disorders.

Psychological and Emotional Changes

The patient's loss of independence and mastery over ADL or other previously assumed roles creates deep narcissistic wounds that will shape his or her adaptation to dependence upon others. Sadness, grief, resentment, and anger may be obstacles to healthy acceptance of such situations.

Dependency and the caretaker's response that it induces have been of wide concern in the literature.[10] Patients may exhibit a "giving up" response, resulting in nonperformance of tasks that could be realistically accomplished and insistence on total assistance in every respect. Such behavior, however draining for the caretaker, is sometimes tolerated and subtly abetted as a means of control. Independent behavior may be ignored or discouraged. In other cases, dependency perceived as willful will lead the caretaker to anger, rejection, neglect, or abuse.

Role changes occur in both the patient and the caretaker. The iron-fisted matriarch or patriarch, for example, must now look up to children or a spouse she or he used to dominate. The locus of control has shifted to persons still intimidated by the strong personality of their now ward. Caretaker spouses must assume duties formerly performed by the patient.[11] Children may have to "mother" their own parents. Support and counseling are needed for both parties to reach an acceptable equilibrium.

Homebound status is per se a source of stress.[12] Living conditions that do not ensure survival and safety drain the adaptive resources of the patients. Dwindling social contacts create boredom and isolation. Inability to perform routine tasks or hobbies decreases self-esteem and robs the patient of pleasurable activities. However, the patient is not immune to new stresses arising from the illness or death of family members and friends, financial constraints, strife within or outside of the nuclear family, cramped living quarters, or other stressful events. The patient's impotence or perceived impotence in participating in crisis resolution adversely affects his or her adaptation. Supportive psychotherapy, grief work, and stress reduction techniques will be useful here, as will knowledge of the patient's past coping style and skills.

Behavioral acting out (this does not mean violent behavior in particular here) may be the patient's way of expressing distress; such behavior includes whining, incessant babbling or uncommunicativeness, cantankerousness, orneriness, oppositional stance, intrusiveness, sulking, or persistent demands. It is important to assess whether this behavior represents an exaggeration of preexisting personality traits or an underlying psychiatric disorder. In the case of a transient maladaptation, counseling, education, and behavioral approaches are of benefit. Wandering off is a common complication of the dementias that respond poorly to such interventions. Safety features such as alarms or automatic doors may have to be installed.

Psychiatric Disorders

Depressive states (major depression, dysthymic disorder) are common complications. These are characterized by sadness, pessimism, crying spells, hopelessness, helplessness, anhedonia, difficulty in concentrating, vegetative signs (such as change in appetite or sleep pattern, constipation), apathy or agitation, and suicidal thoughts. The syndrome may be difficult to diagnose in the severely physically disabled, the poststroke patient, the mildly demented, or the elderly.[13] It may be dismissed as a normal reaction to what many would consider an intolerable situation. Vegetative signs, lack of concentration, and resulting disorientation and memory loss (pseudodementia) may be attributed to underlying illness. In cancer patients, the interactive pain–depression dyad[14] poses a particular challenge. When a definite diagnosis of depression is made, antidepressants combined with supportive or cognitive psychotherapy is an effective approach.

Chronic anxiety and panic attacks may complicate any physical illness. They are particularly common in cardiac, pulmonary, and stroke patients and aggravate the physical symptoms. Experienced clinicians have often witnessed the advent of severe anxiety to be the omen of an otherwise stable patient's demise. In most cases, anxiety can be easily managed with short-acting benzodiazepines (oxazepam, alprazolam, lorazepam).

Hypochondriasis is another condition difficult to diagnose in patients with legitimate physical complaints. When the symptoms claimed are polymorphous, unexplainable, unresponsive to established treatments, or affectively charged, this diagnosis must be entertained. An antidepressant trial may be an effective diagnostic tool and treatment.

It is not unusual for socially isolated, frequently sensorially impaired, or mildly organic patients to develop persecutory delusions. The patient's claims to be harassed or robbed place an onerous burden on the caretakers. The latter may benefit from counseling, but psychotherapy is of little use for the patient, who may benefit from small doses of a major tranquilizer. However, before assuming the patient's claims are not reality based, the possibility of abuse should be considered.

Atkinson[15] found that alcoholism is the third most common mental disorder among elderly men, accounting for 2 to 10% in those over 65. Most often such conditions are diagnosed when the patient needs hospitalization or institutionalization. It may be novel to think that homebound patients would have access to alcohol or drugs, but they do.[16] Caretakers may be in denial of the problem; they may provide alcohol as a means to keep peace while providing some pleasure to the patient's restricted life, or they may be abusers themselves. They may also resort to over-the-counter (OTC) drugs to keep the patient subdued. Any change in mental status indicating depression, unexpected or worsening organicity, or behavioral changes should alert the health professional to this possibility. Interaction of alcohol and OTC drugs with the patient's regular medications may induce a worsening of the condition or new side effects. Street drugs are seldom a problem in the elderly but may be a problem in the younger patient. For example, Mr. B became quadriplegic after an accident during military service. He had an attentive covey of friends. Prodigal with his pension, he financed the purchase of drugs he willingly shared with his courier-friends. A urine screen confirmed the suspicion that his wild mood swings had aroused. In cases such as this, intervention is difficult as the drug connection is enmeshed within the patient's social fabric. However, in most cases, working through denial, education, detoxification, and referral to specialized programs will prove useful. While total abstinence is not required of nonalcoholic or nonsubstance-dependent patients, the use of alcohol or mild sedatives must be monitored.

When a previously alert or mildly cognitively impaired patient starts developing symptoms of an organic brain syndrome (memory loss, disorientation, confusion, sleep disturbance, behavioral changes), various possibilities must be considered (viz., dementia, delirium, or pseudodementia). Laboratory tests (electrolytes, CBC, thyroid function, vitamin levels, liver function tests, and medication levels, to name just a few), a review of the patient's diet and medications with special attention to polypharmacy and drug interactions, and the use of alcohol or OTC preparations are the first lines of investigation. Delirium is a medical emergency that requires hospital care. Dementia may prove to be reversible (for example, B_{12} deficiency) or not, if due to a superimposed brain degeneration. Pseudodementia, as previously mentioned, may mask a severe depression and an antidepressant trial may clinch the diagnosis.

Psychiatric Monitoring of the Homebound

Based upon their observations or the reports of caretakers, visiting health professionals are usually the first to detect mental changes. Checking of orientation alone is not a useful approach.[17] Several tools exist that will give a better understanding of what is happening to the patient. Easily administered, these instruments bring valuable information to the physician regarding treatment approaches. Functional status can be appraised by the Older Adults Resource Survey, developed at Duke University.[18] The Mental Status Questionnaire,[19] Minimental State Exam,[20] Short Portable Mental Status Questionnaire,[21] and Geriatric Depression Scale[22] all are useful tools, when complemented by a medication profile and an alcohol/substance abuse history. Estimation of suicide risk is of capital importance in the elderly, a group at high risk for suicide, particularly when chronic illness, alcohol abuse, and recent losses are involved.

Referral to the patient's physician is a must, and consultation with a psychiatrist and hospitalization are the best approaches to intervention.

Mental Health Issues and Caretakers

A substantial number of homebound patients live alone,[23] but many live with family members; of those who live alone, many usually receive familial support and assistance. The familial relationships and the mental health needs of the caretakers as they preexist or arise in the care of the homebound are considered in this section.

Who Are the Caretakers?

Contrary to a popularly held belief,[24] adult children, particularly daughters, provide substantial care to their parents. The typical caretaker of an elderly person is a middle-aged daughter near the age of retirement or already retired. Sons more rarely assume caretaking, and daughters-in-law often take on the day-to-day responsibilities in such cases. Spouses, usually wives,[10] are second in line. Siblings are less often involved and nowadays so is the extended family. Parents remain the most frequent caretakers when the homebound person is a child or young adult, while companions provide care for many AIDS patients. The caretaker's willingness and ability to care for the homebound patient is influenced by the caretaker's stage in life, familial commitments, physical and mental health, financial situation, and living conditions. Middle-aged children see their postretirement plans affected by the presence of a homebound parent, while younger caretakers juggle duties to their spouse and growing children and see their jobs and social activities affected. Elderly spouses may themselves be in declining health, and assuming tasks previously discharged by the patient (home maintenance, financial arrangements) is stressful. Extended family members may share the burden in a more equitable manner, but squabbles and rivalries may create tensions in the network. The social integration of the caretakers is of import as it impacts their resiliency. A recent study by Mintzer et al.[25] showed that black caretakers may experience fewer psychological consequences than white, even when faced with patients with more severe dysfunctions.

Mental Health Needs of the Caretakers

Preexisting conditions are fertile ground for maladaptive responses of caretakers to their roles. Preexisting depression or anxiety may worsen. More rarely, delusional states (folie a deux) may be imparted to the patient.[26] Alcohol and substance abuse may demand intervention. A clinical vignette will illustrate the latter. Ms. A, a recovering alcoholic, lives several states away from her alcoholic mother (B) and her centenarian grandmother (C). On a recent visit, A found several empty liquor bottles, but the house was otherwise clean and C appeared well cared for, although she complained of B's sudden and sometimes prolonged disappearances to a neighborhood bar. Neither C nor B would consider institutionalization and B denied any problem with alcohol. A was torn between her familial loyalty, her own needs for recovery, and her limited ability to intervene due to distance. Contacting social agencies and the Council on Aging in B and C's locality provided some relief.

Brody[24] has described parent care as a normative family stress that may lead to psychological dysfunction, and Brown[11] has explored issues involving spouses. Jorm[27] has shown that wives were more at risk for depression than husbands, daughters, or other relatives. Psychological maladaptations run the gamut from mild to severe depression or anxiety, irritability to abusive behavior, marital conflict to estrangement, fatigue to exhaustion, and somatic illnesses. Assessment of the coping skills of the caretakers, their mental status, and their support resources is paramount to successful home placement. Financial worries due to patient care expenses (safety measures, respite care, sitters) are sometimes a red herring for more personal issues and need to be addressed in that light.

Mental Health Issues and the Caregivers

Who Are the Caregivers?

Caregivers are defined as the health professionals who visit patients in their homes and are the main providers of formal care. They most often include nurses and social workers.

Caregivers often develop personal and deeply caring relationships with their patients. Developing such an alliance is very satisfying, but it is also fraught with pitfalls. Other chapters in this book have explored these issues, and only those that impact the mental health of patients, their caretakers, and the caregivers themselves will be mentioned here.

Nurses have long been the primary caregivers of the homebound, with the Visiting Nurse Association providing the majority of the care. Their crucial role in assessing the patient's environment, the physical and psychological needs of patients as well as those of their caretakers, in tailoring expectations, and in providing advice, counseling, and support has been well documented. Their knowledge of medications, nutritional regimens, and compliance issues is also of paramount importance. Daudell-Strejc and Murphy[28] have summarized the special expertise of psychiatric nurses. Setting limits, identifying boundaries, and being aware of transference and countertransference phenomena are part of their clinical practice. Nurses need flexibility in assuming an educational versus a counseling role and, as determined by the patient's psychological needs, assessing their function as a surrogate parent. Recognizing dependency and rewarding reasonable efforts toward independence and establishing realistic expectations are essential to a healthy therapeutic alliance. Ensuring compliance with medications, keeping doctor's appointments, and facilitating socialization through referral to community services are other contributions made by nurses. Peplau describes the phases of the relationship from orientation, identification of perceptions and expectations, and exploitation, during which the patient may test the limits and the issues of dependence–independence come to the fore.[29] Resolution is the last phase, the end of treatment. Whether it is due to the patient's institutionalization or death or nurse relocation or retirement, issues of grief and abandonment need to be worked out by all parties.

Social workers[3,30,31] are another group of professionals intimately involved with the homebound. By training, they have special knowledge of the roles of family members, their functions, interactions, homeostasis, and factors that disrupt such. However, this is not their only function. They act as brokers in establishing connections with community agencies, educators, counselors, mediators, advocates, and collaborators.[30] They also impart special skills to the termination process for themselves, the families, and other caregivers.

Other professional caregivers include physical rehabilitation therapists, occupational therapists, and pastoral personnel. In the first two instances, the focus of intervention is more narrow, but their communication with the treatment team is essential. Pastoral counselors and ministers are seldom part of the treatment team. Nonetheless, their input in addressing the patient and family's spiritual needs is far from negligible in our culture.

Another group of caregivers are nonprofessional (i.e., volunteers), hired by an agency or the family for supervision, companionship, respite care, and domestic tasks. This group may encounter difficulties in dealing with problematic behavior, providing stimulating activities, and addressing interpersonal issues. Their needs for training and supervision should not be neglected.[32] A pilot project described by Grossman et al.[33] has used volunteer peer counselors in the care of "frail elderly." Recruited volunteers from the community were screened and trained by the North Carolina Home Care team and provided weekly "social" visits to the homebound. Here again, training and supervision were the necessary ingredients for a successful interaction.

Mental Health Needs of the Caregivers

The care of the chronically or terminally ill may elicit emotional difficulties even in the most professional, well-trained caregivers. Burnout is the generic and perhaps overused term for such situations. Several studies have addressed this issue, as well as job satisfaction.[31,32,35] A positive appraisal of the role of caregivers is most often reported by professionals and nonprofessionals alike, even in the face of identified stressors such as lack of time, lack of resources, and communication difficulties. However, maladaptive responses rank high, including depression, tension, anxiety, psychosomatic symptoms, insomnia, and a sense of futility or isolation. Continuing education, frequent meetings with the health team, and contacts with an experienced and trusted supervisor are useful preventive strategies. Needless to say, "troubled employees' services" should be made available to field workers.[36]

Interventions

Perhaps the most important intervention is a judicious assessment of the potential homebound patient and his or her environment. Abraham et al.[37] have reviewed these issues and the variety of care environments best suited to the Alzheimer's patient. In this section, we will concentrate on psychiatric and family interventions as their need arises during the course of homebound care.

Interventions Primarily Focused and Aimed at the Patient

Monitoring of the Psychiatric Homebound Patient

The primary treatments of psychiatric patients have already been mentioned. In the long-term care of schizophrenic patients, in addition to medication administration which remains the mainstay of treatment, changes in the patient's condition and behavior must be examined in light of the following:

1. **Compliance**—Is the patient taking medication as prescribed, missing doses, or taking too much or too little? Is the caretaker monitoring medications appropriately?
2. **Emergence of side effects**—The early diagnosis of tardive dyskinesia entails examination by a physician. Other side effects (extrapyramidal symptoms, drowsiness, insomnia, etc.) may be due to newly prescribed medications for other conditions or intake of nonprescribed drugs.
3. **Emergence of other psychiatric conditions**—Schizophrenic patients may become depressed as a result of a loss of or change in their environment. Consultation by the treating psychiatrist is a must here.

4. **Emergence of physical conditions**—Chronically ill psychiatric patients are not immune to physical illness, the clinical presentation of which may be altered by their psychiatric condition and medication. A regular yearly physical examination should be routine, but should not preclude referral to the physician in the presence of new complaints.

Management of Psychiatric Conditions Arising During the Homebound Treatment Course

Psychopharmacotherapy—Indications for antidepressants, anxiolytics, and major tranquilizers have already been mentioned. Going into more detail would result in another chapter, if not a book. It is important to emphasize here the general principles of psychopharmacology in the elderly or frail adult. The metabolism of drugs is altered by age and medical illnesses; absorption and elimination are important parameters that will demand individualized dosage and administration schedules. Review of the patient's medical regimen should be frequent and systematic, and one physician should be responsible for its monitoring. Polypharmacy is too frequent and complications from drug interactions are too often "treated" with additional medications. When psychotropic drugs are indicated, such a medication review is a must. Identifying which antidepressant, anxiolytic, or major tranquilizer is indicated should take into consideration the patient's previous response to such drugs, if prior episodes have existed.

Potential side effects are of import. In the treatment of depression, for example, tricyclic antidepressants are extremely effective, but their multiple side effects (blurred vision, tachycardia, sweating, or orthostatic hypotension, which can lead to falls and fractures) may preclude their use in the homebound. Serotonin uptake inhibitors may be better tolerated by the elderly, but again, dose titration must be individualized.

Short-acting benzodiazepines, used in treating anxiety or agitation, are usually well tolerated. The issue of the dependence they may induce must be appraised in light of the patient's past history (a history of drug or alcohol dependence is a red flag) and present condition. If the patient is terminal, the issue is academic. If the patient is chronic but stable, such medications must be closely supervised. Low doses of major tranquilizers for paranoid ideation, sundowning, or agitation are effective and well tolerated. However, whenever the need for medication arises, the expertise of a geriatrician is crucial.[38]

Psychotherapy—This is often a neglected treatment tool in the elderly or the physically ill.[39] Formal psychotherapy in the psychiatrist's office is hardly manageable for these patients and certainly not an option for the homebound. Patient resistance due to a well-implanted belief system that equates need for help with weakness or craziness, the assumption that depression is unavoidable, minimization, and ambivalence are definite obstacles to psychotherapeutic approaches. Counseling at home is a preferred option. Its depth will depend upon the counselor's training and skills, but the following ingredients will at one time or another be of benefit.

An empathetic, encouraging, and respectful attitude; recognition of the patient's physical limitations; a realistic and explicit treatment plan; and setting time limits will facilitate the counselor–patient relationship. Supportive psychotherapy emphasizes ventilation, with advice and help in accepting decreasing capacities. A psychodynamic approach will deal with age and interrelated issues, transference, dependence–independence conflicts, and grief. Self-image and self-esteem enhancement, working through past traumatic events, and adjustment to retirement, widowhood, and changing roles are areas of exploration. Acceptance of mortality is another goal. Cognitive therapy[40] has been shown to be effective in the treatment of depression. It addresses the cognitive fallacies induced by depression (overgeneralization of negative expectations, maladaptive assumptions, automatic negative thoughts). Behavioral techniques aimed at enhancing recent memory may also help.[41] Some other specialized approaches such as stress management techniques[42,43] have been advocated, as have rehabilitative modalities.[44,45]

Patient education is now considered an intrinsic part of treatment for any patient, including the homebound. However, when such patients are mentally impaired, whether organically or psychologically, the issue of how much they can learn is to be considered. Clinically, if their impairment is mild, such patients are educable. For more impaired patients, standard adult intelligence tests may provide a clue, but they tend to give a picture of where the patient is at more than whether he or she can progress. Neuropsychological tests have better predictive potential,[46] but are expensive and not routinely administered. Interestingly, occupational therapists are most helpful. They give instructions for simple tasks and first observe how patients accomplish the tasks and then observe how they can repeat them on their own. However, occupational therapists are not frequently included in the outreach team, but they can be productively utilized when the patient is hospitalized.

Attention to issues such as bowel management[47] or urinary incontinence[48,49] will go a long way in restoring the patient's self-esteem and his or her continued acceptance by caretakers. Incontinence, along with assaultive behavior and wandering off, is often the precursor of institutionalization.[9]

Interventions Focusing on the Caretaker–Patient Dyad

Caretakers are involved at every level of care, not only as care providers but also as people. They bring to their task their strengths, their frailties, their love, and their resentments. Their role is a difficult one and their needs many. The pitfalls inherent in their role were reviewed earlier. Education, counseling, establishing realistic expectations, and coaching in dealing with erratic or violent behavior are most important needs. Many caretakers discharge their tasks without major emotional upheaval, but when their resources are overwhelmed, the caregiver's intervention is needed. Wilson[50] has offered an intervention model tailored to the Alzheimer's caregiver, but other traditional family interventions are helpful. Most often, consideration of patient institutionalization is a critical period: guilt, fatigue, anger, depression, and anxiety are the lot of not only the primary caretaker, but also the rest of the family. Referral to clinical services, including family therapy, may be indicated. Another critical time for caretakers is after the patient has left, through institutionalization or death, when the whole support system has to readjust, not only to daily life but plans for the future.

Social manipulation offers many opportunities to allay the burdens. Respite care, which provides time-limited (but welcome) relief, goes a long way in maintaining stamina. Day-care centers for adults and the elderly[51] are potentially beneficial both for the patient and caretakers, but the Medicare-Medicaid stipulations for reimbursement (that is, leaving the home must be taxing and potentially hazardous) render their frequent use unfeasible for many. Community support or self-help groups also offer an opportunity for ventilation, validation, and coping strategies. Alzheimer family groups are the best established examples of such groups.

Program Evaluation

An in-depth evaluation of homecare programs for the homebound is beyond the scope of this chapter. Therefore, discussion here will be confined to questions raised by the literature. It is commonly assumed that home care is more economical than institutionalization, that it preserves the patient's functional ability, and that is provides a better quality of life. However, studies evaluating home care have yielded mixed results. Depending primarily upon the population studied (elderly, veterans, physically disabled, mentally disabled, demented patients) and the length of follow-up, conclusions fall into the "maybe yes–maybe no" range. The studies by Hicks[52] and Hughes et al.[53] fall on the positive side; those by Simpson et al.,[54] Marks et al.,[55] and Knapp et al.[56] fall on the more negative side. Liang et al.[57] evaluated a rehabilitation component of a home care program for the elderly with moot results.

Studies focusing upon the use of community services by homebound patients do not give a clear picture either. Home care does not seem to decrease the utilization of formal community services.[58–60] In terms of cost, Weinberger et al.[61] contest the widely held belief that home care is cost effective. In fact, their study shows that expenditures assumed by caretakers are substantial. There is, however, consistent agreement, except for the study by Hulsman and Chubou,[62] that the patient's quality of life, measured by satisfaction with care or life situation, is reported as better by patients and sometimes caretakers.

This rather sobering summary should not cast opprobrium on home care and the philosophy upon which it rests. Deeply ingrained in our culture and our psyches is the notion that familial surroundings, being cared for by family members, and maintaining independence to the bitter end are overall positive. Strong disapproval of the "warehousing" of the elderly or the disabled and horrifying reports of institutional abuse are powerful societal forces that frame delivery of care. For many, home care, however imperfect, is preferable to institutionalization. And when we look into our own souls, what do we prefer for ourselves?

Special Issues in the Care of the Homebound

Is Homebound Status Permanent?

Most of the time, homebound status is permanent, until institutionalization or death. There are, however, situations that may lead to its reversal. New treatments or spontaneous remissions may lead to such an outcome. Parkinson's disease vastly improved by fetal tissue injection, multiple sclerosis in remission, paraplegics able to walk, and unexpected response to a new cancer treatment modality are the most common examples.

In such cases, even though "cure" is a most positive event, patients and their caretakers may need assistance with the recovery process. Patients' adaptation to being "normal" again and caretakers' confusion in role changes must be addressed for successful resolution. This issue, in the euphoria of newfound wellness, is often neglected, at the price of destabilized relationships.

Psychological or environmental factors may play a part, as illustrated in the following vignette. Retired master sergeant N and his wife chose a small village in southwest France to spend their golden years. The couple lived modestly in a small but new house and were judged to be of comfortable financial means. Mrs. N, crippled by arthritis, was homebound and seen only when traveling by car for a doctor's visit. Mr. N assumed all household duties, including shopping. Whether because of Mr. N's rugged looks and military bearing or for the smell of money, a young woman started befriending the couple and stole Mr. N's heart. Loaded with ginseng, yohimbine, and other potency enhancers, Mr. N began to behave erratically. Usually reserved but friendly, he became irritable with neighbors and made a spectacle of his new relationship, lavishing expensive gifts on the young woman, buying a red convertible for long rides in the countryside or city, and totally neglecting his wife. Left to her own devices, Mrs. N resumed her long-abandoned household chores and could be seen hobbling to the market or the doctor's office. Abandonment and the looming of poverty were her price for mobility.

Abuse and Neglect

According to Adelman,[63] one out of three persons over 65 who lives alone or with family experiences physical or verbal abuse. Such abuse includes threats, insults, slaps, punches, and shoves, sometimes resulting in bruises, fractures, and/or dislocations. Others are neglected, intentionally or unintentionally, in that they are deprived of assistance in important activities. Malnutrition, soiling, and bed sores are ominous results.

Although statistics are not reliable, a conservative estimate is that 700,000 to 1 million adults nationwide are subjected to such indignities. This does not include financial exploitation or sexual abuse. The most likely abuser is a spouse and, in a surprising reversal from younger age groups, a wife. However, when husbands are the abusers, the wives are more severely injured. Of course, other caretakers, adult children, or siblings may also be involved, and the media have reported multiple examples pinpointing hired help as the perpetrators. Race, socioeconomic status, religion, or educational level are not discriminating factors. Violence tends to increase in frequency and severity over time, with sometimes fatal results. The identification of abuse or neglect is an essential, if difficult, task of the caregiver. Obstacles include the reluctance of victims to report abuse, for fear of retaliation, embarrassment, protection of the abuser, and loathing of legal intervention. Sometimes the caregiver's "ageism" bias will interfere with the assessment of bruises or wounds attributed to falls. The social isolation of the victim due to a shrinking circle of visitors, limitation of outside activities, or, in the worst case, restriction by the abuser (inaccessibility to the telephone being the most frequent) contributes to the invisibility of the problem.

The caregiver should always be alert to the possibility of abuse. The patient must be given an opportunity to be interviewed alone as a matter of routine. If any suspicion exists, questioning of the patient must be persistent and pat answers held as suspicious. Attention must be paid to clustering of telltale signs in patient behavior, unexplained mental changes, and physical findings. Attention must also be directed toward the caretakers, their level of stress, their mental health and drug/alcohol use or abuse, their dependence (emotional or financial) on the patient, and their own social isolation. Whenever abuse or neglect is identified, one must judge whether emergency measures are necessary (removal of the patient, police intervention) or whether referral to social agencies is sufficient. If the latter course is taken, follow-up is essential.

Physical Safety and Restraints

The use of physical restraints to ensure the patient's safety is controversial. Nursing homes and other institutions must abide by strict rules regarding the use and monitoring of physical restrictions. Caretakers do have more leeway, but the treatment team must be attuned to the risk of abuse that such devices entail. Patients who hit themselves, are violent toward others, tend to wander off, or have frequent falls are at greater risk. Interventions aimed at less restrictive means (alarms, card-access doors) and proper attention to unwelcome behavioral triggers are helpful.

Ethical and Legal Considerations

From a legal point of view, any person is considered competent unless declared incompetent through the legal system. Clinical experience, however, indicates otherwise. Patients may be able to manage from day to day but not comprehend all issues relevant to their health care. Their health belief system, minimization, denial, and cognitive deficits may interfere with their appraisal of their true condition.

Physicians have long been familiar with the dilemma of truthful disclosure versus benevolent deception.[64] These issues are of primordial importance when informed consent is needed for new treatment or hospitalization. Of particular interest here is consent for psychiatric interventions.[65,66] Even if only a minority of homebound or elderly with mental disorders are totally refractory to entering treatment, persuasion, tact, and diplomacy are needed to offset the reluctance of many others. Cooperation of the caretakers is needed to ensure compliance with treatment.

Assisted Suicide

Euthanasia and physician-assisted suicide have become inescapable issues in the care of the chronically irremediably disabled and the terminally ill. The purpose of this discussion is not to judge what remains a highly personal decision, shaped by ethical and religious beliefs and subject to legislative edicts. The area of interest here is the psychiatric component as it bears on patients or their guardians' decisions. Chochinov et al.[67] investigated 200 terminally ill patients. While wishes that death would come soon were common, only 8% of the patients reported a will to die. Pain and lack of family support were frequently associated complaints. More than half suffered clinical depression. It is therefore important for caretakers and caregivers to be aware that an expressed suicidal request could overlay a treatable psychiatric condition.

Conclusions

The aging population and increased longevity of persons with chronic illnesses and disabilities will contribute to an increase in homebound care. The mental health needs of this population and their caretakers are not to be neglected; the quality of life of both parties should remain acceptable. Consultations with mental health specialists such as psychiatric nurses and social workers, family therapists, and psychogeriatricians will enhance the therapeutic effectiveness of the treatment team. The caregivers themselves need the support of their team and, in addition, continuing education and supervision to function at their best and avoid burnout.

To the homebound, we offer a short poem:

My home, my cage, my prison, my nest.
I see the walls, but also the sky,
I hear the silence, but also a song,
I feel the cement, but also the wind.
Memories of what I was bring me tears
But also the vibrant joy of having been me.
My world is shrunk, but not my spirit,
Homebound—my heart is free.

Acknowledgments

To my husband, Calvin N. Turns, M.D., who, before his death, edited this manuscript. To the VNA of Southern Indiana for their assistance.

References

1. Benjamin, A. E., An historical perspective on home care policy, *The Milbank Quarterly*, 71:129–166, 1993.
2. Schechter, M. and Butler, R. N., Long term care, in *Comprehensive Textbook of Psychiatry*, 5th edition, Kaplan, H. I. and Sadock, B. J., Eds., Williams & Wilkins, Baltimore, 1989.

3. Axelrod, T. B., Innovative roles for social workers in home care programs, *Health Social Work*, 3:49–67, 1978.

4. O'Brien, J., Down stairs that are never your own: supporting people with developmental disabilities in their own homes, *Mental Retardation*, 32:1–6, 1994.

5. Piette, Y. D., Fleishman, J. A., Stein, M. D., Mor, V., and Mayer, K., Perceived needs and unmet needs for formal services among people with HIV disease, *J. Comm. Health*, 18:11–23, 1993.

6. Cath, S. H., The geriatric patient and his family. The institutionalization of a parent—a nadir of life, *J. Geriat. Psych.*, 5:1–5, 1972.

7. Pollack, M., Sachs, G. S., Tesar, G. E., Shushtari, J., Herman, J. B., Otto, M. W., and Rosenbaum, J. F., Pilot outreach services to homebound agoraphobic patients, *Hosp. Comm. Psych.*, 42:315–317, 1991.

8. Oatley, K. and Hodgson, D., Influence of husbands on the outcome of their agoraphobic wives' therapy, *Br. J. Psych.*, 150:380–386, 1987.

9. Morycz, R. K., Caregiving strain and the desire to institutionalize family members with Alzheimer's disease, *Res. Aging*, 7:329–361, 1985.

10. Baltes, M. M. and Wahl, H. W., The dependency-support script in institutions: generalization to community settings, *Psychol. Aging*, 7:409–418, 1992.

11. Brown, P. L., The burden of caring for a husband with Alzheimer's disease, *Home Healthcare Nurse*, 9:33–38, 1991.

12. Allen, M. E., Homebound aging women and the management of stress, *Home Healthcare Nurse*, 8:30–33, 1990.

13. Buschman, M. B. T., Dixon, M. A., and Tichy, A. M., Geriatric depression, *Home Healthcare Nurse*, 13:47–56, 1995.

14. Spiegel, D., Sands, S., and Koopman, C., Pain and depression in patients with cancer, *Cancer*, 74:2570–2578, 1994.

15. Atkinson, R., Alcoholism in the elderly population, *Mayo Clin. Proc.*, 63:825–828, 1988.

16. Cutezo, E. A. and Dellasega, C., Substance abuse in the homebound elderly, *Home Healthcare Nurse*, 10:19–23, 1992.

17. Dellasega, C. and Cutezo, E., Strategies used by home health nurses to assess the mental status of homebound elderly, *J. Comm. Health Nurs.*, 11:129–138, 1994.

18. Duke University, *Multidimensional Functional Assessment: The OARS Methodology,* 2nd edition, Durham NC Center for the Study of Aging and Human Development, 1978.

19. Kahn, R., Goldfarb, A., Pollack, M., and Peck, A., Brief objective measures for the determination of the mental status in the aged, *Am. J. Psychiatry*, 117:326–328, 1960.

20. Folstein, M. F., Folstein, S. E., and McHugh, P. R., "Mini mental state," a practical method for grading the cognitive state of patients for the clinician, *J. Psychiatr. Res.*, 12:189–198, 1975.

21. Pfeiffer, E., A short portable mental status questionnaire for the assessment of organic brain deficit in elderly patients, *J. Am. Geriat. Soc.*, 23:433–441, 1975.

22. Krach, P., Assessment of depressed older persons living in a home setting, *Home Healthcare Nurse*, 13:61–64, 1995.

23. Dey, A. N., Characteristics of elderly men and women discharged from home health care services: United States, 1991–1992, Advance Data No. 259, U.S. Department of Health and Human Services, Washington, D.C., 1995.

24. Brody, E. M., Parent care as a normative family stress, *The Gerontologist*, 25:19–28, 1985.

25. Mintzer, J. E., Knapp, R. S., Nietert, P., Herman, K. C., and Walters, T. H., Differences in the care giving experience between black and white caregivers of demented elderly patients, presented at the 148th Annual Meeting of the APA, Miami, May 20–25, 1995.

26. Lasègue, C. and Faret, J., La Folie à deux (ou folie communiquee), *Ann. Med. Psychol.*, 18:321–355, 1877.

27. Jorm, A. F., Henderson, S., Scott, R., Mackinnon, A. J., Korten, A. E., and Christensen, H., The disabled elderly living in the community: care received from family and formal services, *Med. J. Australia*, 158:383–386, 1993.

28. Daudell-Strejc, D. and Murphy, C., Emerging clinical issues in home health psychiatric nursing, *Home Healthcare Nurse*, 13:17–21, 1995.

29. Peplau, H. E., *Interpersonal Relations in Nursing*, Putnams' Sons, New York, 1952.

30. Sar, B. K. and Phillips, I., The role of the social worker in home care, in *Home Health Care: Principles and Practices*, Spratt, J. S., Hawley, R. L., and Hoye, R. E., Eds., St. Lucie Press, Delray Beach, Florida, 1997, chap. 9.

31. Jacobs, P. E. and Lurie, A., A new look at home care and the hospital social worker, in *Gerontological Social Work in Home Health Care*, The Hayworth Press, New York, 1984.

32. Bjorkhem, K., Olsson, A., Hallberg, I. R., and Norberg, A., Caregivers' experience of providing care for demented persons living at home, *Scand. J. Prim. Health Care*, 10:53–59, 1992.

33. Grossman, E. H., Rizzols, P. J., and Atkinson, V., Geriatric peer counseling—pilot project provides support for the homebound elderly, *NC Med. J.*, 53:296–298, 1992.

34. Audini, B., Marks, I. M., Lawrence, R. E., Connolly, J., and Watts, V., Home-based versus out-patient/in-patient care for people with serious mental illness, *Br. J. Psychiatry*, 165:204–210, 1994.

35. Beck-Friis, B., Strang, P., and Sjoden, P. O., Caring for severely ill cancer patients: a comparison of working conditions in hospital-based home care and in hospitals, *Support Care Can.*, 1:145–151, 1993.

36. Muldary, T. W., *Burnout and Health Professional's Manifestations and Management*, Appleton-Century-Crofts, New York, 1983.

37. Abraham, I. L., Onega, L., Chalifoux, L., and Maes, M. J., Care environment for patients with Alzheimer's disease, *Nurs. Clin. North Am.*, 29:157–172, 1994.

38. Rossman, I., The geriatrician and the homebound patient, *Perspect. Am. Geriat. Soc.*, 36:348–354, 1988.

39. Lazarus, L. W., Psychotherapy with the elderly, in *Comprehensive Textbook of Psychiatry*, 5th edition, Kaplan, H. I. and Saddock, B. J., Eds., Williams & Wilkins, Baltimore, 1989.

40. Beck, A. T., Rush, A. J., and Emery, G., *Cognitive Therapy of Depression*, Guilford Press, New York, 1979.

41. Small, G., Alzheimer's disease and other dementing disorders, in *Comprehensive Textbook of Psychiatry*, 5th edition, Kaplan, H. I. and Sadock, B. J., Eds., Williams & Wilkins, Baltimore, 1989, pp. 2028–2033.

42. Lachman, V. D., *Stress Management—A Manual for Nurses*, Grune & Stratton, New York, 1983.

43. Meichenbaum, D., *Stress Inoculation Training*, Pergamon Press, New York, 1986.

44. Levine, R. E. and Gitlin, L. N., Home adaptation for persons with chronic disabilities: an educational model, *Am. J. Occup. Ther.*, 44:923–929, 1990.

45. Liang, M. H., Rational home care based on the disability model, *Scand. J. Rheumatol. Suppl.*, 82:19–23, 1989.

46. Levin, H. S., Benton, A. L., Fletcher, J. M., and Satz, P., Neuropsychiatric and intellectual assessment of adults, in *Comprehensive Textbook of Psychiatry*, 5th edition, Kaplan, H. I. and Sadock, B. J., Eds., Williams & Wilkins, Baltimore, 1989, pp. 496–512.

47. Ellickson, E. B., Bowel management plan for the homebound elderly, *J. Gerontol. Nurs.*, 14:16–19, 1988.

48. Rose, M. A., Baigis-Smith, J., Smith, D., and Newman, D., Behavioral management of urinary incontinence in homebound older adults, *Home Healthcare Nurse*, 8:10–15, 1990.

49. Newman, D. K. and Smith, O. A. J., Incontinence in elderly homebound patients, *Holistic Nurs. Prac.*, 4:52–60, 1989.

50. Wilson, H. S., Family caregiving for a relative with Alzheimer's dementia: coping with negative choices, *Nurs. Res.*, 38:94–98, 1989.

51. Reifler, B., Adult day centers: new opportunities for geropsychiatrists, *Psychiatr. News*, 30:15–17, 1995.

52. Hicks, B., The triage experiment in coordinated care for the elderly, *Am. J. Public Health*, 71:991, 1981.

53. Hughes, S. L., Cummings, J., Weaver, F., Manheim, L. M., Conrad, K. J., and Nash, K., A randomized trial of Veterans Administration home care for severely disabled veterans, *Medical Care*, 28:135–145, 1990.

54. Simpson, C. J., Seager, C. P., and Robertson, J. A., Homebound care and standard hospital care for patients with severe mental illness: a randomized controlled trial, *Br. J. Psychiatry*, 162:239–243, 1993.

55. Marks, I. M., Connolly, J., Muijen, M., Audini, B., McNamee, G., and Lawrence, R. E., Home based versus hospital based care for people with serious mental illness, *Br. J. Psychiatry*, 165:179–194, 1994.

56. Knapp, M., Beecham, J., Koutsogeorgopoulou, V., Hallam, A., et al., Service use and costs of home based versus hospital based care for people with serious mental illness, *Br. J. Psychiatry*, 165:195–203, 1994.

57. Liang, M. H., Partridge, A. J., Gall, V., and Taylor, J., Evaluation of a rehabilitation component of home care for homebound elderly, *Am. J. Prev. Med.*, 2:30–34, 1986.

58. Edelman, P. and Hughes, S., The impact of community care on provision of

informal care to homebound elderly persons, *J. Gerontol. Soc. Sci.*, 45:S74–S84, 1990.

59. Fredericks, C. M. A., Wierik, M. J. M., Visser, A. P., and Sturmans, F., The functional status and utilization of care of elderly people living at home, *J. Comm. Health*, 15:307–317, 1990.

60. Kempen, G. I. J. M. and Suurmeijer, T. P. B. M., Factors influencing professional home care utilization among the elderly, *Soc. Sci. Med.*, 32:77–81, 1991.

61. Weinberger, M., Gold, D. T., Divine, G. W., Cowper, P. A., Hodgson, L. G., et al., Expenditures in caring for patients with dementia who live at home, *Am. J. Public Health*, 83:338–341, 1993.

62. Hulsman, B. and Chubou, S. J., A comparison of disabled adults' perceived quality of life in nursing facilities and home settings, *Public Health Nurs.*, 6:141–146, 1989.

63. Adelman, R. D., Elder abuse and neglect, in *Comprehensive Textbook of Psychiatry*, 5th edition, Kaplan, H. I. and Sadock, B. J., Eds., Williams & Wilkins, Baltimore, 1989.

64. Eth, S. and Mills, M. J., Ethical and legal considerations, in *Comprehensive Textbook of Psychiatry,* 5th edition, Kaplan, H. I. and Sadock, B. J., Eds., Williams & Wilkins, Baltimore, 1989.

65. DeVries, J., Consent and the geriatric psychiatry home team (letter to editor), *Can. J. Psychiatry*, 38:301–302, 1993.

66. Grauer, H., Kravitz, H., Davis, E., and Rodrigue, C., Homebound aged: the dilemma of psychiatric intervention, *Can. J. Psychiatry*, 36:497–501, 1991.

67. Chochinov, H. M., Wilson, K. G., Enns, M., Mowchun, N., et al., Desire for death in the terminally ill, *Am. J. Psychiatry*, 152:1185–1191, 1995.

Oral Health Management in Chronically Ill Patients

18

Margaret Hill, D.M.D. and
Regan L. Moore, D.D.S., M.S.D.

Introduction

Prevention of dental disease is the key to optimum oral health for all patients. In patients who are experiencing health problems, prevention of dental diseases is critical to maintain oral comfort and to minimize potential oral complications. For some patients, especially those whose immune systems are compromised, such as cancer or AIDS patients, dental problems can become life threatening.[1]

Some simple oral care techniques, performed daily by patients or by caregivers, can give maximal benefits for minimal effort. Common dental problems such as tooth decay and gum diseases can be controlled or prevented by meticulous daily attention to oral hygiene. A healthy, functional dentition can greatly improve quality of life for patients who are chronically ill.[2] Preventing and controlling oral infections are also essential in these patients. Reducing the discomfort that can occur with problems in the mouth is critical for patients who often have pain from other medical conditions. Maintaining good nutrition is easier when the patient can chew food efficiently and without pain.[3]

This chapter will discuss prevention of oral diseases, with suggestions for modification of the usual methods to accommodate special problems that may occur in patients with chronic illnesses. It will also discuss oral conditions that occur commonly in chronically ill patients and suggest treatment options that can be used by the home care provider for prevention and treatment of these common oral problems.

What Causes Dental Diseases?

Tooth decay and gum diseases are two common dental problems. Both are caused primarily by dental plaque, which is a sticky, colorless, almost invisible microbial film that constantly forms on teeth, soft tissues, restorations, and oral appliances. Plaque contains many different types of bacteria. Some species have been identified with specific oral conditions. Many of these plaque bacteria produce toxic by-products that are harmful to the teeth and gums. These include substances that can induce inflammation, cause direct tissue damage, and affect the body's defense mechanisms.[4,5]

Tooth decay, or dental caries, begins when acidic by-products of plaque bacteria attack the enamel that makes up the outer layer of the tooth. The enamel is demineralized by the acids and becomes soft. Bacteria then invade dentin, the softer material beneath the enamel, and the decay process proceeds rapidly.[6] If not treated, the decay eventually reaches the pulp of the tooth and kills it, causing necrosis. A necrotic pulp can cause an abscess that spreads beyond the tooth, into the bone. Treatment for an abscessed tooth involves root canal therapy or extraction. Dental abscesses can be very painful, and if infections develop and are not treated promptly, they can spread to other areas of the head and neck, including the brain. These advanced infections are difficult to control and have severe morbidity and mortality potential.[6]

Root caries is another insidious form of tooth decay. Root surfaces often become exposed due to recession or gum disease. The outer coating of the root surface, called cementum, is thinner and not as highly mineralized as enamel. This type of decay can progress rapidly through cementum and the root to the pulp. Root caries is also difficult to treat due to the inaccessibility of the decay.[7]

Gingival and periodontal diseases are also plaque related. As dental plaque forms at or under the gum line, the acidic toxins produced by the bacteria irritate the gum tissue, or gingiva. The gingiva becomes red, swollen, and bleeds easily. This inflammatory response is called gingivitis.[8] Minimal discomfort is associated with gingivitis, especially in otherwise healthy patients, and it is easy to ignore the seemingly minor symptoms. Left untreated, the condition can become progressively more severe. In some patients, gingivitis can eventually lead to periodontitis, an infection of the supporting structures of the teeth. These tissues, including the bone, can be progressively destroyed by direct and indirect actions of the plaque bacterial by-products and by the body's own immune response. If untreated, the teeth can become loose, leading to tooth loss. Abscesses may form around the teeth, and the infections can spread in much the same patterns as infections resulting from decayed teeth.[8]

This progression of oral diseases occurs even in relatively healthy patients. In patients with chronic health problems, oral diseases can occur very quickly, and the infections can be aggressive and devastating. The sequelae of dental diseases can range from problems such as minor discomfort and inconvenience to death from infections. Most of these conditions, however, can be prevented or controlled by following a few good health habits. Daily thorough plaque removal by brushing and flossing, good dietary habits, elimination of tobacco use, and regular dental maintenance by a dental professional seem like simple actions, but they can help maintain good dental health for everyone, especially chronically ill patients.

Oral Hygiene

Tooth Brushing

Thorough daily removal of dental plaque deposits is simple with the proper tools and the appropriate application of these tools. The most familiar plaque removal tool is the toothbrush. Soft nylon bristles, a small-sized head, and a straight handle are the standard elements of an acceptable toothbrush choice for most patients.[9] The bristles should be rounded and polished to prevent damage to teeth and gums. The brush head should be small enough to reach all the easily accessible surfaces of the teeth: facial, lingual/palatal, and occlusal surfaces.

Variations on conventional toothbrush designs range from flat trimmed bristles mounted on a straight plastic handle to multilayered variations of bristle patterns on ergonomically designed handles. Bristles can be trimmed at varying lengths and arranged in patterns that attempt to reach posterior and interproximal surfaces more effectively. Handles are positioned in a variety of angles, also attempting to increase access. If a patient perceives a benefit from a particular brush design, use of that toothbrush should be encouraged.[10]

Toothbrushes should be replaced when they start to show signs of wear, such as spreading of bristles. This time varies from patient to patient, but the usual recommendation for replacement is 3 months.[10]

Powered toothbrushes are as effective as conventional toothbrushes in plaque removal for healthy patients[11] and may be more effective than manual brushes for patients with disabilities or for caregivers who provide oral care.[12] Powered toothbrushes have large handles, which make them easier to manipulate, both for patients with limited dexterity and for caregivers. Brush head designs vary greatly in powered toothbrushes. Conventional multitufted nylon bristles are available, along with some unique designs. They range from a single tuft that rotates, to ten independently counter-rotating tufts, to a round multitufted brush head that rotates in a circular back-and-forth motion.[9]

The perception of the time spent brushing is commonly overestimated. A timer acts as a reminder to spend the needed time for thorough plaque removal. A well-lit mirror is essential for proper visualization of toothbrush placement.

If the patient or caregiver uses glasses for reading, they should also be used for oral hygiene sessions. Visualization of the teeth during plaque removal is important. The teeth are not aligned in straight rows, and the angle of the toothbrush head or handle may need to be varied slightly to adapt to the positions of the teeth. Watching the bristles as they contact each tooth surface is very helpful to ensure complete plaque removal.

Toothpaste

The effective ingredients in regular toothpaste are detergents, abrasives, and fluoride. Other additives are for texture, consistency, and taste. Several special toothpaste formulations are marketed for consumers who have special needs. Some toothpastes include chemicals that decrease sensitivity for patients who have exposed root surfaces. Because these products must be used over a period of weeks to be effective, a formulation that includes fluoride may be a wise selection since exposed roots are prone to decay rapidly. Tartar-control toothpastes use chemicals to prevent plaque left on teeth from mineralizing to become tartar, or calculus. These calcified deposits must be professionally removed with dental instruments. Tartar-control toothpastes may be associated with increased sensitivity.[13] If plaque is removed daily by brushing and flossing and regular professional cleaning is performed, calculus will not form quickly, and the additional chemicals are not needed. Toothpastes that claim to whiten teeth either use chemical whiteners such as peroxide or are high in abrasives to remove stain. With good oral hygiene and periodic professional cleaning, these additives are not needed. Many manufacturers have recently added baking soda to toothpaste, but these formulations do not offer any advantages in plaque removal over other types of toothpastes. A tooth-cleaning regimen using baking soda and peroxide was shown to be no more effective than conventional oral hygiene techniques.[14]

Mouthwashes

Mouthwash manufacturers have made many claims to sell their products—from halitosis cures to bacteria killers. In many formulations, the ingredients may act only temporarily to mask breath odors. For a few, the claims of plaque control has been proven by controlled clinical studies. Listerine® is an over-the-counter, safe and effective chemical plaque-control agent. Studies show that plaque reduction averages 25 to 35%. The alcohol content is high, which may be irritating to soft tissues, especially if they are inflamed.[13,15]

Chlorhexidine-containing mouthwashes are the mainstays of chemical plaque control. These are available by prescription in a 0.12% rinse in the United States.

Chlorhexidine has a broad spectrum of antimicrobial activity, including Gram-positive and Gram-negative organisms and fungi.[15] Chlorhexidine exhibits substantivity, the ability to bind to a substrate and release slowly. This quality may explain the high antimicrobial activity of the chemical intraorally, since chlorhexidine is slowly released from the surfaces of oral tissues, creating a constant level of antibacterial activity. Studies show up to 60% plaque reduction with rinsing. Chlorhexidine use is not a substitute for mechanical plaque removal, but in patients who for any reason cannot perform adequate plaque removal, it is a useful adjunct to brushing and flossing. It does have some side effects, including staining, increased calculus deposition, and taste alteration.[13,15] The stain and calculus can be removed with professional cleaning, but may permanently stain some anterior restorative materials. The taste alteration subsides gradually, so food should be eaten prior to use of chlorhexidine.

Flossing

Even the most thorough tooth brushing cannot remove all dental plaque from the teeth. The surfaces where the teeth touch, called the interproximal or interdental surfaces, are not accessible to toothbrush bristles, especially if the gum tissue completely fills the area between the teeth. Dental floss is commonly recommended to remove plaque from the sides of the teeth.[10] Many different types of dental floss are available, from wide dental tapes to thin multistranded nylon. Floss can be waxed or unwaxed. Some varieties have flavors or additives such as baking soda. Teeth with tight contacts, especially those that shred floss, can be easily cleaned with waxed, Teflon®, or Teflon®-coated floss. All varieties of floss are used in essentially the same way, and they are all effective when used properly.[10]

A floss holder can be helpful for patients with dexterity problems or for caregivers. Floss holders, however, can be difficult to manipulate, especially when changing the floss.[16] Flossing technique should be monitored to be sure the floss is not damaging the gum tissue. Sawing motions tend to cut the tissue, and snapping the floss through the contact point can also injure the gingiva.

Other Oral Hygiene Aids

Many other tools are used for plaque removal when a toothbrush and floss cannot reach specific areas. If the gum tissue between the teeth has pulled away from the teeth, a small interproximal brush is effective in plaque removal on the interdental surfaces of the teeth. These brushes resemble bottle brushes and come in several shapes and sizes. The brushes are available attached directly to handles or in a replaceable type that inserts into a handle. Either way, they wear out quickly and need to be replaced regularly. They are used by sliding the brush between the teeth and gently scrubbing to remove plaque. Using the brush from both the facial and lingual surfaces results in the most effective plaque removal.

Other plaque removal devices include end-tufted brushes, handles for round toothpicks, and rubber tip stimulators. These tools are particularly useful in areas where roots are exposed when gum tissue and bone are lost in periodontitis. These areas can be difficult to clean because of problems with accessibility.

Frequency of Plaque Removal

Most patients are familiar with a routine that includes brushing their teeth two or three times during the day, usually in the morning and before bedtime. One of these tooth brushing times should be designated as a total plaque removal session, complete with flossing and other needed oral hygiene devices. This routine can be very effective in maintaining oral health.[10] Plaque removal is often associated with the bathroom sink, but some plaque removal devices such as floss or toothpicks can be used effectively in other places. Sufficient time must be allowed for brushing and flossing to be effective in plaque removal. Bedtime is usually an optimal opportunity for total plaque removal, but any time that an effective, unhurried effort can be made is good.

Oral Complications in Cancer Treatment

Patients undergoing treatment for cancer are especially vulnerable to oral complications. Medical management of cancer patients is complex and constantly changing. It often includes procedures such as radiation, chemotherapy, or bone marrow transplants. These procedures all have potential oral complications; many are similar, and some are unique to the particular treatment.[17] These complications can be the result of both direct and indirect effects of the treatment.[18] The more aggressive the malignancy and the more potent the treatment, the greater the incidence of oral complications.[19] Oral status before initiation of cancer treatment, type of treatment administered, diet, age, and support systems may act as predictors of type and severity of oral complications.[20,21] Creating a clean healthy oral environment before the onset of therapy can prevent or lessen the severity of many of these oral problems.[22,23]

Chemotherapy

The pretreatment stage of dental management of chemotherapy patients should begin as soon as possible after diagnosis. The dentist, in conjunction with the oncologist, should complete baseline examination and determine treatment needs. The goals include elimination of existing infections and elimination of any oral conditions that could produce infections, such as large carious lesions or teeth with periapical abscesses.[22] Once immunosuppression begins, the clinical signs and symptoms of inflammation are diminished and may not indicate the severity of oral infections.[24]

Maximizing the patient's comfort level by eliminating or minimizing effects of chemotherapy on oral soft tissues is critical. This includes treatment of any areas that might be irritating to soft tissues, such as fractured or rough restorations and ill-fitting dentures.[22] Areas that are plaque retentive should also be addressed to make oral hygiene procedures, both mechanical and chemical, more effective.[25] Care should also be directed toward maximizing oral comfort so that eating is not painful and the patient's nutritional status can be maintained.

Initiation of an oral hygiene program that will help the patient or caregiver maintain excellent plaque control is also imperative at this time. The goal is to teach gentle but effective techniques. Use of chemical plaque control and topical fluoride should also be considered. As a part of the process of evaluation, the patient and caregiver should be educated about the ongoing nature of the patient's oral care needs and the potential oral complications that may arise. Home care techniques can be suggested to manage appropriate conditions.[26]

Hematologic Considerations

The dentist and the oncologist must communicate clearly concerning the specific guidelines of the relationship between the hematologic status of the patient and the timing of dental care.[27] The ideal time for definitive dental treatment is before initiation of chemotherapy if possible. Any indicated extractions, restorations, periodontal therapy, or other definitive treatment that can be done before chemotherapy will reduce the occurrence of oral infections and decrease the need for dental treatment during chemotherapy.[28] If delay of initiation of chemotherapy is not possible, the most appropriate time for dental treatment is between chemotherapy cycles, when the patient's hematologic status permits treatment.[29]

Each patient's hematologic status must be considered individually by the oncologist and the dentist, but general guidelines include consideration of neutrophil count and platelet count. Absolute neutrophil counts less than 1000 to 2000 per cubic millimeter present a high risk of infection for the patient. Platelet counts of less than 40,000 to 50,000 per cubic millimeter present a high risk of hemorrhage.[3,27] Elective dental procedures should not be performed when these test results are at high-risk levels. Emergency care should only be performed after consultation with the oncologist. Antibiotic coverage, platelet replacement, or other prophylactic treatment may be necessary before dental care is initiated.[30]

When the hematologic status is at high-risk levels for infection or hemorrhage, daily plaque control measures should be modified to be as gentle as possible and may include chemical plaque control.[26] Tooth brushing is stopped and damp gauze wrapped around a finger is used to remove as much plaque as possible. Flossing and use of sharp objects such as toothpicks must also be ceased until the hematologic status has improved.[22] Another alternative may be the use of a foam toothbrush dipped in chlorhexidine solution. The foam brush alone is not as effective as a toothbrush in plaque removal, but when used as an applicator for a measured amount of chlorhexidine solution, the foam brush has been found to be effective in plaque removal.[31]

Antibiotic Coverage

Another consideration when planning invasive dental care for chemotherapy patients includes administration of appropriate antibiotic coverage. Prophylactic premedication is not indicated for routine daily care, but is used when a procedure may cause bleeding. The usual indications apply for prophylactic premedication for prevention of bacterial endocarditis: conditions such as prosthetic heart valves, valvular disfunction, or other cardiac abnormalities.[32] Premedication may also be indicated if the patient has an indwelling catheter for intravenous drug administration. These devices are susceptible to infection from bacteria that enter the bloodstream during invasive dental procedures.[30] The American Heart Association's recommendations for antibiotic premedication to prevent subacute bacterial endocarditis are also appropriate in these patients, but each case must be considered individually by the oncologist.

Plaque Control Modifications

After the chemotherapy stage is initiated, careful plaque removal should be performed at least daily by the patient or caregiver. Techniques for plaque removal may need to be varied according to the hematologic status of the patient. Oral complications may also compromise plaque-control measures, especially if the patient has a painful condition, such as an oral mucositis. Softening toothbrush bristles with very hot water or use of an extremely soft bristle brush may be helpful. Use of topical anesthetics may make tooth brushing less painful and allow more thorough plaque removal.[3] Foam toothbrushes, gauze, and cotton-tipped applicators do not remove plaque completely. Lemon-glycerine swabs do not remove plaque well and are also contraindicated due to the anhydrous quality of the glycerine and the acidity of the lemon flavor.[29] Bland flavors of fluoride toothpaste may be tolerated; an alternative is a thick paste of baking soda and water.[26] Supplementation with a chemical plaque control agent such as 0.12% chlorhexidine rinse may be helpful but does not replace mechanical plaque control.[3] The chlorhexidine rinse contains alcohol and may not be tolerated at full strength by patients with mucositis. Chlorhexidine maintains some effectiveness in plaque control even in a diluted form. Other methods of application, such as foam brushes or cotton-tipped applicators, may be accepted better than rinsing.

A solution of 1 to 2 teaspoons baking soda and $^1/_2$ teaspoon salt dissolved in 1 quart water can be used as an oral rinse, followed by a plain water rinse. This solution is prepared fresh to be used as an oral rinse at least four times per day. This solution of baking soda and saline is useful for neutralizing the acids in the mouth following episodes of emesis and should be used after emesis and before tooth brushing to prevent enamel etching.[3]

Removable oral appliances such as partial dentures, complete dentures, or orthodontic retainers require special care. These appliances should be carefully evaluated by a dental professional. If they do not fit properly, the appliances should be eliminated or remade to be as nonirritating to oral soft tissues as possible. If worn during the chemotherapy phase, the appliances require daily brushing with a denture brush for plaque removal and nightly soaking in an antimicrobial cleanser, such as chlorhexidine.[33,34] Removal of the appliances at night can prevent additional mucosal irritation.[3]

Xerostomia

Saliva production is often diminished during chemotherapy. Dry mouth, or xerostomia, may create many associated problems.[35] Discomfort from the sensation of dry oral tissues and difficulties in chewing, swallowing, and speaking are only a few examples of the effects of xerostomia. Dry tissues are also more susceptible to bacterial and fungal infections.[36] Several saliva substitutes are available as over-the-counter products. These sprays may provide temporary relief from xerostomia.[26] Cool water for sipping can also be helpful to relieve the discomfort associated with a dry mouth. Salivary stimulants such as a bolus of paraffin, sugarless gum, or candy may be helpful in increasing saliva production temporarily. Foods with a high water content such as gelatins and flavored frozen treats can be added to the diet.[37] Some medications, such as topical antifungals, can be used in a frozen form,[38] combining the comfort of cool liquid with the administration of the medication.

The use of a cool mist humidifier during sleep may also provide a level of increased comfort. It is important to ensure that the humidifier does not become contaminated with bacteria that could become airborne. The lips also can become dry, cracked, and painful. Lanolin or cocoa-butter-based products are superior to petrolatum-based lip preparations due to the hygroscopic properties of petrolatum.[3] Water-based gels are also available to coat dry oral tissues and may be useful, especially during sleep. Some positive results have been seen in xerostomic patients using pilocarpine as a salivary gland stimulant.[39]

Another side effect of xerostomia is demineralization of tooth structure, leading to development of caries. Saliva has decay-fighting antimicrobial properties and acts to cleanse the tooth surfaces. For patients who experience long-term saliva reduction, daily application of a fluoride gel will reduce problems with demineralization and subsequent tooth and root decay.[3] Application of a 1.1% neutral sodium fluoride gel or a 0.4% stannous fluoride gel is preferable to application of a fluoride rinse.[40] Acidulated fluorides are contraindicated if the patient has porcelain restorations and may not be tolerated well if oral tissues are ulcerated.[3] Brushing with a gel is an acceptable method of application for transient xerostomia, but use of a custom-made applicator tray is ideal, especially in patients with long-term xerostomia, compliance problems, or active caries.[3]

Mucositis

A clinical condition sometimes called stomatitis, but more accurately described as mucositis, occurs commonly in chemotherapy patients. The incidence of mucositis is increased with use of specific chemotherapy regimens, and it may occur more frequently in patients on intravenous hyperalimentation therapy.[41] Mucositis varies from a clinical presentation of slight redness of mucosal tissues associated with a burning sensation to bright red tissue with ulcerations, bleeding, and yellowish pseudomembrane formation. The lips, cheeks, soft palate, tongue, and floor of the mouth may be involved.[42] In the more severe form, the patient complains of severe pain and is often unable to eat solid or liquid foods. The ulcerated tissues are vulnerable to infections. Many studies address the occurrence of mucositis and possible preventive and treatment methods.[43–46] Treatment is traditionally directed toward pain relief and infection control, but prevention of the condition is highly desirable. Patients who practice excellent plaque control seem to develop less mucositis during treatment.[38] Many researchers have studied chlorhexidine as a possible preventive agent.[47–53] Some studies have demonstrated the effects of other antifungal medications in prevention and control of mucositis.[46,54–56]

Effective treatment of mucositis mostly involves palliative measures. Meticulous oral hygiene and lubricants, antimicrobials, systemic analgesics, anti-inflammatory drugs, topical anesthetics, and coating agents have been used to treat mucositis.[57] The use of the previously mentioned baking soda/saltwater rinsing solution can be modified to exclude the salt if it is not well tolerated. Baking soda rinses may act as a mucolytic emollient[18] and act to increase the pH of the inflamed tissues.[54] If rinsing is too painful, the solution can be hung in an intravenous bag and allowed to flow through the mouth.[3] Peroxide rinses are acidic and should be avoided. Topical anesthetics can be used to provide temporary pain control and may allow the patient to eat or to perform oral hygiene procedures more comfortably.[58]

Elixirs of diphenhydramine and kaolin with pectin can be used as a mouth rinse to help alleviate the discomfort of mucositis.[42] Viscous lidocaine hydrochloride can be used as a topical anesthetic.[29] Sucralfate suspensions have been found to reduce pain and weight loss in patients with mucositis.[57] The drug acts by binding to damaged mucosal surfaces and forming a protective coating over ulcers.[59] Neutral flavoring agents can be added to the suspension to avoid aggravating nausea.[60]

Tissues affected with mucositis are sensitive to temperature and pressure. Dietary modifications may be needed to maintain an appropriate nutritional intake. A bland, semisoft, cool diet will usually be tolerated. Liquid nutritional supplements may be alternatives if the patient cannot eat solid foods. Alcohol consumption and tobacco use are irritating to inflamed tissues and should be discontinued.[29]

Radiation Therapy

Many of the oral complications associated with radiation therapy, especially head and neck radiation therapy, are similar to the oral complications that occur with chemotherapy.[40] Some of these conditions may be permanent, and treatment should be planned for long-term application.[61] Radiation mucositis and xerostomia are caused by the direct effects of the radiation on tissues in the oral cavity and can be managed as previously discussed. Some decrease in the incidence and severity of xerostomia may be possible if the salivary glands can be protected from direct exposure with special shielding during radiation treatments. This possibility should be considered by the dentist and radiation oncologist, since radiation to the salivary glands destroys them and the xerostomia becomes a permanent condition. Radiation caries can occur as a result of the xerostomia.[62] Daily fluoride application as previously described, using a custom tray for maximum contact with tooth surfaces, is essential in radiation patients and should continue throughout life.[3]

There are a number of oral complications that are unique to radiation therapy patients. Diminished ability to taste tends to occur during radiation therapy, but ability tends to return a few months after radiation has been discontinued.[63] Tightening, or trismus, of the facial muscles can occur with direct radiation exposure. Gentle daily exercise of the muscles may help decrease the tightening. The use of stacked tongue blades placed in the mouth several times daily to stretch the muscles can help maintain normal mouth opening and allow for easier oral access.[1]

The most serious oral complication of head and neck radiation therapy is osteoradionecrosis. Direct exposure of the maxilla and mandible to radiation affects the blood supply to the bone in these areas. The healing capacity of the bone is limited and infections can occur, resulting in devastating necrosis.[1] The head and neck radiation patient continues to be at high risk for developing osteoradionecrosis throughout life. Sometimes this will occur spontaneously, but it is more likely caused by trauma to oral tissues, such as dental extractions. It is imperative that definitive dental treatment is performed before radiation therapy to prepare the patient to be able to maintain a healthy oral environment. Regular and frequent professional dental maintenance should be instituted early in treatment for reinforcement of oral hygiene procedures and early detection of dental problems that could lead to extractions.[40,61]

HIV-Infected Patients: Special Oral Problems

In all patients with impaired immune systems, oral lesions occur frequently. In HIV-infected patients, the oral findings are similar to other immune-compromised patients, but a few conditions occur commonly in HIV-positive patients. Periodontal diseases found in these patients can vary from an atypical presentation of gingivitis to a severe form of necrotizing periodontitis.[64] HIV-positive patients with preexisting periodontal diseases have more severe oral complications.[65] Periodontal lesions may be seen as the earliest signs of HIV infection in an otherwise asymptomatic patient.[66] The unique form of gingivitis found in HIV-positive patients is linear gingival erythema (LGE). It appears as a distinct 2- to 3-mm-wide band at the gingival margin. The tissue tends to bleed easily, sometimes spontaneously. The cheek tissue, or alveolar mucosa, may be bright red. Very little discomfort is associated with this condition.[67] LGE does not respond well to conventional therapy. Even after treatment, it often continues to present the same clinical appearance.[68] Identification of the disease and attempts to control it are critical; however, it may be a precursor to a more severe periodontal condition found in HIV-positive patients, necrotizing ulcerative periodontitis, or NUP. This condition exhibits similar characteristics as seen in LGE but is associated with severe deep pain, spontaneous bleeding, soft tissue necrosis, ulceration, and exposure of bone.[67,69] NUP can occur in either a generalized form or a localized form described as islands of disease surrounded by relatively normal tissue.[70,71]

Treatment of these lesions involves both therapy administered by a dental professional and an aggressive home care regimen.[37] An initial debridement is performed with use of 10% povidone-iodine if the patient reports a negative history of an allergy to iodine.[70,71] The povidone-iodine acts as an antimicrobial and an anesthetic, allowing the operator to debride the necrotic tissue. It also helps control the bleeding that occurs during the procedure. After the initial debridement, the patient is instructed to irrigate between the teeth with the povidone-iodine at least five times per day. Plaque removal can then be performed at home due to the anesthetic effect and the bleeding control offered by the solution. The irrigation with povidone-iodine is continued for several weeks, until healing has progressed significantly. Twice daily rinsing with 0.12% chlorhexidine is then substituted for the povidone-iodine. The 0.12% chlorhexidine is not used in initial treatment of these lesions; the alcohol content is not well tolerated due to the soft tissue necrosis and exposure of bone. Studies show that patients maintained on chlorhexidine rinses have less recurrence of NUP over time than patients maintained on povidone-iodine.[64,70,71]

Oral hygiene procedures need to concentrate on total plaque removal. This can be difficult to accomplish due to the pain, necrotic tissue, ulcerations, and bleeding that occur in the acute stages of the disease. The anesthetic effect provided by the povidone-iodine irrigation can help relieve the pain and bleeding during plaque removal. Topical anesthetics may also be helpful. A soft bristle toothbrush, softened further by holding under hot water before use, can be used on the surfaces that are accessible, but the interproximal areas can be difficult to clean. Interproximal brushes can be helpful, especially in cratered areas.[71] Larger diameter floss products or yarn may also be useful in performing plaque removal between teeth.

Antibiotics are only used in severe cases that cannot be managed locally with other treatment. Fungal infections can be life threatening to HIV-positive patients, and the risk of candidal overgrowth with the use of most antibiotics is high.[68] When an antibiotic is indicated for treatment of a periodontal problem in these patients, metronidazole can be used due to its specificity for anaerobic bacteria and the low risk of candidal colonization.[72]

Other oral manifestations of HIV infection can also occur. One common condition seen in HIV-positive patients is thrush, also known as a yeast infection. Caused by the *Candida* organism, it can be seen as an oral or esophageal infection.[73] Candidiasis may occur as a creamy coating on cheeks or gums that can be scraped off, a red lesion on the palate or tongue, or an irritation in the corners of the mouth.[74] If a yeast infection is suspected, consultation with a dentist or physician should be immediate. The diagnosis needs to be confirmed by smears and cultures and antifungal therapy initiated as soon as possible.[1]

Viral lesions are also common in HIV-positive patients. Several different types of warts caused by viruses can occur in the mouths of these patients. Herpes viruses can also cause painful recurrent ulcerations on the lips and palate and painful eruptions on the skin commonly known as shingles.[73] Epstein-Barr virus causes hairy leukoplakia, a white vertical lesion usually seen on the lateral borders of the tongue.[74] All these viral conditions should be seen by a dentist or physician for diagnosis and treatment, often with antiviral medications like acyclovir.

Oral Care Issues in Disabled and Elderly Patients

A disability is any impairment restricting or limiting daily activities in some way. Developmental disabilities are recognized early in life and include such conditions as cerebral palsy and Down's syndrome. Acquired disabilities can occur at any time, although they usually occur later in life, and include, for example, neurological conditions, traumatic injuries, and psychiatric disorders.[2] Patients with disabilities may also have medical conditions that must be considered in management of their general health care. Especially in these types of patients, early intervention with preventive oral care can keep oral complications from occurring.

Many oral care philosophies and techniques that are appropriate for disabled patients are also applicable to elderly patients. Modifications of plaque-control tools and techniques and the training of caregivers to perform oral care are examples of areas that are common to both groups.[2,75] In all situations, patients should be involved as much as is practical in their own oral care. Encouraging independence, preserving dignity, and fostering a sense of well-being are critical and can be accomplished very effectively with some patients in their oral care efforts.

Management of patients with cognitive and physical disabilities can be complicated by the level of cooperation that can be obtained. Physical resistance to treatment may be encountered in all types of disabilities, regardless of age, including developmental disabilities, neurological disorders, severe psychiatric disorders, and neuromuscular disorders.[76,77]

When developing an oral health care plan for these patients, educating the patient, family, or caregiver about the importance of preventive dental care must be considered along with the routine professional disease control and maintenance.[78] Disabled and elderly patients are susceptible to the same dental diseases as any patient, but the consequences of developing these chronic oral problems are magnified, adding additional complications to already disabling mental or physical conditions. These patients often receive liquid medications that have a high sugar content, which promotes the development of tooth decay, or caries.[79] The diets of these patients are also often high in sugar content, and in some cases, sweet treats are used for behavioral modification, increasing the development of dental problems.[2] Elderly patients may have compromised oral hygiene due to exposed roots and existing dental work that is difficult to keep clean, problems with vision and dexterity, and decreased salivary flow.[80] Dental caries and periodontal diseases must be controlled using whatever methods are necessary. As much as possible, these preventive care techniques should be integrated into activities of daily living.[2] If these activities can become habits, they will be practiced for a lifetime.

Tooth Brushing Techniques and Modifications

Using a toothbrush to efficiently remove plaque from tooth surfaces is an acquired skill. It requires dexterity and cognitive ability of a fairly high level to be effective.[34] Supervision and assistance are recommended for all children until they develop the maturity to master and apply tooth brushing skills, usually at 6 to 12 years old.[81] Tooth brushing is the only method of oral care practiced consistently by older adults.[82] For disabled patients, the techniques that can be used to teach tooth brushing range from simple oral instructions and demonstrations given to the patients themselves to professionally produced programs for parents or caregivers to learn how to administer appropriate care with special toothbrushes.

Creative and appropriate modifications of the standard methods are the keys to successful implementation of daily plaque-control programs. Dental professionals and caregivers should be observant and willing to try new ideas to achieve the highest level of care possible.[78]

If a conventional manual toothbrush can be effectively manipulated by the patient, it is the least expensive and most practical option. Simple modifications to a conventional toothbrush may make it easier to use. Bending the handle of a straight toothbrush may help the patient gain access to posterior areas in the mouth. Using devices to enlarge the handle of a conventional toothbrush can be one of the easiest and most effective modifications. Many patients can manipulate the toothbrush very well if given a larger handle to grasp. Options include anything that works, from a plastic bicycle handle slid onto the toothbrush handle to a rubber ball with a hole through the middle for the toothbrush. Pipe insulation can be modified to adapt to a toothbrush. Duct tape wound onto the toothbrush handle has been used for minor enlargements. A custom handle can be fabricated from dental acrylic. Specially designed toothbrushes are also produced by manufacturers and are available through catalogues of adaptive aids.[80] Toothbrushes are available that have multiple heads, allowing removal of plaque on more than one surface of the tooth as the brush is moved in the mouth. Another brush has straight, short bristles in the middle of the brush, with longer curved bristles on the sides. It allows the toothbrush to be placed on the occlusal, or biting, surface of the teeth and moved back and forth, removing plaque from the facial and lingual surfaces as well as the occlusal. In one study, this style of manual toothbrush was preferred by both patients and brushers over foam brushes, conventional brushes, and a powered toothbrush. It was reported to be easier to manipulate, more comfortable, and inexpensive.[83] An appliance with filament-like projections has been studied in disabled children. The device is inserted into the mouth and the patient is instructed to chew. It requires no manual dexterity and is effective in plaque removal, especially on the lingual surfaces.[84]

Powered toothbrushes are also an excellent alternative for plaque removal. A number of studies have found powered toothbrushes to be more effective than manual toothbrushes in plaque removal in disabled or elderly patients.[12] Compliance may be improved with powered toothbrushes when their use is perceived as simple and timesaving.[85] The handles are larger and manipulation may be easier. Fine motor skills are not needed since the toothbrush moves itself. The only requirement for manipulation is guiding the toothbrush along the surfaces of the teeth to be brushed. These qualities make the use of powered toothbrushes easier for patients and for caregivers. There are several powered toothbrushes that are available, with different types of head designs for different needs. Disadvantages include expense, durability, and infection-control problems if the powered toothbrush is used by more than one person.

Other oral hygiene aids, like floss, can be modified to make manipulation easier. Floss holders are useful and if the handle is enlarged may be easier to control. Other interproximal aids, like small brushes, can also be used more effectively with modified, larger handles. Creativity and sensitivity to the patient or caregiver's individual needs, combined with thoughtful observation of the use of oral hygiene devices by the patient or caregiver, can offer solutions that are easily incorporated into the activities of daily living.

Delivery of Chemotherapeutic Agents

Sometimes, mechanical plaque control like tooth brushing and flossing cannot be performed by either the patient or the caregiver to a level that is sufficient to maintain oral health. In these situations, chemical plaque control may be indicated to augment mechanical plaque control. Antiplaque and anticariogenic agents are useful in these patients. These are not a substitute for but an adjunct to mechanical plaque control, since even the best chemotherapeutic agents kill the bacteria but do not completely eliminate plaque mass. There are also side effects associated with chemical plaque-control agents, although in severely disabled patients, they are outweighed by the benefits of use.[86]

Chlorhexidine is recognized as an excellent chemical plaque-control agent[87] and has been studied in the disabled and elderly populations in a number of delivery systems. Use of fluoride to prevent or control decay in these patients is also often desirable. Mouth rinsing is the most common form of delivery of chlorhexidine and fluoride, but not all patients can rinse and expectorate. Alternatives to rinsing have been explored; gel delivery in trays, intraoral sprays, and application of solutions with a foam brush are examples of systems that have been studied. Gel delivery in a tray was very effective but not well accepted by patients and caregivers.[88,89] Foam brush application of chlorhexidine and fluoride is also effective and well accepted.[31,90] Another delivery system is the spray pump method. It has been used to administer several medications, including chlorhexidine and stannous fluoride, and is a useful method in both disabled and elderly patients, especially in cases when the patient is unable to cooperate with oral care activities.[91–93]

Side effects associated with chlorhexidine use include staining and taste alteration. These side effects may be minimized by some of the alternate delivery systems such as the spray pump method. Another side effect is increased tartar, or calculus deposition. Mechanical plaque control to remove the soft deposits before they mineralize is helpful, but regular professional cleaning will remove both the stain and the calculus. Fluorosis, or staining of developing teeth, is a concern in children, and so care must be taken that the patient does not swallow excess amounts of fluoride. Access to fluoride should be limited to parents or caregivers to avoid accidental ingestion, especially with pleasant-tasting formulations.[94,95]

Medical Conditions with Special Oral Complications

Some common medical conditions and the medications used to treat them have associated oral complications.[96] Seizure disorders are a common occurrence that can be idiopathic or associated with other medical conditions such as stroke or traumatic injury. Phenytoin, or Dilantin®, is one of several medications used to treat seizure disorders. A common oral complication associated with Dilantin® is gingival overgrowth, or hyperplasia.[1] The gingiva may show only minor swelling or enlarge until the crowns of the teeth are barely visible, and surgical resection may be the only option. Meticulous plaque control before the hyperplasia begins can control or decrease the severity of the hyperplasia.[97]

Diabetes is another medical condition that has obvious oral signs and symptoms. Oral complications of diabetes include xerostomia, poor healing, increased incidence and severity of periodontal diseases, and burning mouth syndrome. Most of these problems are related to poorly controlled diabetes.[1] Meticulous plaque control is essential, especially to prevent periodontal diseases. Uncontrolled or poorly controlled diabetes is associated with an increased incidence of oral infections.[98]

Several medical conditions require dental intervention prior to treatment or progression of the disease. Dental treatment before cancer therapy has been discussed previously. Many of the same principles of treatment apply in other situations. Any time the immune system will be compromised, comprehensive dental treatment should be done as soon as possible. Organ transplant patients require many of the same considerations as chemotherapy patients, with efforts directed at oral disease control and prevention before transplantation and the immunosuppression that is necessary to prevent rejection.[1]

Patients with neurological disorders,[99,100] especially those with some progressive form of dementia, such as Alzheimer's disease, may have special dental treatment needs. As dementia progresses, patients gradually lose the ability to perform oral hygiene. The combined effects of memory loss, confusion, and loss of motor skills make all activities of daily living at first difficult and then impossible.[101] These patients should be brought to an optimum level of oral health and placed on a preventive program while they are still responsive, to retain oral function for as long as possible. Fixed prosthetic replacements, such as bridges, are preferred to removable dentures.[101] If removable appliances must be used, the patient's name can be permanently placed on the appliance when it is fabricated for identification. It is helpful for caregivers who may be working with more than one patient to be able to easily identify the patient's dentures.

Studies of terminally ill patients show a high prevalence of oral signs and symptoms. Complaints about fit of dentures are common because the fit changes as patients lose weight. Candidal, or yeast, infections are also a common oral finding.[102] Any interceptive treatment that can reduce or prevent oral complications is appropriate and should be administered as early as possible in the disease process.

Resource Materials

Oral Management of the Cancer Patient by Gerry J. Barker, R.D.H., M.A., Bruce F. Barker, D.D.S., and Ronald E. Gier, D.M.D., M.S.D., is available as both a manual and a slide show for presentations or instruction. Address orders and inquiries to: Instructional Resources Librarian, UMKC School of Dentistry, 650 East 25th Street, Kansas City, MO 64108-2795, phone (816) 235-2064. Another excellent resource is *Practical Considerations in Special Patient Care, The Dental Clinics of North America,* Volume 38, Number 3, July 1994, edited by John S. Rutkauskas, M.S., D.D.S. The publisher is W.B. Saunders Company, Philadelphia.

References

1. Little, J. W. and Falace, D. A., *Dental Management of the Medically Compromised Patient*, Mosby-Year Book, St. Louis, 1993.
2. Tesini, D. A. and Fenton, S. J., Oral health needs of persons with physical or mental disabilities, *Dent. Clin. North Am.,* 38(3):483–497, 1994.
3. Barker, G. J., Barker, B. F., and Gier, R. E., *Oral Management of the Cancer Patient. A Guide for the Health Care Professional*, Oncology Education, University of Missouri–Kansas City, Kansas City, Missouri, 1992.
4. Schluger, S., Yuodelis, R. A., and Page, R. C., *Periodontal Disease*, Lea and Febiger, Philadelphia, 1978.
5. Carranza, F. A., *Glickman's Clinical Periodontology,* W.B. Saunders, Philadelphia, 1990.
6. Shafer, W. G., Hine, M. K., and Levy, B. M., *A Textbook of Oral Pathology,* W.B. Saunders, Philadelphia, 1983.
7. Grant, D. A., Stern, I. B., and Listgarten, M. A., *Periodontics in the Tradition of Gottlieb and Orban,* C.V. Mosby, St. Louis, 1988.
8. Caton, J., Periodontal diagnosis and diagnostic aids, in *Proceedings of the World Workshop in Clinical Periodontics,* American Academy of Periodontology, Chicago, 1989, pp. I-1–I-32.
9. Murtomaa, H. and Meurmann, J., Mechanical aids in the prevention of dental diseases in the elderly, *Int. Dent. J.,* 42(5):365–372, 1992.
10. Schmid, M. O. and Perry, D. A., Plaque control, in *Glickman's Clinical Periodontology,* Carranza, F. A., Ed., W.B. Saunders, Philadelphia, 1990, pp. 684–711.
11. Axelsson, P. and Lindhe, J., The effect of a preventive programme on dental plaque, gingivitis, and caries in school-children: results after one and two years, *J. Clin. Periodontol.,* 1:126–132, 1974.
12. Blahut, P., A clinical trial of the Interplak® powered toothbrush in a geriatric population, *Compend. Contin. Educ. Dent. Suppl.,* 16:S606–S610, 1993.
13. Ciancio, S. G., Non-surgical periodontal treatment, in *Proceedings of the World Workshop in Clinical Periodontics,* Academy of Periodontology, Chicago, 1989, pp. II-1–II-21.
14. Greenwell, H. et al., Clinical and microbiologic effectiveness of Keyes' method of oral hygiene on human periodontitis treated with and without surgery, *J. Am. Dent. Assoc.,* 106:457–461, 1983.
15. Ciancio, S. G., Pharmacology of oral antimicrobials, in *Perspectives on Oral Antimicrobial Therapeutics*, American Academy of Periodontology, PSG Publishing, Littleton, Mississippi, 1987.
16. Casamassimo, P. S. and Griffen, A. L., Prevention for the physically and mentally handicapped and the medically compromised patient, *in Clark's Clinical Dentistry*, Hardin, J. F., Ed., J.B. Lippincott, Philadelphia, 1994, pp. 1–13.
17. Dahllof, G. et al., Oral health in children treated with bone marrow transplantation: a one-year follow-up, *J. Dent. Child.,* May–June:196–200, 1988.

18. Peterson, D. E. and D'Ambrosio, J. A., Nonsurgical management of head and neck cancer patients, *Dent. Clin. North Am.,* 38(3):425–445, 1994.

19. Dreizen, S., Bodey, G. P., and Valdivieso, M., Chemotherapy-associated oral infections in adults with solid tumors, *Oral Surg. Oral Med. Oral Pathol.,* 55(2):113–120, 1983.

20. Casamassimo, P. S., Oral complications of cancer therapy, *Pediatric Dent.,* 12:232, 1990.

21. Maier, H. et al., Dental status and oral hygiene in patients with head and neck cancer, *Otolaryngol. Head Neck Surg.,* 108:655–661, 1993.

22. McClure, D., Barker, G., Barker, B., and Feil, P., Oral management of the cancer patient. Part 1. Oral complications of chemotherapy, *Compend. Contin. Educ. Dent.,* 8(1):41–50, 1987.

23. DeBeule, F., Bercy, P., and Ferrant, A., The effectiveness of a preventive regimen on the periodontal health of patients undergoing chemotherapy for leukemia and lymphoma, *J. Clin. Periodontol.,* 18:346–347, 1991.

24. Overholser, C. D. et al., Periodontal infection in patients with acute nonlymphocytic leukemia, prevalence of acute exacerbations, *Arch. Intern. Med.,* 142:551–554, 1982.

25. Bergmann, O. J. et al., Gingival status during chemical plaque control with or without prior mechanical plaque removal in patients with acute myeloid leukemia, *J. Clin. Periodontol.,* 19:169–173, 1992.

26. Wright, W. E. et al., An oral disease prevention program for patients receiving radiation and chemotherapy, *J. Am. Dent. Assoc.,* 110:43–47, 1985.

27. Patton, L. L. and Ship, J. A., Treatment of patients with bleeding disorders, *Dent. Clin. North Am.,* 38(3):465–482, 1994.

28. Williams, L. T., Peterson, D. E., and Overholser, C. D., Leukemia and dental treatment, *Dent. Hyg.,* April:29–33, 1981.

29. Fattore, L., Baer, R., and Olsen, R., The role of the general dentist in the treatment and management of oral complications of chemotherapy, *Gen. Dent.,* Sept.–Oct.:374–377, 1987.

30. Lockhart, P. B. and Schmidtke, M. A., Antibiotic considerations in medically compromised patients, *Dent. Clin. North Am.,* 38(2):381–402, 1994.

31. Epstein, J. B. et al., Enhancing the effect of oral hygiene with the use of a foam brush with chlorhexidine, *Oral Surg. Oral Med. Oral Pathol.,* 77:242–247, 1994.

32. Dajani, A. S. et al., Prevention of bacterial endocarditis, *JAMA,* 264(22):2919–2922, 1990.

33. Carl, W. and Schaaf, N. G., Dental care for the cancer patient, *J. Surg. Oncol.,* 43:293–310, 1974.

34. Al-Tannir, M. A. and Goodman, H. S., A review of chlorhexidine and its use in special populations, *Spec. Care Dent.,* 14(3):116–122, 1994.

35. Krywulak, M. L., Dental considerations for the pediatric oncology patient, *J. Am. Dent. Assoc.,* 58(2):125–130, 1992.

36. Sreebny, L. M. et al., The preparation of an autologous saliva for use with patients undergoing therapeutic radiation for head and neck cancer, *J. Oral Maxillofac. Surg.,* 53:131–139, 1995.

37. Aldous, J. A. and Aldous, S. G., Management of oral health for the HIV-infected patient, *J. Dent. Hyg.*, March–April:143–145, 1991.

38. Lindquist, S. F., Hickey, A. J., and Drane, J. B., Effect of oral hygiene on stomatitis in patients receiving cancer chemotherapy, *J. Prosth. Dent.*, 40(3):312–314, 1978.

39. Greenspan, D. and Daniels, T. E., Effectiveness of pilocarpine in post radiation xerostomia, *Cancer*, 59:1123–1125, 1987.

40. McClure, D. et al., Oral management of the cancer patient. Part II. Oral complication of radiation therapy, *Compend. Contin. Educ. Dent.*, 8(2):88–93, 1987.

41. Hickey, A. J. and Lindquist, S. B., Effect of intravenous hyperalimentation and oral care on the development of oral stomatitis during cancer chemotherapy, *J. Prosth. Dent.*, 47(2):188–193, 1982.

42. Dental Management of the Cancer Patient, AAOMS Surgical Update, Summer 1992, pp. 2–6.

43. Weisdorf, D. J. et al., Oropharyngeal mucositis complication bone marrow transplantation: prognostic factors and the effect of chlorhexidine mouth rinse, *Bone Mar. Transpl.*, 4:84–95, 1989.

44. Barrett, A. P., Clinical characteristics and mechanisms involved in chemotherapy-induced oral ulceration, *Oral Surg. Oral Med. Oral Pathol.*, 63:424–428, 1987.

45. Berkowitz, R. J. et al., Stomatologic complications of bone marrow transplantation in a pediatric population, *Pediatr. Dent.*, 9(2):105–110, 1987.

46. Berkowitz, R. J. et al., Oral complications associated with bone marrow transplantation in a pediatric population, *Am. J. Pediatr. Hematol./Oncol.*, 5(1):53–57, 1983.

47. Toljanic, J. A. et al., Evaluation of the substantivity of a chlorhexidine oral rinse in irradiated head and neck cancer patients, *J. Oral Maxillofac. Surg.*, 50:1055–1059, 1992.

48. McGaw, W. T. and Belch, A., Oral complications of acute leukemia: prophylactic impact of a chlorhexidine mouth rinse regimen, *Oral Surg. Oral Med. Oral Pathol.*, 60:275–280, 1985.

49. Rutkauskas, J. S. and Davis, J. W., Effects of chlorhexidine during immunosuppressive chemotherapy, a preliminary report, *Oral Surg. Oral Med. Oral Pathol.*, 76:441–448, 1993.

50. Ferretti, G. A. et al., Control of oral mucositis and candidiasis in marrow transplantation: a prospective. Double-blind trial of chlorhexidine digluconate oral rinse, *Bone Mar. Transpl.*, 3:483–493, 1988.

51. Ferretti, G. A. et al., Chlorhexidine for prophylaxis against oral infections and associated complications in patients receiving bone marrow transplants, *J. Am. Dent. Assoc.*, 114:461–467, 1987.

52. Ferretti, G. A. et al., Chlorhexidine prophylaxis for chemotherapy- and radiotherapy-induced stomatitis: a randomized double-blind trial, *Oral Surg. Oral Med. Oral Pathol.*, 69:331–338, 1990.

53. Spijkervet, F. K. L. et al., Effect of chlorhexidine rinsing on the oropharyngeal ecology in patients with head and neck cancer who have irradiation mucositis, *Oral Surg. Oral Med. Oral Pathol.*, 67:154–161, 1989.

54. Carl, W. and Higby, D. J., Oral manifestations of bone marrow transplantation, *Am. J. Clin. Oncol. (CCT),* 8:81–87, 1985.

55. DeGregorio, M. W., Lee, W. M. F., and Ries, C. A., Candida infections in patients with acute leukemia: ineffectiveness of nystatin prophylaxis and relationship between oropharyngeal and systemic candidiasis, *Cancer,* 50:2780–2784, 1982.

56. Epstein, J. B. et al., Efficacy of chlorhexidine and nystatin rinses in prevention of oral complications in leukemia and bone marrow transplantation, *Oral Surg. Oral Med. Oral Pathol.,* 73:682–689, 1992.

57. Barker, G. et al., The effects of sucralfate suspension and diphenhydramine syrup plus kaolin-pectin on radiotherapy-induced mucositis, *Oral Surg. Oral Med. Oral Pathol.,* 71:288–293, 1991.

58. Graser, G. N., The efficacy of topical anesthetics in reducing intraoral discomfort, *J. Prosth. Dent.,* 58:42–46, 1984.

59. Shenep, J. L. et al., Efficacy of oral sucralfate suspension in prevention and treatment of chemotherapy-induced mucositis, *J. Pediatr.,* 113:758–763, 1988.

60. Pfeiffer, P. et al., Effect of prophylactic sucralfate suspension on stomatitis induced by cancer chemotherapy, *Acta Oncol.,* 29:171–173, 1990.

61. Cacchillo, D., Barker, G. J., and Barker, B. F., Late effects of head and neck radiation therapy and patient/dentist compliance with recommended dental care, *Spec. Care Dent.,* 13(4):159–162, 1993.

62. Epstein, J. B. et al., Chlorhexidine rinse in prevention of dental caries in patients following radiation therapy, *Oral Surg. Oral Med. Oral Pathol.,* 68:401–405, 1989.

63. Peterson, D., Dental care of the cancer patient, *Compend. Contin. Educ. Dent.,* 4(2):115–120, 1983.

64. Grassi, M. et al., Management of HIV-associated periodontal lesions, in *Perspectives on Oral Manifestations of AIDS,* Robertson, P. B. and Greenspan, J. S., Eds., American Academy of Periodontology, PSG Publishing, Littleton, Mississippi, 1988.

65. Yeung, S. C. H. et al., Progression of periodontal disease in HIV seropositive patients, *J. Periodontol.,* 64:651–657, 1993.

66. Sciubba, J., Recognizing the oral manifestations of AIDS, *Oncology,* 6:64–70, 1992

67. Winkler, J. R. et al., Diagnosis and management of HIV-associated periodontal lesions, *J. Am. Dent. Assoc.,* Suppl. (Nov.):25-S–34-S, 1989.

68. Periodontal Consideration in the HIV-Positive Patient, Position paper of the American Academy of Periodontology, Chicago, 1994.

69. Murray, P. A., HIV disease as a risk factor for periodontal disease, *Compend. Contin. Educ. Dent.,* 15(8):1052–1063, 1994.

70. Greenspan, J. S., Greenspan, D., Winkler, J. R., and Murray, P. A., Acquired immunodeficiency syndrome: oral and perioral changes, in *Contemporary Periodontics,* Genco, R. J., Goldman, H. M., and Cohen, D. W., Eds., C.V. Mosby, St. Louis, 1990, pp. 298–322.

71. Winkler, J. R. and Robertson, P. B., Periodontal disease associated with HIV infection, *Oral Surg. Oral Med. Oral Pathol.,* 73:145–150, 1992.

72. Loesche, W. et al., Metronidazole therapy for periodontitis, *J. Periodontal. Res.,* 22(3):224–226, 1987.

73. Barr, C. E., Dental management of HIV-associated oral mucosal lesions, in *Perspectives on Oral Manifestations of AIDS,* Robertson, P. B. and Greenspan, J. S., Eds., American Academy of Periodontology, PSG Publishing, Littleton, Mississippi, 1988, pp. 77–95.

74. Barr, C. E., Practical considerations in the treatment of the HIV-infected patient, *Dent. Clin. North Am.,* 38(3):403–423, 1994.

75. Weyant, R. J. et al., Oral health status of a long-term-care, veteran population, *Community Dent. Oral Epidemiol.,* 21:227–233, 1993.

76. Henry, R. G. and Ceridan, B., Delivering dental care to nursing home and homebound patients, *Dent. Clin. North Am.,* 38(3):537–551, 1994.

77. Shuman, S. K. and Bebeau, M. J., Ethical and legal issues in special patient care, *Dent. Clin. North Am.,* 38(3):553–575, 1994.

78. Glassman, P. et al., A preventive dentistry training program for caretakers of persons with disabilities residing in community residential facilities, *Spec. Care Dent.,* 14(4):137–143, 1994.

79. Felder, R. S. and Millar, S. B., Dental care of the polymedication patient, *Dent. Clin. North Am.,* 38(3):525–536, 1994.

80. Shay, K., Identifying the needs of the elderly dental patient, *Dent. Clin. North Am.,* 38(3):499–523, 1994.

81. Recommendations for Preventive Pediatric Dental Care, American Academy of Pediatric Dentistry, May 1992.

82. Payne, B. J. and Locker, D., Oral self-care behaviors in older dentate adults, *Community Dent. Oral Epidemiol.,* 20:376–380, 1992.

83. Kambhu, P. P. and Levy, S. M., An evaluation of the effectiveness of four mechanical plaque-removal devices when used by a trained care-provider, *Spec. Care Dent.,* 13(1):9–14, 1993.

84. Kritsineli, M., Venetikidou, A., and Grigorakis, G., The Myo as an oral prophylactic device used by motor skill functionally disabled patients, *J. Clin. Pediatr. Dent.,* 16(3):159–161, 1992.

85. Hellstadius, K. et al., Improved maintenance of plaque control by electrical tooth brushing in periodontitis patients with low compliance, *J. Clin. Periodontol.,* 20:235–237, 1993.

86. Storhaug, K., Hibitane in oral disease in handicapped patients, *J. Clin. Periodontol.,* 4:102, 1977.

87. Grossman, E. et al., A clinical comparison of antibacterial mouthrinses: effects of chlorhexidine, phenolics, and sanguinarine on dental plaque and gingivitis, *J. Periodontol.,* 60(8):435–440, 1989.

88. Francis, J. R., Hunter, B., and Addy, M., A comparison of three delivery methods of chlorhexidine in handicapped children. I. Effects on plaque, gingivitis, and toothstaining, *J. Periodontol.,* 58(7):451–455, 1987.

89. Francis, J. R., Addy, M., and Hunter, B., A comparison of three delivery methods of chlorhexidine in handicapped children. II. Parent and house-parent preferences, *J. Periodontol.,* 58(7):456–459, 1987.

90. Saunders, R. H. et al., The effectiveness of sponge-type intraoral applicators for applying topical fluorides in institutionalized older adults, *Spec. Care Dent.*, 14(6):224–228, 1994.

91. Kalaga, A., Addy, M., and Hunter, B., The use of 0.2% chlorhexidine spray as an adjunct to oral hygiene and gingival health in physically and mentally handicapped adults, *J. Periodontol.*, 60(7):381–385, 1989.

92. Kalaga, A., Addy, M., and Hunter, B., Comparison of chlorhexidine delivery by mouthwash and spray on plaque accumulation, *J. Periodontol.*, 60(3):127–130, 1989.

93. Chikte, U. M. et al., Evaluation of stannous fluoride and chlorhexidine sprays on plaque and gingivitis in handicapped children, *J. Clin. Periodontol.*, 18:281–286, 1991.

94. Chan, J. T., Wyborny, L. E., and Kula, K., Clinical applications of fluorides, in *Clark's Clinical Dentistry,* Hardin, J. F., Ed., J.B. Lippincott, Philadelphia, 1994, pp. 1–25.

95. Flynn, A. A., Counseling special populations on oral health care needs, *Am. Pharm.*, NS33(9):33–39, 1993.

96. Arneberg, P. et al., Remaining teeth, oral dryness and dental health habits in middle-aged Norwegian rheumatoid arthritis patients, *Community Dent. Oral Epidemiol.*, 20:292–296, 1992.

97. Pihlstrom, B. L., Prevention and treatment of dilantin-associated gingival enlargement, *Compend Contin. Educ. Dent. Suppl.,* 14:S506–S510, 1990.

98. Rees, T. D., The diabetic dental patient, *Dent. Clin. North Am.*, 38(3):447–463, 1994.

99. Persson, M. et al., Influence of Parkinson's disease on oral health, *Acta Odontol. Scand.*, 50:37–42, 1992.

100. Lucas, V. S., Association of psychotropic drugs, prevalence of denture-related stomatitis, and oral candidosis, *Community Dent. Oral Epidemiol.*, 21:313–316, 1993.

101. Sigal, M. J. and Levine, N., Down syndrome and Alzheimer's disease, *J. Can. Dent. Assoc.*, 59(10):824–829, 1993.

102. Aldred, M. J. et al., Oral health in the terminally ill: a cross-sectional pilot survey, *Spec. Care Dent.*, 11(2):59–62, 1991.

Home Health Care for Cardiac Patients

19

Albert G. Goldin, M.D., F.A.C.P.

Rationale for Home Care

Cardiovascular diseases are responsible for the largest number of health problems and disabilities in the United States. Despite a significant nationwide effort to modify risk factors, the incidence of coronary artery disease morbidity and mortality has declined rather little over the past 10 years. Current estimates of the annual deaths from coronary artery disease are still in the range of 500,000, and it is also estimated that 5.6 million persons in the United States have angina.[1]

The economic burden of such an extensive health problem is straining the financial capability of those who must pay the bills. These payors include government agencies (mainly Medicare and Medicaid), insurance companies including health maintenance organizations, and private payors. As a response to the dilemma, home care has grown rapidly in an effort to reduce hospital stays (and thus costs) and still provide excellent case management to those in need. This applies to cardiac patients as well as to those with various other medical problems. It is thought that substantial savings in medical costs will result. Studies now under way should determine if this hypothesis is correct.

Complicating the analysis of potential savings is the fact that with the diagnosis-related group system of reimbursement to hospitals, shorter stays mean more profit to the hospital because the remuneration from the payor is fixed according to the diagnostic category and not (with certain exceptions) to the length of stay. Earlier discharge, then, means earlier involvement by the home health care agency, with the result that there may be little overall savings. For example, daily hospital charges may range from $550 to $750 or more depending upon use of intensive care and operating room usage. If a fixed amount is allowed by the insurer (based upon the stated charges), hospitals make more money with shorter stays. Charges for home care include visits by a registered nurse, currently at a rate of $90 to $100 per visit. In addition, there may be visits by home care aides at $45 to $50 per trip and visits by a social worker, physical therapist, and occupational therapist at $100 to $110 per call. These rates and charges apply to the Louisville, Kentucky area and will vary in different regions of the country.

Efforts to guard against overutilization of home care include the requirement that the treatments be reasonable and necessary. Also, the number of visits allowed for various categories and diagnoses is subject to limitations. There is also pending legislation in Congress to require a modest co-payment for Medicare recipients, which will likely reduce utilization to some extent. It must be clear that the main impact on reducing health care costs appears to lie in the prevention of repeated hospitalizations, which is typical of chronic cardiovascular problems. Studies to confirm this are being undertaken.[4]

The Home Visit

The initial visit by the home health nurse is made shortly after the patient is discharged from the hospital and after appropriate consultations between the attending physician and the hospital discharge planner. At this first visit, the nurse evaluates the home situation to determine whether or not the environment is satisfactory for the patient's convalescence. This evaluation includes such factors as the bedroom and bathroom facilities, adequacy of heating and air conditioning, and ventilation in general. The nurse also makes an estimate of the intellectual resources of the caregivers to judge whether or not they can follow instructions and learn such procedures as taking vital signs, administering injections, cleansing wounds, and changing dressings if needed. The financial resources of the family also have to be considered from the standpoint of purchasing drugs and supplies and special dietary needs, as many of these items are not reimbursed by Medicare or other insurance.

Assessment of the patient from the standpoint of performance of activities of daily living and exercise tolerance is very important. Skilled observation, teaching and training for self-care, and instruction of home caregivers are deemed reimbursable by Medicare regulations.[2]

Assuming that the evaluation is satisfactory, it is then necessary to establish parameters for when to call the nurse, the doctor, or 911 emergency. It it important to keep in mind that the attending physician is ultimately responsible for the patient's care; therefore, he or she must work closely with the nurses and home caregivers. However, attention has been called to the legal implications for the home health nurse and the need to be well informed in all aspects of the medical problem being attended, as well as in rendering nonnegligent care.[8]

Cardiovascular Problems Amenable to Home Care

Hypertension

Accurate measurement and proper recording of blood pressure are essential for evaluating response to therapy and for assessing possible need for changes in regimen. Postural lightheadedness or even syncope is a frequent problem, especially in elderly and chronically ill patients, and should be noted. Other side effects of medical regimens include electrolyte changes (with diuretics), pulse rate and rhythm alterations (with beta and calcium channel blockers and digitalis), sexual dysfunction, edema, dehydration, fatigue and lethargy, and mental changes. These and any other problems, such as allergic reactions or gastrointestinal complaints, should be noted and reported to the attending physician for appropriate action. Hypertensive encephalopathy and acute pulmonary edema are examples of situations that require urgent or emergency attention.

An illustrative case report is that of a 42-year-old diabetic man in chronic renal failure who had been on renal dialysis for approximately 10 years but remained hypertensive. His shunt thrombosed and required surgical intervention as well as placement of another shunt. Infection developed in the original shunt site. When satisfactorily controlled, he was discharged from the hospital and home care nurses were called in. Daily dressing changes were carried out initially by the home care nurses, and the family caregivers were taught to perform these tasks as well. Strong emphasis was placed on dietary and medication compliance. Blood sugars, blood pressures, and electrolytes were appropriately monitored. The wounds healed and home care nursing was terminated within 8 weeks. Involvement of the home care nurse resulted in improved compliance and blood pressure control. Potential complications and rehospitalizations were believed to have been avoided. This case also illustrates the multiple problems that home care cases entail even though one aspect or presenting complaint may predominate.

Ischemic Heart Disease

This category includes angina pectoris, myocardial infarction, and postoperative coronary artery bypass. In cases of angina, the home care nurse has an important educational role. Evaluating compliance with medication, discovering precipitating factors, and modifying lifestyle behaviors which are deleterious (including dietary and exercise regimens) are necessary areas of concern to the home health nurse. Other risk factors such as smoking, alcohol use, associated hypertension and/or diabetes mellitus, obesity, family history, and lipid derangements are essential items in the educational curriculum for the patient and family. The goal is to stabilize and minimize the anginal episodes and hopefully induce regression of plaques in the coronary vessels, as some studies suggest is possible.

A case presentation illustrates many of the above-described factors. An 86-year-old man lived at home with his 81-year-old wife. Both were physically frail but mentally very alert. He had been experiencing angina pectoris of a stable exertionally induced type for 3 to 4 years. These pains were readily relieved by sublingual nitroglycerine until the angina became unstable. He was then hospitalized. Medications were readjusted, and he was returned home with the new regimen plus oxygen at night and as needed during the day. Home nurses were called in to implement and supervise the new dietary, drug, and oxygen program. An aide for personal care was also required, as some daily activities such as bathing would induce angina.

Home nursing visits, initially daily, were tapered to twice weekly. End-stage care was not taught, as the patient did not want his frail wife to be burdened with such chores and activities or to be confronted with his death at home. After several months, when he developed chest pains unrelieved by three nitroglycerine tablets and oxygen, he was hospitalized and expired in the coronary care unit within 36 hours. It appears that with the provision of home nursing care, this gentleman avoided being placed in a nursing home, was able to stay at home with his wife, and an earlier demise was avoided.

Myocardial Infarction

When the ischemic process has progressed to coronary occlusion, myocardial damage may be variable, depending upon the amount and location of the heart muscle destruction. In England, there has been an attempt to treat some of these cases at home, especially in very elderly and debilitated patients with poor prognosis. In the United States, the usual venue for care of acute myocardial infarction is the hospital. With newer methods for reestablishing coronary blood flow using thrombolytic agents and invasive procedures such as balloon and laser angioplasty, as well as bypass surgery, hospital stays for this illness have been considerably shortened. The role of the home health nurse thus becomes quite important, not only in education but in monitoring convalescence. Supervision of compliance with medication and diet, observation of vital signs, and checking for edema, neck vein distention, and pulmonary congestion are some of the duties during the home visit. Inquiries are made as to the recurrence of chest pain. The goal is prevention of rehospitalization as well as awareness of any developments which will dictate readmission.[10]

A case history in this category is a 72-year-old man, nonsmoker, normotensive, and of normal weight but with high LDL and total cholesterol levels. He sustained a myocardial infarction which led to a three-vessel coronary artery bypass graft. He was discharged from the hospital 10 days postoperation. Home care nursing services were requested. Attention was directed to modifiable lifestyle activities, in this case mainly dietary changes emphasizing low-fat, low-cholesterol, and low-sodium foods. A walking program was developed suitable to his home area. He was seen three times a week for 3 weeks, then twice a week for 2 weeks, and was then discharged to begin an outpatient cardiac rehabilitation program. The home care nursing was thought to have facilitated the convalescence and may have prevented complications.

Congestive Heart Failure

This complication of heart problems from varying etiologies has common symptoms brought on by the inadequate pumping action of the myocardium, resulting in impaired perfusion of tissues. The decrease in cardiac output results in changes in blood pressure (usually a fall) and in heart rate (usually a rise), dyspnea, possibly rales at the lung bases, edema of the legs (or of the back if the patient is bedfast), and mental changes due to decrease in cerebral perfusion. The home care nurse should be alert to these developments and notify the attending physician promptly so that remedial measures can be taken. Hopefully, with a good response to diuretic agents, oxygen if necessary, reevaluation of medicines which may have negative inotropic or other adverse effects, and more rigid sodium restriction, the process may be arrested and reversed and thus hospitalization avoided.[3] There have been some efforts to improve inotropic action of the myocardium using dobutamine infusions in the home setting. This drug is usually administered intravenously via an infusion pump over a period of several hours two to three times a week. This therapy requires very close collaboration of the entire caregiving team.[6]

An example of a patient in this category is a 77-year-old diabetic female with cardiomyopathy considered to be NYHA class IV. Her ejection fraction was 18%. She was not responding very well to various diuretics. Home nursing care was requested and began on a three times per week schedule. At these times, vital signs, weight, and pulmonary status were assessed. Pulse oximetry was checked at each visit. Blood was drawn for laboratory tests weekly. Transtelephonic EKG monitoring was available for arrhythmia evaluation, as she had developed atrial fibrillation. Adherence to dietary and medicine regimens was emphasized. This patient did not require hospitalization during 9 months of home nursing care, whereas in the 6-week period prior to referral she was hospitalized six times. The benefit of home nursing care in this case is quite obvious.

Cardiac Rehabilitation

Home care for patients recovering from myocardial infarction, cardiac surgery, or congestive failure may involve a rehabilitation program. This will require cooperation between the physical therapist, occupational therapist, and home nurse in scheduling activities deemed appropriate. Active consultation with the cardiologist is important. Extensive teaching of the patient and family as to activities to be undertaken and necessary monitoring measures is required. Home-based rehabilitation may be more convenient and less expensive than hospital-based programs but requires a team approach, with the home care cardiac nurse acting as a case manager in carrying out the plan developed by the various disciplines concerned.[7]

An example of this situation, briefly presented, is a 70-year-old man discharged from the hospital 8 days after a triple aortocoronary bypass operation. He had been very sedentary, spending most of his time watching television prior to his surgery, supposedly due to his easily induced exertional angina. His total and LDL cholesterol levels were elevated and his HDL levels were low. His wife was the primary home caregiver but was limited by moderately severe arthritis in the knees and hands. A cardiac home care nurse was requested, and a home exercise program was developed in consultation with the cardiologist. This consisted chiefly of a gradually increasing walking program, which emphasized time walked instead of distance. Stretching exercises and range of motion exercises for the extremities were taught. Medication and dietary compliance was also supervised. Educational materials including a videotape were made available. Daily visits were made during the first week and gradually tapered to weekly visits. After 1 month, the patient was ready to advance to the hospital outpatient rehabilitation center, where more strenuous and monitored exercises could be instituted. Home nursing care facilitated postoperative rehabilitation and may have prevented complications.

Pacemakers

In addition to the considerations described above, the pacemaker patient may have additional concerns. Since most of these patients are elderly and often have other chronic and debilitating conditions, the need for reassurance and education is very important. Some education about pacemaker functioning must be provided. How to take a pulse, pacemaker malfunction, and battery failure must be explained in a nonanxiety-producing manner. Electromagnetic interference with pacemaker signals, as from microwave ovens, is no longer a significant problem; however, power-transmitting lines and radio, television, and radar towers may cause interference with pacemaker signals. Knowing when to contact the nurse or doctor is an important part of the educational plan. Telephonic checking of pacemaker function is readily available via transmitting units over the home telephone and is done at approximately 1- to 2-month intervals or for urgent or emergency evaluations. A very recent development in bioelectronic medicine is the implantable cardioverter-defibrillator, which can sense ventricular tachycardia or fibrillation and promptly deliver an electric shock sufficient to abolish the malignant rhythm. The implications for home care in these cases are essentially the same as for pacemakers, namely education of the patient and family and close liaison with the cardiologist. Teaching family members how to perform cardiopulmonary resuscitation is also important in case of malfunction of the defibrillator.

Illustrative of the multiple and complex problems which may be encountered when dealing with home nursing care in this category is the case of a bedridden 78-year-old female with left hemiparesis, requiring gastric tube feedings and Foley catheter. When hospitalized with her stroke, she was found to have a complete heart block, which was treated with a fixed-rate demand pacemaker. Home nursing care was arranged for her at discharge. Daily visits were made for the first week, then three times a week, and gradually tapered to a visit every 2 weeks. During the home visits, her daughter was taught to administer the tube feedings and to perform skin care and bed care. The pacemaker was checked telephonically once a month. In addition to the nurse, the services of a home health aide, a social worker, and a dietician were utilized. The patient lived for another 2.5 years and did not need to be rehospitalized.

Postoperative States

The conditions most frequently encountered in this category are coronary artery bypass, carotid endarterectomy, and peripheral vascular surgical procedures involving the lower extremities. Cases of abdominal aortic aneurysm and cerebral vascular surgery are encountered less frequently and cardiac transplantation even less often. In addition to the usual monitoring and educational aspects associated with home care, the nurse must be especially alert to potential postoperative problems such as bleeding, wound infection, cardiac arrhythmias, and pulmonary complications such as atelectasis and pneumonitis. In the case of transplants, adverse effects of immunosuppressive drugs, particularly renal toxicity and hypertension, must be identified.

A patient in this category is a 72-year-old woman discharged from the hospital after a 21-day stay for a five-vessel aortocoronary bypass operation. She was also a diabetic and arthritic. Postoperatively she had developed staphylococcus infection at the femoral puncture sites and in the sternal incision, requiring 10 days of intravenous vancomycin. Upon discharge, home care nurses were called upon for twice daily visits to change dressings and to try to teach the family caregivers how to dress the wounds and give medications. Instructions for diet and exercises were also attempted. Because the family members were reluctant to learn (they were fearful that they might make errors), the home nursing visits were continued twice a day for several weeks, until healing progressed satisfactorily. The visits were then tapered to weekly and later biweekly. A social worker was involved in the care, but offers of home health aides and physical therapy were refused by the family. Nevertheless, readmission was avoided in this case due to the involvement of the home care nursing service.

Strokes

The incidence of stroke has declined somewhat in the past 10 years due, it is thought, to the major effort undertaken to detect and control high blood pressure in the general population. Surveys have revealed that there were about 145,000 deaths from stroke in 1992 and that about one-half million Americans suffer strokes each year.[1] The impact on the stroke victim and family remains devastating and requires the utmost sympathetic attention and skill of the home care nurse. The home care nurse assesses the neurologic deficits and limitations of function incurred by the cerebral vascular disease process. Risk factors, similar to those for other cardiovascular problems, are identified and efforts to modify them are instituted in coordination with the attending physician and other members of the health care team. Education of the family caregivers is a vital part of the home care program.[5] Exercise regimens are prescribed by the physiatrist and the physical therapist but require the attention of the home care nurse for compliance and progress evaluation. Concomitant medical problems such as diabetes mellitus, coronary artery disease, or peripheral vascular conditions require surveillance. Being alert to potential problems and initiating prompt action will often prevent a return to the hospital. Independence in activities of daily living as far as possible is the measure of success in rehabilitation, and usually the degree of recovery is attained within 6 months after onset.[11]

A condensed description of a representative case in this category is a 52-year-old single mother with four teenage daughters at home. She had longstanding hypertension and had sustained a stroke 10 years earlier, resulting in left hemiparesis. Just prior to the present hospitalization, she had developed a transient ischemic episode. After 3 days, she was discharged and home nursing care began. The daughters were instructed in basic bed and skin care and in encouraging range of motion exercises and ambulation. Dietary instructions were given and supervised, as was medication compliance. Initially, blood was drawn weekly for prothrombin time determinations. After some difficulty in stabilizing the warfarin dosages, the patient was regulated and the phlebotomies were rescheduled to monthly intervals. Without the availability of home nursing care, this patient would have faced a hospital stay of 2 to 3 weeks.

Peripheral Vascular Disease

Home care of peripheral vascular problems begins with a careful appraisal of symptoms and physical evaluation. Attention to risk factors and compliance with corrective measures are of utmost importance, especially with regard to smoking and diabetes control. Blood pressure control and dietary and medication compliance are also essential. Assessment of improvement or decline in exercise tolerance will measure the effectiveness of the program being followed and serve as a guide to whether or not modifications in the regimen are required. Situations involving deep venous thrombosis may also be followed by the home care nurse, in which case serial determinations of prothrombin times and/or other anticoagulant measures will be necessary. As in the other conditions discussed previously, the ultimate goal is to restore as much function as possible and to prevent or delay progression to the point that hospitalization and surgery are required. The home care nurse serves a vital role in education and surveillance in these cases.

A patient illustrating some aspects of this category of illness is a 60-year-old very obese woman with chronic venous stasis ulcers at both ankles. After a brief hospitalization to control edema and infection, she was discharged to the care of home nurses. With the physician's directives, Unna boots were applied twice a week for 4 weeks, then weekly. In addition, the patient's diet was supervised and smoking cessation was encouraged. Physical activity was also encouraged. Within 5 months, the ulcers had healed completely and the patient had lost about 20 pounds. Without home nursing care, it is quite certain that the patient would have developed recurrent sepsis and the ulcers would not have healed. Rehospitalization was not necessary in this case.

Pulmonary Disease

In many home care organizations, pulmonary problems are included under the umbrella of the cardiovascular department. The most common problems in this area are chronic obstructive disease with pulmonary insufficiency, often requiring home oxygen use. Pulmonary infections and postoperative states are also frequently encountered. In these situations, the same principles that relate to monitoring and patient and family education pertain. Exercise tolerance is assessed at intervals, as are arterial blood gas determinations. Compliance with the multiple medications often used in pulmonary problems as well as proper use of inhaled medications are important areas of concern to the home care nurse.[9] Close liaison with the respiratory therapist and attending physician should be maintained in order to note and address any deterioration and thereby prevent return to the hospital if possible.

Illustrating the complexities that may be seen in this condition is the case of a 46-year-old man who was paraplegic following an automobile accident several years earlier. He was confined to a wheelchair, overweight, and smoked heavily. He lived alone, but many family members visited frequently to check on him. Following a bout of severe pneumonia, he required a tracheostomy, and upon discharge from the hospital, home nursing care was instituted. Initially, daily visits were made, tracheostomy care was given, and compliance with medications and diet was encouraged. Finally, after much encouragement, he did stop smoking. A home health aide came daily to assist with personal care, including bowel and catheter care. Nursing visits were tapered to once every 2 weeks. The benefit of the home nursing care consisted of helping him maintain a semblance of independence and avoid nursing home care. Undoubtedly, rehospitalization was also avoided.

Acknowledgments

I wish to acknowledge with thanks the assistance of Sheila Kirk, R.N., M.S.N., executive manager of the cardiopulmonary program for the Louisville Visiting Nurse Association, in discussing the materials in and reviewing the manuscript for this chapter.

References

1. Fact Sheet on Heart Attack, Stroke and Risk Factors, American Heart Association, 1995.
2. Neal, L. J., Activities of daily living and the cardiac client who is homebound, *Home Healthcare Nurse*, 13:70–71, 1995.
3. Singh, P., Managing chronic congestive heart failure in the home, *Home Healthcare Nurse*, 13:11–13, 1995.
4. Kornowski, R., Zeeli, D., Averbuch, M., et al., Intensive home care surveillance prevents hospitalization and improves morbidity rates among elderly patients with severe congestive heart failure, *Am. Heart J.*, 129:762–766, 1995.

5. Evans, R. L., Bishop, D. S., and Haselkorn, J. K., Factors predicting satisfactory home care after stroke, *Arch. Phys. Med. Rehabil.*, 72:144–147, 1991.

6. Coffin, M. R., Dobutamine infusion for the treatment of congestive heart failure in the home setting, *J. Intravenous Nurs.*, 17:145–150, 1994.

7. Green, K. and Lydon, S., Home health cardiac rehabilitation, *Home Healthcare Nurse*, 13:29–39, 1995.

8. Brent, N. J., Legal implications for the home healthcare nurse, *Home Healthcare Nurse*, 13:8–9, 1995.

9. Powell, S. G., Medication compliance of patients with COPD, *Home Healthcare Nurse*, 12:44–50, 1994.

10. Osguthorpe, S. G. and Woods, S. L., Myocardial ischemia and infarction, in *Cardiac Nursing*, 3rd edition, Woods, S. L., Sivarajan Froelicher, E. S., Halpenny, C. J., and Motzer, S. U., Eds., J.B. Lippincott, Philadelphia, 1995, chap. 26.

11. Gresham, G. E., Stroke outcome research, *Stroke*, 17:358–360, 1986.

Index

A

Abdominal radiation, 297–299
Abscesses, 37
Abuse, 330–331
Abuse reporting statutes, 197
Access devices, 40, 42
Accreditation, for home care organizations
    that provide food and nutrient therapies,
    102–107
Accrediting bodies, 213
Acetaminophen, 39, 66
Acetate, 93–94, 95, 96
Actinomycin D, 281
Activities of daily living, 10, 11, 61, 63, 316,
    318, 319
  communicative disorders and, 129
  rehabilitation and, 111, 113, 117, 118, 122
Acupuncture, 72
Acute pulmonary edema, 363
ADL, see Activities of daily living
Adolescents, pain control in, 74–75
Advance directives, 198–200
Advocate, social worker as, 178
Aerosolized antimicrobial therapy, 263–264
Agencies, see Home care agencies
Agoraphobia, 316, 318
Agranulocytosis, 317
Aid to Families with Dependent Children, 182
Aide, see Home health aide
AIDS, 51, 151, 169, 316
  intravenous antibiotic therapy, 38, 39–40
  pain control, 77
  pediatric, 237
Aids for daily living, 119
Albumin, 96, 97

Alcoholism, 320
Allogeneic bone marrow transplant, 278, 282
Alloplastic maxillofacial prosthetics, 305
Alprazolam, 320
Alzheimer's disease, 127, 133, 151, 316, 318,
    354
American Academy of Pediatrics, 236, 238
American Medical Association, 1–2
American Society for Parenteral and Enteral
    Nutrition, 102
American Society of Health-System
    Pharmacists, 102
Aminess, 95
Amino acids, 92, 96, 98
Aminoglycoside, 43
Aminosyn, 93, 95
Amphotericin B, 39, 43
Amputation, 113
Amyotrophic lateral sclerosis, 127, 133, 151
Analgesia, 62–63, 64, 66, 70, 71, 72, 75
Anaphylactic reactions, 45
Anemia, 96, 277
Angina pectoris, 363
Anoxia, 84, 127
Antacids, 299
Antibiotic barrier cream, 294
Antibiotic therapy
  for cystic fibrosis, 263
  intravenous, see Intravenous antibiotic
    therapy
Anticonvulsants, 66
Antidepressants, 66, 318, 320
Antiemetics, 63, 298–299
Anti-inflammatory agents, 265, 300
Antimicrobial therapy, 263–264
Antineoplastic therapies, 66